Instructor's Manual to Accompany

3-2-1 Code It!

Third Edition

Michelle A. Green, MPS, RHIA, FAHIMA, CPC
SUNY Distinguished Teaching Professor
Department of Physical & Health Sciences,
Alfred State College, Alfred, NY

Contributing Authors
Judith E. Fields, CCS, CCS-P, CPC, CPC-H
Adjunct Instructor Medical Coding Program
Southeast Kentucky Community &
Technical College, Harlan, KY

Erica S. Matteson, RHIA
Instructional Support Assistant
Department of Physical & Health Sciences
Alfred State College, Alfred, NY

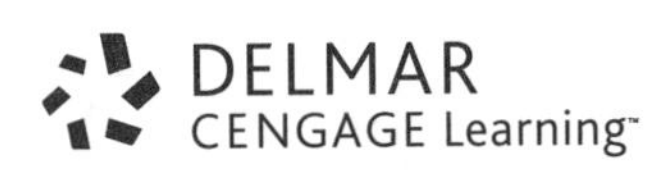

Australia • Brazil • Japan • Korea • Mexico • Singapore • Spain • United Kingdom • United States

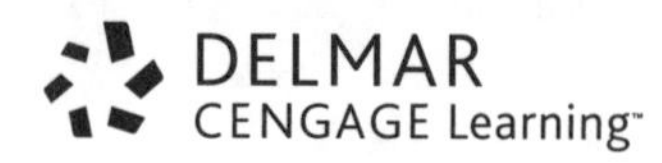

Instructor's Manual to Accompany
3-2-1 Code It! Third Edition
Michelle A. Green, Judith Fields,
and Erica Matteson

Vice President, Editorial: Dave Garza

Director of Learning Solutions: Matthew Kane

Executive Editor: Rhonda Dearborn

Managing Editor: Marah Bellegarde

Senior Product Manager: Jadin Babin-Kavanaugh

Editorial Assistant: Lauren Whalen

Vice President, Marketing: Jennifer Baker

Executive Marketing Manager: Wendy Mapstone

Senior Marketing Manager: Nancy Bradshaw

Marketing Coordinator: Erica Ropitzky

Production Director: Carolyn Miller

Production Manager: Andrew Crouth

Senior Content Project Manager: Stacey Lamodi

Senior Art Director: Jack Pendleton

For product information and technology assistance, contact us at
Cengage Learning Customer & Sales Support, 1-800-354-9706

For permission to use material from this text or product,
submit all requests online at **cengage.com/permissions**
Further permissions questions can be emailed to
permissionrequest@cengage.com

Library of Congress Control Number: 2010932347

ISBN-13: 978-1-111-54060-9

ISBN-10: 1-111-54060-8

Delmar
5 Maxwell Drive
Clifton Park, NY 12065-2919
USA

Cengage Learning is a leading provider of customized learning solutions with office locations around the globe, including Singapore, the United Kingdom, Australia, Mexico, Brazil, and Japan. Locate your local office at **international.cengage.com/region**

Cengage Learning products are represented in Canada by Nelson Education, Ltd.

To learn more about Delmar, visit www.cengage.com/delmar

Purchase any of our products at your local college store or at our preferred online store **www.cengagebrain.com**

NOTICE TO THE READER

Publisher does not warrant or guarantee any of the products described herein or perform any independent analysis in connection with any of the product information contained herein. Publisher does not assume, and expressly disclaims, any obligation to obtain and include information other than that provided to it by the manufacturer. The reader is expressly warned to consider and adopt all safety precautions that might be indicated by the activities described herein and to avoid all potential hazards. By following the instructions contained herein, the reader willingly assumes all risks in connection with such instructions. The publisher makes no representations or warranties of any kind, including but not limited to, the warranties of fitness for particular purpose or merchantability, nor are any such representations implied with respect to the material set forth herein, and the publisher takes no responsibility with respect to such material. The publisher shall not be liable for any special, consequential, or exemplary damages resulting, in whole or part, from the readers' use of, or reliance upon, this material.

Printed in the United States of America
1 2 3 4 5 6 7 14 13 12 11

Contents

Preface

This Instructor's Manual is organized into seven sections:

- Section I: Preparing Your Course
- Section II: Answer Keys to Chapter Exercises and Reviews
- Section III: Chapter Exams and Answer Keys to Chapter Exams
- Section IV: Answer Keys to Workbook Assignments and Reviews
- Section V: Answer Keys to Workbook Appendices A-D: Coding Patient Records
    - Answer Key to Appendix A: Coding Ambulatory Care Surgery Patient Records
    - Answer Key to Appendix B: Coding Emergency Department Patient Records
    - Answer Key to Appendix C: Coding Physician Office Records
    - Answer Key to Appendix D: Coding Hospital Inpatient Records
- Section VI: Answer Key to Workbook Appendix E: Mock Certified Professional Coder (CPC) Certification Examination
- Section VII: Answer Key to Workbook Appendix F: Mock Certification Coding Specialist-Physician (CCS-P) Certification Examination
- Section VIII: Answer Key to Workbook Appendix G: Mock Certified Coding Specialist (CCS) Certification Examination

Section I (Preparing Your Course) assists instructors in the organization of the course. Sample semester plans are provided along with policies for administering exams and grading assignments and exams. The purpose of creating lesson plans is discussed, and chapter lesson plans that can be modified for individual use are included. Section II (Answer Keys to Chapter Exercises and Reviews), Section III (Chapter Exams and Answer Keys to Chapter Exams), and Section IV (Answer Keys to Workbook Assignments and Reviews) are organized according to chapter. Detailed feedback is located below answers to clarify assigned codes. Section V (Answer Keys to Workbook Appendices A–D: Coding Patient Records) is organized according to patient case number, and detailed feedback is included below answers to clarify assigned codes. Section VI (Answer Key to Workbook Appendix E: Mock Certified Professional Coder [CPC] Certification Examination), Section VII (Answer Key to Workbook Appendix F: Mock Certification Coding Specialist-Physician [CCS-P] Certification Examination), and Section VIII (Answer Key to Workbook Appendix G: Mock Certified Coding Specialist [CCS] Certification Examination) contains answers to the mock exams.

Note:

Chapter exams (and answers) in this Instructor's Manual contain questions that are different from those found in the computerized test bank on the Instructor Resources CD-ROM. The chapter exams are the same as those included in the WebTutor™, which provides detailed feedback for the answers.

Teaching Tip:

For ease of reference in locating the sections in the Instructor's Manual, consider placing a sticky note as a tab at the beginning of each section.

STUDYWARE

StudyWARE allows students to review concepts learned in each chapter and to assign codes to practice cases. Login instructions for StudyWARE are located in the textbook Preface and on the Printed Access Card.

Teaching Tip:

StudyWARE is an automated study guide for students. Instead of publishing (and selling!) a separate study guide of questions for students to complete, Delmar Cengage Learning bundles StudyWARE with the textbook. Your students will notice that all types of questions are included in StudyWARE (e.g., multiple choice, matching, true/false, fill-in-the-blank, and "open" coding). The software organizes the questions in a game format (e.g., fill-in-the-blank as hangman and crossword puzzles), which makes it fun for students to use.

ENCODER PRO

Ingenix's www.EncoderPro.com is a powerful medical coding solution that allows you to look up ICD-9-CM, CPT, and HCPCS Level II codes quickly and accurately. In addition, an ICD-10-CM crosswalk displays the ICD-10-CM code(s) that correspond to an ICD-9-CM code. This software can be used to assign codes to any of the exercises in the *3-2-1 Code It!* textbook and workbook. (Be sure to check with your instructor before activating your username and password at **www.EncoderPro.com** because the software expires 59 days after installation.)

STUDENT COMPANION

Additional resources can be found online at **http://www.cengagebrain.com**. Login instructions for the Student Companion are located in the textbook Preface and on the Printed Access Card.

Items listed as Instructor Resources are password-protected. To access the protected instructor resources, go to www.cengagebrain.com to create a unique single-user sign-on. Contact your sales representative for more information:

Teaching Tip:

The Instructor Companion site also contains revision files, which include changes to be made in the textbook and/or Instructor's Manual after publication (e.g., revised code numbers due to coding updates). You are welcome to e-mail the authors at delmarauthor@yahoo.com with questions or comments. The authors will respond to your e-mails, and appropriate corrections will be posted to provide clarification about textbook and workbook content.

INSTRUCTOR RESOURCES CD-ROM

The Instructor Resources CD-ROM contains an electronic version of this Instructor's Manual, a computerized test bank (CTB), and instructor's slides in PowerPoint®. Go to **http://www.delmarhealthcare.com** or contact your Cengage Delmar Learning sales representative to order the Instructor Resources CD-ROM. These same supplements are also located at the password-protected Instructor's Resources link at the Instructor Companion site.

Teaching Tip:

- *The CTB contains true/false, short answer, completion, multiple choice, and matching questions. ExamView® software is also included on the Instructor Resources CD-ROM as well as the Instructor Companion site to allow you to generate exams quickly, which can be printed or web-enabled. This means that you can create different versions of the same exam for large classes of students (when students cannot be separated from each other by an empty desk).*
- *For online courses, presentations prepared using Microsoft PowerPoint® can be web-enabled. Just use Microsoft's PowerPoint® software to open a presentation; click "File," then "Save as Web Page." Upload the *.mht file you created to your online course or to the web. Students do not need Microsoft PowerPoint® software installed on their computer to view the presentation. (If your students have Microsoft PowerPoint® software installed on their computers, you can just upload the *.ppt files to your online course or the web.)*
- *An* Insurance, Billing, and Coding Curriculum Guide *is also located at the Instructor Companion site to assist you in developing new academic programs and in modifying existing programs. The guide contains information about the job outlook and salaries for coders, available professional certification examinations, and curriculum coordination (e.g., marketing, student advising, teaching, professional practices, program approval, and program assessment). Content taught in a coding curriculum is linked to AAPC, AHIMA, and AMBA educational standards. Content is also linked to Cengage Delmar Learning products to assist you in selecting textbooks for instruction. Course outlines and course syllabi are included as samples, and they can be modified for your program. (In Adobe Reader, click on "File," then "Save as Text" to convert the guide to a document that can be opened in word processing software. All of the formatting will be lost, but you can scroll through the document to locate the content you want to cut/paste and modify to reformat. You might find it easier to print pages from the guide, edit them, and then keyboard new documents for your use.)*

WEBTUTOR™

WebTutor™ is available as a downloadable course cartridge or e-Pack for schools that use Blackboard, eCollege, WebCT, or another platform (e.g., Angel, Desire2Learn, Educator) as an online learning management system. Go to **http://webtutor.cengage.com** to order WebTutor™.

Teaching Tip:

- *WebTutor™ can be used to teach a course entirely online or to web-enhance an on-campus course. (Your textbook author teaches entirely online; but if she ever has an opportunity to teach a face-to-face course again, she will use WebTutor™ to administer all quizzes and exams* outside of class time *in her college's testing center because that will add five hours or more of teaching time to her courses.)*
- *Chapter exams in this Instructor's Manual contain the same questions as those included in WebTutor™. Detailed feedback is provided for incorrect answers when students take exams using WebTutor™. (Administering quizzes and exams* outside of class time *is possible because students are provided with detailed feedback once they submit their quiz or exam. The instructor can delay viewing of detailed feedback until all students have submitted the quiz or exam. For a face-to-face course, the instructor can devote part of a class to discussing the exam results and questions about difficult exam items. For an online course, students can e-mail the instructor or post discussion comments about exam issues.)*

SECTION I

Preparing Your Course

3-2-1 Code It! is a comprehensive textbook that covers all coding systems, and its content is written to prepare medical assistants and other health care professionals for beginner or entry-level coding positions. The third edition embeds ICD-10-CM and ICD-10-PCS in a side-by-side format next to ICD-9-CM content in textbook Chapters 2–6 (except for ICD-10-PCS content located in Chapter 5, which is located at the end of the chapter). The textbook is organized so that content can be taught in parts (Table 1) in one course as well as in two (or more) courses. Your academic program and course requirements will determine the sections that should be taught to students.

EXAMPLE 1

A sequence of two-semester coding courses could include Parts I and II in an ICD-9-CM and ICD-10-CM/PCS coding course. Then Parts III and IV could be taught in a HCPCS/CPT coding course. Many medical assistant and coding programs also teach a separate insurance and reimbursement course, eliminating the need to require Part V in either coding course. However, if your program does not have a separate course, consider adding Part V to one of your coding courses (or to an entirely different course, such as Introduction to Health Information Management).

EXAMPLE 2

A one-semester coding course taught in a medical assistant (MA) or medical office administration (MOA) program could include Parts II, III, and IV, eliminating Chapter 5 from Part II. You could also consider eliminating Chapters 10, 17, and 18 from the course syllabus (and assigning them outside of class or offer them as an independent study course).

Many MA and MOA programs teach a separate insurance and reimbursement course, eliminating the need to include Part V in the coding course. If the program doesn't offer a separate insurance and reimbursement course, consider adding Part V content to a different course (e.g., Administrative Medical Assisting or Introduction to Health Information Management).

Table 1 Organization of *3-2-1 Code It!*

Part	Title	Chapter
I	Coding Overview	Chapter 1: Overview of Coding
II	ICD-9-CM, ICD-10-CM, and ICD-10-PCS Coding Systems	Chapter 2: Introduction to ICD-9-CM and ICD-10-CM/PCS Coding Chapter 3: ICD-9-CM and ICD-10-CM/PCS Coding Conventions Chapter 4: ICD-9-CM and ICD-10-CM Coding Guidelines Chapter 5: ICD-9-CM and ICD-10-CM/PCS Hospital Inpatient Coding Chapter 6: ICD-9-CM and ICD-10-CM Outpatient and Physician Office Coding
III	Health Care Procedure Coding System (HCPCS), Level II National Coding System	Chapter 7: HCPCS Level II National Coding System
IV	Current Procedural Terminology (CPT) Coding System	Chapter 8: Introduction to CPT Coding Chapter 9: CPT Evaluation and Management Chapter 10: CPT Anesthesia Chapter 11: CPT Surgery I Chapter 12: CPT Surgery II Chapter 13: CPT Surgery III Chapter 14: CPT Surgery IV Chapter 15: CPT Surgery V Chapter 16: CPT Radiology Chapter 17: CPT Pathology and Laboratory Chapter 18: CPT Medicine
V	Insurance and Reimbursement Overview	Chapter 19: Insurance and Reimbursement

SEMESTER PLANS

The one-semester plan (Table 2) assumes 45 hours of classroom lecture (or 3 hours per week for 15 weeks). Your course may also include an additional 45 hours of laboratory during the semester, for which corresponding workbook chapters can be assigned. The final examination is not included in the 45-hour plan.

Some educators prefer to use this textbook for a two-semester sequential course, teaching ICD-9-CM and ICD-10-CM/PCS in one course and HCPCS/CPT in another course. If that is the method you prefer, refer to the two-semester plan (Table 3).

Table 2 One-Semester Plan

Week	Chapter
1-2	Chapter 1: Overview of Coding Chapter 2: Introduction to ICD-9-CM and ICD-10-CM/PCS Coding Exam 1
3-4	Chapter 3: ICD-9-CM and ICD-10-CM/PCS Coding Conventions Chapter 4: ICD-9-CM and ICD-10-CM Coding Guidelines Exam 2
5-6	Chapter 5: ICD-9-CM and ICD-10-CM Hospital Inpatient Coding Chapter 6: ICD-9-CM and ICD-10-CM Outpatient and Physician Office Coding Exam 3
NOTE: If teaching in a medical assistant or medical office administration program, consider eliminating Chapter 5: ICD-9-CM and ICD-10-CM/PCS Inpatient Coding.	
7	Chapter 7: HCPCS Level II National Coding System Exam 4
8	Chapter 8: Introduction to CPT Coding Chapter 10: CPT Anesthesia Exam 5
NOTE: If teaching in a medical assistant or medical office administration program, consider requiring Chapter 10: CPT Anesthesia as an outside-of-class assignment.	
9	Chapter 9: CPT Evaluation and Management Exam 6
10-12	Chapters 11-15: CPT Surgery I-V Exam 7
NOTE: If teaching in a medical assistant or medical office administration program, consider covering just those portions of Chapters 11-15: CPT Surgery I-V that pertain to your academic program's *community of interest*. A *community of interest* includes employers who hire an academic program's graduates; the employers should be surveyed to determine the level of CPT Surgery coding required of graduates. For example, medical assistants might be required to assign codes for simple and intermediate repairs in the CPT Integumentary subsection (but not for skin grafts and flaps, which are often performed in a hospital ambulatory surgery or inpatient setting and coded by hospital outpatient and inpatient coding specialists).	
13-14	Chapter 16: CPT Radiology Chapter 17: CPT Pathology and Laboratory Chapter 18: CPT Medicine Chapter 19: Insurance and Reimbursement Exam 8
15	Review of Chapters 1-19 for final examination
Finals Week	Comprehensive Final Examination (Chapters 1-19)

Table 3 Two-Semester Plan

First Semester

Week	Chapter
1-2	Chapter 1: Overview of Coding Exam 1
3-4	Chapter 2: Introduction to ICD-9-CM and ICD-10-CM/PCS Coding Exam 2
5-6	Chapter 3: ICD-9-CM and ICD-10-CM/PCS Coding Conventions Exam 3
7-8	Chapter 4: ICD-9-CM and ICD-10-CM Coding Guidelines Exam 4
9-12	Chapter 5: ICD-9-CM and ICD-10-CM/PCS Hospital Inpatient Coding Exam 5
NOTE: If teaching in a medical assistant or medical office administration program, consider eliminating Chapter 5: ICD-9-CM and ICD-10-CM/PCS Hospital Inpatient Coding (and from Week 15, Review of Chapters 1-6 for final examination and Comprehensive Final Examination).	
13-14	Chapter 6: ICD-9-CM and ICD-10-CM Outpatient and Physician Office Coding Exam 6
15	Review of Chapters 1-6 for final examination
Finals Week	Comprehensive Final Examination (Chapters 1-6)

Second Semester

Week	Chapter
1	Chapter 7: HCPCS Level II National Coding System Exam 1
2	Chapter 8: Introduction to CPT Coding Exam 2
3-4	Chapter 9: CPT Evaluation and Management Exam 3
5	Chapter 10: CPT Anesthesia Exam 4
6-10	Chapters 11-15: CPT Surgery I-V Exam 5
11	Chapter 16: CPT Radiology Exam 6
12	Chapter 17: CPT Pathology and Laboratory Exam 7
13	Chapter 18: CPT Medicine Exam 8
14	Chapter 19: Insurance and Reimbursement Exam 9
NOTE: If a separate insurance and reimbursement course is taught in your program, consider eliminating Chapter 19: Insurance and Reimbursement (and from Week 15, Review of Chapters 7-19 for final examination and Comprehensive Final Examination).	
15	Review of Chapters 7-19 for final examination
Finals Week	Comprehensive Final Examination (Chapters 7-19)

ADMINISTERING EXAMS

Administer short quizzes that cover definitions, coding conventions, and so on, to ensure that students keep up with reading assignments. Unit exams include theory and coding practice. If time permits, you may want to include content from the chapter(s) covered in the last unit on the final examination (instead of administering a separate unit exam).

Teaching Tip:

Consider using WebTutor™ to administer quizzes and exams, whether your course is offered entirely online or face-to-face. The detailed feedback for incorrect answers in WebTutor™ will prove helpful to students. If you teach face-to-face, you can administer the online exams in a classroom setting or use your college's testing center. Then devote part of a class to answering students' questions about the exam so they have a good understanding about the concepts they hadn't mastered.

The textbook author enjoys this discussion with students, and she encourages students to challenge the authenticity of questions and answers as a critical thinking activity. When students convince her that a question was badly written or there could have been more than one answer, she rewards them by adding appropriate points to their exam grade. Then, of course, she revises that exam item for future use! This turns what can be an intimidating process, especially for a new instructor, into a fun learning activity for all. Students learn to think critically, new instructors don't dread discussing exam results, and everyone benefits because exam items are revised and perfected each time the course is taught. (As an aside, it can take up to five years for a new instructor to feel totally comfortable discussing exam results. Embracing students' questions and criticisms is a way to jump-start the "road to comfort.")

GRADING ASSIGNMENTS AND EXAMS

It is important to communicate your grading policy for coding assignments and exams. Refer to the suggested grading policies for ICD-9-CM, ICD-10-CM, ICD-10-PCS, and HCPCS/CPT coding assignments and exams below.

ICD-9-CM, ICD-10-CM, and ICD-10-PCS Coding

Assign one point for each correct ICD-9-CM code, including required fourth and fifth digits for diagnosis codes (and required third and fourth digits for procedure codes). Deduct one-half point for each additional code listed that is not required by ICD-9-CM coding guidelines (e.g., student assigns a code to an inpatient qualified diagnosis and assigns individual codes to its signs and symptoms).

Assign one point for each correct ICD-10-CM code, including required fourth through seventh digits. Deduct one-half point for each additional code listed that is not required by ICD-10-CM coding guidelines.

Assign one point for each correct ICD-10-PCS code, each of which require seven characters *without a decimal*. Deduct one-half point for each additional code listed that is not required by ICD-10-PCS coding guidelines.

HCPCS and CPT Coding

Assign one point for each correct code, plus one point for each required modifier. Deduct one-half point for each additional code or modifier that is not required by CPT/HCPCS guidelines and notes.

LESSON PLANS

Lesson plans assist instructors in preparing for class so that specific activities and objectives are accomplished. Lesson plans for each textbook chapter have been created to assist you in organizing your course. Just complete the information in the Time row for each chapter; then enter the class and lab numbers to set up your course. (The lesson plans can be used for a one- or two-semester coding course.)

Chapter 1: Overview of Coding		
Time:	• Instructor preparation (_____ hours) • Introduction to course (1/2 hour) • In-class lecture (_____ hours) • In-class lab (if laboratory component is included as part of course) (_____ hours)	
Topics:	• Career as a Coder • Professional Associations and Discussion Boards • Coding Overview • Documentation as Basis for Coding • Health Data Collection	
Overview:	This chapter focuses on coding career opportunities in health care, the importance of joining professional associations and obtaining coding credentials, the impact of networking with other coding professionals, and the development of opportunities for career advancement. A coding overview provides students with an introduction to coding concepts, including the role patient record documentation plays in accurate coding.	
Objectives:	• Define key terms. • Explain coding career opportunities and the coding credentialing process. • Identify professional associations and describe the benefits of membership. • Clarify student responsibilities during a coding internship. • Identify coding systems used for reimbursement, and indicate the relationship between patient record documentation and accurate coding.	
	Task	**Resource**
Prior to class:	• Read textbook and prepare lecture notes. • Review answers to chapter review. • Select workbook assignments for homework. • Prepare course syllabus. • Prepare chapter quiz.	• *3-2-1 Code It!*, Chapter 1 • *Instructor's Manual to Accompany 3-2-1 Code It!*, Chapter 1 • *Workbook to Accompany 3-2-1 Code It!*, Chapter 1 • *Instructor's Manual to Accompany 3-2-1 Code It!*, Introduction • *Instructor's Manual to Accompany 3-2-1 Code It!*, Chapter 1
Class # ___:	• Distribute and explain course syllabus. • Point out major features of textbook. • Review WebTutor™ features (if applicable). • Assign Chapter 1 as reading assignment. • Lecture on Chapter 1 content. • Encourage students to create flash cards. • Assign chapter review as homework.	• Prepared course syllabus • *3-2-1 Code It!*, Preface • *3-2-1 Code It!*, Preface • *3-2-1 Code It!*, Chapter 1 • Lecture notes prepared from *3-2-1 Code!*, Chapter 1 • *3-2-1 Code It!*, Chapter 1 • *3-2-1 Code It!*, Chapter 1
Class # ___:	• Review previous class lecture and answer students' questions about chapter content. • Continue lecture on Chapter 1 content. • Collect homework (and grade). • Administer chapter quiz. • Assign Chapter 1 as reading assignment.	• Ask students to identify key topics and issues from previous class lecture. • *3-2-1 Code It!*, Chapter 1 • *Instructor's Manual to Accompany 3-2-1 Code It!*, Chapter 1 • *Instructor's Manual to Accompany 3-2-1 Code It!*, Chapter 1 • *3-2-1 Code It!*, Chapter 2
Lab # ___:	• Point out major features of workbook. • Communicate assignments to be accomplished during lab and explain how each is to be completed. • Rotate among students as they complete lab assignments to provide individual assistance. • Consider reviewing rough draft work during lab and allowing students to submit final draft at the beginning of the next lab class. • Assign additional workbook assignments for homework.	• *Workbook to Accompany 3-2-1 Code It!*, Preface • *Workbook to Accompany 3-2-1 Code It!*, Chapter 1
Assessment:	• Homework assignments • Chapter quiz • In-class participation • Lab assignments	

Chapter 2: Introduction to ICD-9-CM and ICD-10-CM/PCS Coding		
Time:	• Instructor preparation (______ hours) • In-class lecture (______ hours) • In-class lab (if laboratory component is included as part of course) (______ hours)	
Topics:	• Overview of ICD-9-CM and ICD-10-CM/PCS • ICD-9-CM Tabular List of Diseases and ICD-10-CM Tabular List of Diseases and Injuries • ICD-9-CM Index to Diseases and ICD-10-CM Index to Diseases and Injuries • ICD-9-CM Tabular List of Procedures and Index to Procedures • ICD-10-PCS Index and Tables • Official ICD-9-CM and ICD-10-CM/PCS Guidelines for Coding and Reporting	
Overview:	This chapter focuses on the organization of the ICD-9-CM, ICD-10-CM, and ICD-10-PCS coding systems and the official guidelines for coding and reporting.	
Objectives:	• Define key terms. • Explain the organization of the ICD-9-CM Tabular List of Diseases, Index to Diseases, and Tabular List of Procedures and Index to Procedures. • Explain the organization of the ICD-10-CM Index to Injuries and Diseases and the Tabular List of Diseases and Injuries. • Explain the organization of the ICD-10-PCS Index and Tables. • List and describe the guidelines for coding and reporting ICD-9-CM and ICD-10-CM/PCS. • Interpret ICD-9-CM and ICD-10-CM/PCS guidelines for coding and reporting. • Apply guidelines for coding and reporting when assigning ICD-9-CM and ICD-10-CM/PCS codes.	
	Task	**Resource**
Prior to class:	• Read textbook and prepare lecture notes. • Review answers to chapter review. • Select workbook assignments for homework. • Prepare course syllabus. • Prepare chapter quiz.	• *3-2-1 Code It!*, Chapter 2 • *Instructor's Manual to Accompany 3-2-1 Code It!*, Chapter 2 • *Workbook to Accompany 3-2-1 Code It!*, Chapter 2 • *Instructor's Manual to Accompany 3-2-1 Code It!*, Introduction • *Instructor's Manual to Accompany 3-2-1 Code It!*, Chapter 2
Class # ___:	• Distribute and explain course syllabus. • Point out major features of textbook. • Review WebTutor™ features (if applicable). • Assign Chapter 2 as reading assignment. • Lecture on Chapter 2 content. • Encourage students to create flash cards. • Assign chapter review as homework.	• Prepared course syllabus • *3-2-1 Code It!*, Preface • *3-2-1 Code It!*, Preface • *3-2-1 Code It!*, Chapter 2 • Lecture notes prepared from *3-2-1 Code!*, Chapter 2 • *3-2-1 Code It!*, Chapter 2 • *3-2-1 Code It!*, Chapter 2
Class # ___:	• Review previous class lecture and answer students' questions about chapter content. • Continue lecture on Chapter 2 content. • Collect homework (and grade). • Administer chapter quiz. • Assign Chapter 2 as reading assignment.	• Ask students to identify key topics and issues from previous class lecture. • *3-2-1 Code It!*, Chapter 2 • *Instructor's Manual to Accompany 3-2-1 Code It!*, Chapter 2 • *Instructor's Manual to Accompany 3-2-1 Code It!*, Chapter 2 • *3-2-1 Code It!*, Chapter 2
Lab # ___:	• Point out major features of workbook. • Communicate assignments to be accomplished during lab and explain how each is to be completed. • Rotate among students as they complete lab assignments to provide individual assistance. • Consider reviewing rough draft work during lab and allowing students to submit final draft at the beginning of the next lab class. • Assign additional workbook assignments for homework.	• *Workbook to Accompany 3-2-1 Code It!*, Preface • *Workbook to Accompany 3-2-1 Code It!*, Chapter 2
Assessment:	• Homework assignments • Chapter quiz • In-class participation • Lab assignments	

Chapter 3: ICD-9-CM and ICD-10-CM/PCS Coding Conventions		
Time:	• Instructor preparation (_____ hours) • In-class lecture (_____ hours) • In-class lab (if laboratory component is included as part of course) (_____ hours)	
Topics:	• Format and Typeface • Eponyms • Abbreviations • Punctuation • Boxed Notes • Tables • Includes and Excludes Notes and Inclusion Terms • Other, Other Specified, and Unspecified Codes • Etiology and Manifestation Rules • And • Due to • In • With • Cross-References	
Overview:	This chapter focuses on ICD-9-CM and ICD-10-CM/PCS coding conventions, which are the rules used when assigning codes.	
Objectives:	• Define key terms. • List ICD-9-CM and ICD-10-CM/PCS coding conventions. • Explain ICD-9-CM and ICD-10-CM/PCS coding conventions. • Interpret ICD-9-CM and ICD-10-CM/PCS coding conventions to assign codes accurately.	
	Task	**Resource**
Prior to class:	• Read textbook and prepare lecture notes. • Review answers to chapter review. • Select workbook assignments for homework. • Prepare course syllabus. • Prepare chapter quiz.	• *3-2-1 Code It!*, Chapter 3 • *Instructor's Manual to Accompany 3-2-1 Code It!*, Chapter 3 • *Workbook to Accompany 3-2-1 Code It!*, Chapter 3 • *Instructor's Manual to Accompany 3-2-1 Code It!*, Introduction • *Instructor's Manual to Accompany 3-2-1 Code It!*, Chapter 3
Class # ___:	• Distribute and explain course syllabus. • Point out major features of textbook. • Review WebTutor™ features (if applicable). • Assign Chapter 3 as reading assignment. • Lecture on Chapter 3 content. • Encourage students to create flash cards. • Assign chapter review as homework.	• Prepared course syllabus • *3-2-1 Code It!*, Preface • *3-2-1 Code It!*, Preface • *3-2-1 Code It!*, Chapter 3 • Lecture notes prepared from *3-2-1 Code!*, Chapter 3 • *3-2-1 Code It!*, Chapter 3 • *3-2-1 Code It!*, Chapter 3
Class # ___:	• Review previous class lecture and answer students' questions about chapter content. • Continue lecture on Chapter 3 content. • Collect homework (and grade). • Administer chapter quiz. • Assign Chapter 3 as reading assignment.	• Ask students to identify key topics and issues from previous class lecture. • *3-2-1 Code It!*, Chapter 3 • *Instructor's Manual to Accompany 3-2-1 Code It!*, Chapter 3 • *Instructor's Manual to Accompany 3-2-1 Code It!*, Chapter 3 • *3-2-1 Code It!*, Chapter 3
Lab # ___:	• Point out major features of workbook. • Communicate assignments to be accomplished during lab and explain how each is to be completed. • Rotate among students as they complete lab assignments to provide individual assistance. • Consider reviewing rough draft work during lab and allowing students to submit final draft at the beginning of the next lab class. • Assign additional workbook assignments for homework.	• *Workbook to Accompany 3-2-1 Code It!*, Preface • *Workbook to Accompany 3-2-1 Code It!*, Chapter 3
Assessment:	• Homework assignments • Chapter quiz • In-class participation • Lab assignments	

Chapter 4: ICD-9-CM and ICD-10-CM Coding Guidelines		
Time:	• Instructor preparation (_____ hours) • In-class lecture (_____ hours) • In-class lab (if laboratory component is included as part of course) (_____ hours)	
Topics:	• ICD-9-CM and ICD-10-CM Official Guidelines for Coding and Reporting • General ICD-9-CM and ICD-10-CM Diagnosis Coding Guidelines • ICD-9-CM Chapter-Specific Coding Guidelines with ICD-10 Alerts	
Overview:	This chapter focuses on the interpretation of the *Guidelines for Coding and Reporting Using ICD-9-CM* and the *Guidelines for Coding and Reporting Using ICD-10-CM,* including general ICD-9-CM diagnosis coding guidelines, and ICD-9-CM chapter-specific coding guidelines.	
Objectives:	• Define key terms. • Explain HIPAA's impact on the adherence to *ICD-9-CM Official Guidelines for Coding and Reporting* and *ICD-10-CM Official Guidelines for Coding and Reporting.* • Describe the content of each section of the *ICD-9-CM Official Guidelines for Coding and Reporting* and the *ICD-10-CM Official Guidelines for Coding and Reporting* (see Appendix II located at the Student Companion site at www.cengagebrain.com). • Apply general ICD-9-CM and ICD-10-CM coding guidelines when assigning codes to diagnoses. • Apply chapter-specific ICD-9-CM and ICD-10-CM coding guidelines when assigning codes to diagnoses.	
	Task	**Resource**
Prior to class:	• Read textbook and prepare lecture notes. • Review answers to chapter review. • Select workbook assignments for homework. • Prepare course syllabus. • Prepare chapter quiz.	• *3-2-1 Code It!*, Chapter 4 • *Instructor's Manual to Accompany 3-2-1 Code It!*, Chapter 4 • *Workbook to Accompany 3-2-1 Code It!*, Chapter 4 • *Instructor's Manual to Accompany 3-2-1 Code It!*, Introduction • *Instructor's Manual to Accompany 3-2-1 Code It!*, Chapter 4
Class # ___:	• Distribute and explain course syllabus. • Point out major features of textbook. • Review WebTutor™ features (if applicable). • Assign Chapter 4 as reading assignment. • Lecture on Chapter 4 content. • Encourage students to create flash cards. • Assign chapter review as homework.	• Prepared course syllabus • *3-2-1 Code It!*, Preface • *3-2-1 Code It!*, Preface • *3-2-1 Code It!*, Chapter 4 • Lecture notes prepared from *3-2-1 Code!*, Chapter 4 • *3-2-1 Code It!*, Chapter 4 • *3-2-1 Code It!*, Chapter 4
Class # ___:	• Review previous class lecture and answer students' questions about chapter content. • Continue lecture on Chapter 4 content. • Collect homework (and grade). • Administer chapter quiz. • Assign Chapter 4 as reading assignment.	• Ask students to identify key topics and issues from previous class lecture. • *3-2-1 Code It!*, Chapter 4 • *Instructor's Manual to Accompany 3-2-1 Code It!*, Chapter 4 • *Instructor's Manual to Accompany 3-2-1 Code It!*, Chapter 4 • *3-2-1 Code It!*, Chapter 4
Lab # ___:	• Point out major features of workbook. • Communicate assignments to be accomplished during lab and explain how each is to be completed. • Rotate among students as they complete lab assignments to provide individual assistance. • Consider reviewing rough draft work during lab and allowing students to submit final draft at the beginning of the next lab class. • Assign additional workbook assignments for homework.	• *Workbook to Accompany 3-2-1 Code It!*, Preface • *Workbook to Accompany 3-2-1 Code It!*, Chapter 4
Assessment:	• Homework assignments • Chapter quiz • In-class participation • Lab assignments	

Chapter 5: ICD-9-CM and ICD-10-CM/PCS Hospital Inpatient Coding		
Time:	• Instructor preparation (_____ hours) • In-class lecture (_____ hours) • In-class lab (if laboratory component is included as part of course) (_____ hours)	
Topics:	• Acute Care Facilities (Hospitals) • Inpatient Diagnosis Coding Guidelines • Inpatient Procedure Coding Guidelines • ICD-9-CM Procedure Coding • ICD-10-PCS Procedure Coding	
Overview:	This chapter focuses on inpatient acute care settings (e.g., hospitals) and includes an interpretation of guidelines for sequencing diagnoses and procedures, which are published in the *Guidelines for Coding and Reporting Using ICD-9-CM* and in the *Guidelines for Coding and Reporting Using ICD-9-CM*, and are used as a companion to the official version of ICD-9-CM and ICD-10-CM, respectively.	
Objectives:	• Define key terms. • List and explain differences among acute care inpatient settings. • Interpret inpatient diagnosis and procedure coding and reporting guidelines. • Assign ICD-9-CM and ICD-10-CM/PCS diagnosis and/or procedure codes for acute care inpatient cases.	
	Task	**Resource**
Prior to class:	• Read textbook and prepare lecture notes. • Review answers to chapter review. • Select workbook assignments for homework. • Prepare course syllabus. • Prepare chapter quiz.	• *3-2-1 Code It!*, Chapter 5 • *Instructor's Manual to Accompany 3-2-1 Code It!*, Chapter 5 • *Workbook to Accompany 3-2-1 Code It!*, Chapter 5 • *Instructor's Manual to Accompany 3-2-1 Code It!*, Introduction • *Instructor's Manual to Accompany 3-2-1 Code It!*, Chapter 5
Class # ___:	• Distribute and explain course syllabus. • Point out major features of textbook. • Review WebTutor™ features (if applicable). • Assign Chapter 5 as reading assignment. • Lecture on Chapter 5 content. • Encourage students to create flash cards. • Assign chapter review as homework.	• Prepared course syllabus • *3-2-1 Code It!*, Preface • *3-2-1 Code It!*, Preface • *3-2-1 Code It!*, Chapter 5 • Lecture notes prepared from *3-2-1 Code!*, Chapter 5 • *3-2-1 Code It!*, Chapter 5 • *3-2-1 Code It!*, Chapter 5
Class # ___:	• Review previous class lecture and answer students' questions about chapter content. • Continue lecture on Chapter 5 content. • Collect homework (and grade). • Administer chapter quiz. • Assign Chapter 5 as reading assignment.	• Ask students to identify key topics and issues from previous class lecture. • *3-2-1 Code It!*, Chapter 5 • *Instructor's Manual to Accompany 3-2-1 Code It!*, Chapter 5 • *Instructor's Manual to Accompany 3-2-1 Code It!*, Chapter 5 • *3-2-1 Code It!*, Chapter 5
Lab # ___:	• Point out major features of workbook. • Communicate assignments to be accomplished during lab and explain how each is to be completed. • Rotate among students as they complete lab assignments to provide individual assistance. • Consider reviewing rough draft work during lab and allowing students to submit final draft at the beginning of the next lab class. • Assign additional workbook assignments for homework.	• *Workbook to Accompany 3-2-1 Code It!*, Preface • *Workbook to Accompany 3-2-1 Code It!*, Chapter 5
Assessment:	• Homework assignments • Chapter quiz • In-class participation • Lab assignments	

Chapter 6: ICD-9-CM and ICD-10-CM Outpatient and Physician Office Coding		
Time:	• Instructor preparation (_____ hours) • In-class lecture (_____ hours) • In-class lab (if laboratory component is included as part of course) (_____ hours)	
Topics:	• Outpatient and Physician Office Care • Diagnostic Coding and Reporting Guidelines for Outpatient Services: Hospital-Based and Physician Office • Coding Guidelines for Outpatient Diagnostic Tests	
Overview:	This chapter focuses on outpatient care and physician office settings and interprets the *Diagnostic Coding and Reporting Guidelines for Outpatient Services: Hospital-Based and Physician Office.*	
Objectives:	• Define key terms. • List and explain differences among outpatient and physician office health care settings. • Interpret outpatient diagnosis coding and reporting guidelines. • Assign ICD-9-CM and ICD-10-CM diagnosis codes for outpatient and physician office care.	
	Task	Resource
Prior to class:	• Read textbook and prepare lecture notes. • Review answers to chapter review. • Select workbook assignments for homework. • Prepare course syllabus. • Prepare chapter quiz.	• *3-2-1 Code It!*, Chapter 6 • *Instructor's Manual to Accompany 3-2-1 Code It!*, Chapter 6 • *Workbook to Accompany 3-2-1 Code It!*, Chapter 6 • *Instructor's Manual to Accompany 3-2-1 Code It!*, Introduction • *Instructor's Manual to Accompany 3-2-1 Code It!*, Chapter 6
Class # ___:	• Distribute and explain course syllabus. • Point out major features of textbook. • Review WebTutor™ features (if applicable). • Assign Chapter 6 as reading assignment. • Lecture on Chapter 6 content. • Encourage students to create flash cards. • Assign chapter review as homework.	• Prepared course syllabus • *3-2-1 Code It!*, Preface • *3-2-1 Code It!*, Preface • *3-2-1 Code It!*, Chapter 6 • Lecture notes prepared from *3-2-1 Code!*, Chapter 6 • *3-2-1 Code It!*, Chapter 6 • *3-2-1 Code It!*, Chapter 6
Class # ___:	• Review previous class lecture and answer students' questions about chapter content. • Continue lecture on Chapter 6 content. • Collect homework (and grade). • Administer chapter quiz. • Assign Chapter 6 as reading assignment.	• Ask students to identify key topics and issues from previous class lecture. • *3-2-1 Code It!*, Chapter 6 • *Instructor's Manual to Accompany 3-2-1 Code It!*, Chapter 6 • *Instructor's Manual to Accompany 3-2-1 Code It!*, Chapter 6 • *3-2-1 Code It!*, Chapter 6
Lab # ___:	• Point out major features of workbook. • Communicate assignments to be accomplished during lab and explain how each is to be completed. • Rotate among students as they complete lab assignments to provide individual assistance. • Consider reviewing rough draft work during lab and allowing students to submit final draft at the beginning of the next lab class. • Assign additional workbook assignments for homework.	• *Workbook to Accompany 3-2-1 Code It!*, Preface • *Workbook to Accompany 3-2-1 Code It!*, Chapter 6
Assessment:	• Homework assignments • Chapter quiz • In-class participation • Lab assignments	

Chapter 7: HCPCS Level II National Coding System		
Time:	• Instructor preparation (_____ hours) • In-class lecture (_____ hours) • In-class lab (if laboratory component is included as part of course) (_____ hours)	
Topics:	• Overview of HCPCS • Assigning HCPCS Level II Codes • Determining Payer Responsibility	
Overview:	This chapter focuses on the HCPCS level II national coding system, which contains alphanumeric codes that were developed to complement the *Current Procedural Terminology* (CPT) coding system.	
Objectives:	• Define key terms. • List the HCPCS levels and their components. • Assign HCPCS level II procedure and services codes for outpatient care. • Identify situations in which both HCPCS levels I and II codes are assigned. • Assign claims to primary Medicare administrative contractor (MACs) or Durable Medical Equipment MACs according to HCPCS level II code number.	
	Task	**Resource**
Prior to class:	• Read textbook and prepare lecture notes. • Review answers to chapter review. • Select workbook assignments for homework. • Prepare course syllabus. • Prepare chapter quiz.	• *3-2-1 Code It!*, Chapter 7 • *Instructor's Manual to Accompany 3-2-1 Code It!*, Chapter 7 • *Workbook to Accompany 3-2-1 Code It!*, Chapter 7 • *Instructor's Manual to Accompany 3-2-1 Code It!*, Introduction • *Instructor's Manual to Accompany 3-2-1 Code It!*, Chapter 7
Class # ___:	• Distribute and explain course syllabus. • Point out major features of textbook. • Review WebTutor™ features (if applicable). • Assign Chapter 7 as reading assignment. • Lecture on Chapter 7 content. • Encourage students to create flash cards. • Assign chapter review as homework.	• Prepared course syllabus • *3-2-1 Code It!*, Preface • *3-2-1 Code It!*, Preface • *3-2-1 Code It!*, Chapter 7 • Lecture notes prepared from *3-2-1 Code!*, Chapter 7 • *3-2-1 Code It!*, Chapter 7 • *3-2-1 Code It!*, Chapter 7
Class # ___:	• Review previous class lecture and answer students' questions about chapter content. • Continue lecture on Chapter 7 content. • Collect homework (and grade). • Administer chapter quiz. • Assign Chapter 7 as reading assignment.	• Ask students to identify key topics and issues from previous class lecture. • *3-2-1 Code It!*, Chapter 7 • *Instructor's Manual to Accompany 3-2-1 Code It!*, Chapter 7 • *Instructor's Manual to Accompany 3-2-1 Code It!*, Chapter 7 • *3-2-1 Code It!*, Chapter 7
Lab # ___:	• Point out major features of workbook. • Communicate assignments to be accomplished during lab and explain how each is to be completed. • Rotate among students as they complete lab assignments to provide individual assistance. • Consider reviewing rough draft work during lab and allowing students to submit final draft at the beginning of the next lab class. • Assign additional workbook assignments for homework.	• *Workbook to Accompany 3-2-1 Code It!*, Preface • *Workbook to Accompany 3-2-1 Code It!*, Chapter 7
Assessment:	• Homework assignments • Chapter quiz • In-class participation • Lab assignments	

<table>
<tr><th colspan="3">Chapter 8: Introduction to CPT Coding</th></tr>
<tr><td>Time:</td><td colspan="2">• Instructor preparation (_____ hours)
• In-class lecture (_____ hours)
• In-class lab (if laboratory component is included as part of course) (_____ hours)</td></tr>
<tr><td>Topics:</td><td colspan="2">• History of CPT
• Overview of CPT
• Organization of CPT
• CPT Index
• CPT Appendices
• CPT Symbols
• CPT Sections, Subsections, Categories, and Subcategories
• CPT Modifiers
• National Correct Coding Initiative (NCCI)</td></tr>
<tr><td>Overview:</td><td colspan="2">This chapter introduces the Current Procedural Terminology (CPT) coding system (or HCPCS level I).</td></tr>
<tr><td>Objectives:</td><td colspan="2">• Define key terms.
• Explain the organization, format, and content of CPT.
• Interpret CPT section guidelines, coding notes, and modifiers.
• Assign CPT procedure and service codes for outpatient care.
• Add CPT and/or HCPCS level II modifiers to codes as appropriate.</td></tr>
<tr><td></td><td>Task</td><td>Resource</td></tr>
<tr><td>Prior to class:</td><td>• Read textbook and prepare lecture notes.
• Review answers to chapter review.
• Select workbook assignments for homework.
• Prepare course syllabus.
• Prepare chapter quiz.</td><td>• 3-2-1 Code It!, Chapter 8
• Instructor's Manual to Accompany 3-2-1 Code It!, Chapter 8
• Workbook to Accompany 3-2-1 Code It!, Chapter 8
• Instructor's Manual to Accompany 3-2-1 Code It!, Introduction
• Instructor's Manual to Accompany 3-2-1 Code It!, Chapter 8</td></tr>
<tr><td>Class # ___:</td><td>• Distribute and explain course syllabus.
• Point out major features of textbook.
• Review WebTutor™ features (if applicable).
• Assign Chapter 8 as reading assignment.
• Lecture on Chapter 8 content.
• Encourage students to create flash cards.
• Assign chapter review as homework.</td><td>• Prepared course syllabus
• 3-2-1 Code It!, Preface
• 3-2-1 Code It!, Preface
• 3-2-1 Code It!, Chapter 8
• Lecture notes prepared from 3-2-1 Code!, Chapter 8
• 3-2-1 Code It!, Chapter 8
• 3-2-1 Code It!, Chapter 8</td></tr>
<tr><td>Class # ___:</td><td>• Review previous class lecture and answer students' questions about chapter content.
• Continue lecture on Chapter 8 content.
• Collect homework (and grade).
• Administer chapter quiz.
• Assign Chapter 8 as reading assignment.</td><td>• Ask students to identify key topics and issues from previous class lecture.
• 3-2-1 Code It!, Chapter 8
• Instructor's Manual to Accompany 3-2-1 Code It!, Chapter 8
• Instructor's Manual to Accompany 3-2-1 Code It!, Chapter 8
• 3-2-1 Code It!, Chapter 8</td></tr>
<tr><td>Lab # ___:</td><td>• Point out major features of workbook.
• Communicate assignments to be accomplished during lab and explain how each is to be completed.
• Rotate among students as they complete lab assignments to provide individual assistance.
• Consider reviewing rough draft work during lab and allowing students to submit final draft at the beginning of the next lab class.
• Assign additional workbook assignments for homework.</td><td>• Workbook to Accompany 3-2-1 Code It!, Preface
• Workbook to Accompany 3-2-1 Code It!, Chapter 8</td></tr>
<tr><td>Assessment:</td><td colspan="2">• Homework assignments
• Chapter quiz
• In-class participation
• Lab assignments</td></tr>
</table>

Chapter 9: CPT Evaluation and Management		
Time:	• Instructor preparation (_____ hours) • In-class lecture (_____ hours) • In-class lab (if laboratory component is included as part of course) (_____ hours)	
Topics:	• Overview of Evaluation and Management Section • Evaluation and Management Section Guidelines • Levels of Evaluation and Management Services • Evaluation and Management Categories and Subcategories	
Overview:	This chapter focuses on CPT evaluation and management codes, which generate most of the revenue for the physician's office.	
Objectives:	• Define key terms. • Explain the organization, format, and content of the CPT Evaluation and Management section. • Interpret CPT Evaluation and Management section guidelines, coding notes, and modifiers. • Select CPT evaluation and management levels of service for documented patient care. • Assign CPT evaluation and management service codes for patient care. • Add CPT and/or HCPCS level II modifiers to codes as appropriate.	
	Task	**Resource**
Prior to class:	• Read textbook and prepare lecture notes. • Review answers to chapter review. • Select workbook assignments for homework. • Prepare course syllabus. • Prepare chapter quiz.	• *3-2-1 Code It!*, Chapter 9 • *Instructor's Manual to Accompany 3-2-1 Code It!*, Chapter 9 • *Workbook to Accompany 3-2-1 Code It!*, Chapter 9 • *Instructor's Manual to Accompany 3-2-1 Code It!*, Introduction • *Instructor's Manual to Accompany 3-2-1 Code It!*, Chapter 9
Class # ___:	• Distribute and explain course syllabus. • Point out major features of textbook. • Review WebTutor™ features (if applicable). • Assign Chapter 9 as reading assignment. • Lecture on Chapter 9 content. • Encourage students to create flash cards. • Assign chapter review as homework.	• Prepared course syllabus • *3-2-1 Code It!*, Preface • *3-2-1 Code It!*, Preface • *3-2-1 Code It!*, Chapter 9 • Lecture notes prepared from *3-2-1 Code!*, Chapter 9 • *3-2-1 Code It!*, Chapter 9 • *3-2-1 Code It!*, Chapter 9
Class # ___:	• Review previous class lecture and answer students' questions about chapter content. • Continue lecture on Chapter 9 content. • Collect homework (and grade). • Administer chapter quiz. • Assign Chapter 9 as reading assignment.	• Ask students to identify key topics and issues from previous class lecture. • *3-2-1 Code It!*, Chapter 9 • *Instructor's Manual to Accompany 3-2-1 Code It!*, Chapter 9 • *Instructor's Manual to Accompany 3-2-1 Code It!*, Chapter 9 • *3-2-1 Code It!*, Chapter 9
Lab # ___:	• Point out major features of workbook. • Communicate assignments to be accomplished during lab and explain how each is to be completed. • Rotate among students as they complete lab assignments to provide individual assistance. • Consider reviewing rough draft work during lab and allowing students to submit final draft at the beginning of the next lab class. • Assign additional workbook assignments for homework.	• *Workbook to Accompany 3-2-1 Code It!*, Preface • *Workbook to Accompany 3-2-1 Code It!*, Chapter 9
Assessment:	• Homework assignments • Chapter quiz • In-class participation • Lab assignments	

Chapter 10: CPT Anesthesia		
Time:	• Instructor preparation (_____ hours) • In-class lecture (_____ hours) • In-class lab (if laboratory component is included as part of course) (_____ hours)	
Topics:	• Anesthesia Terminology • Overview of Anesthesia Section • Anesthesia Section Guidelines • Anesthesia Subsections	
Overview:	This chapter focuses on CPT anesthesia codes, which are reported for services related to the administration of anesthesia (including general and regional), the supplementation of local anesthesia, and other supportive anesthesia services.	
Objectives:	• Define key terms. • Explain the organization, format, and content of the CPT Anesthesia section. • Interpret CPT anesthesia section guidelines, coding notes, and modifiers. • Assign CPT evaluation and management service codes. • Add CPT and/or HCPCS level II modifiers to codes as appropriate. • Calculate anesthesia fees.	
	Task	Resource
Prior to class:	• Read textbook and prepare lecture notes. • Review answers to chapter review. • Select workbook assignments for homework. • Prepare course syllabus. • Prepare chapter quiz.	• *3-2-1 Code It!*, Chapter 10 • *Instructor's Manual to Accompany 3-2-1 Code It!*, Chapter 10 • *Workbook to Accompany 3-2-1 Code It!*, Chapter 10 • *Instructor's Manual to Accompany 3-2-1 Code It!*, Introduction • *Instructor's Manual to Accompany 3-2-1 Code It!*, Chapter 10
Class # ___:	• Distribute and explain course syllabus. • Point out major features of textbook. • Review WebTutor™ features (if applicable). • Assign Chapter 10 as reading assignment. • Lecture on Chapter 10 content. • Encourage students to create flash cards. • Assign chapter review as homework.	• Prepared course syllabus • *3-2-1 Code It!*, Preface • *3-2-1 Code It!*, Preface • *3-2-1 Code It!*, Chapter 10 • Lecture notes prepared from *3-2-1 Code!*, Chapter 10 • *3-2-1 Code It!*, Chapter 10 • *3-2-1 Code It!*, Chapter 10
Class # ___:	• Review previous class lecture and answer students' questions about chapter content. • Continue lecture on Chapter 10 content. • Collect homework (and grade). • Administer chapter quiz. • Assign Chapter 10 as reading assignment.	• Ask students to identify key topics and issues from previous class lecture. • *3-2-1 Code It!*, Chapter 10 • *Instructor's Manual to Accompany 3-2-1 Code It!*, Chapter 10 • *Instructor's Manual to Accompany 3-2-1 Code It!*, Chapter 10 • *3-2-1 Code It!*, Chapter 10
Lab # ___:	• Point out major features of workbook. • Communicate assignments to be accomplished during lab and explain how each is to be completed. • Rotate among students as they complete lab assignments to provide individual assistance. • Consider reviewing rough draft work during lab and allowing students to submit final draft at the beginning of the next lab class. • Assign additional workbook assignments for homework.	• *Workbook to Accompany 3-2-1 Code It!*, Preface • *Workbook to Accompany 3-2-1 Code It!*, Chapter 10
Assessment:	• Homework assignments • Chapter quiz • In-class participation • Lab assignments	

Chapter 11: CPT Surgery I		
Time:	• Instructor preparation (_____ hours) • In-class lecture (_____ hours) • In-class lab (if laboratory component is included as part of course) (_____ hours)	
Topics:	• Overview of Surgery Section • Surgery Guidelines • General Subsection • Integumentary System Subsection	
Overview:	This chapter provides an overview of the CPT Surgery section and covers its guidelines. The chapter also focuses on the CPT Surgery General and Integumentary System subsections.	
Objectives:	• Define key terms. • Explain the organization, format, and content of the CPT Surgery section. • Interpret CPT Surgery section guidelines and modifiers • Interpret CPT surgery coding notes for the General and Integumentary System subsections. • Assign CPT surgery codes from the General and Integumentary System subsections. • Add CPT and/or HCPCS level II modifiers to codes as appropriate.	
	Task	**Resource**
Prior to class:	• Read textbook and prepare lecture notes. • Review answers to chapter review. • Select workbook assignments for homework. • Prepare course syllabus. • Prepare chapter quiz.	• *3-2-1 Code It!*, Chapter 11 • *Instructor's Manual to Accompany 3-2-1 Code It!*, Chapter 11 • *Workbook to Accompany 3-2-1 Code It!*, Chapter 11 • *Instructor's Manual to Accompany 3-2-1 Code It!*, Introduction • *Instructor's Manual to Accompany 3-2-1 Code It!*, Chapter 11
Class # ___:	• Distribute and explain course syllabus. • Point out major features of textbook. • Review WebTutor™ features (if applicable). • Assign Chapter 11 as reading assignment. • Lecture on Chapter 11 content. • Encourage students to create flash cards. • Assign chapter review as homework.	• Prepared course syllabus • *3-2-1 Code It!*, Preface • *3-2-1 Code It!*, Preface • *3-2-1 Code It!*, Chapter 11 • Lecture notes prepared from *3-2-1 Code!*, Chapter 11 • *3-2-1 Code It!*, Chapter 11 • *3-2-1 Code It!*, Chapter 11
Class # ___:	• Review previous class lecture and answer students' questions about chapter content. • Continue lecture on Chapter 11 content. • Collect homework (and grade). • Administer chapter quiz. • Assign Chapter 11 as reading assignment.	• Ask students to identify key topics and issues from previous class lecture. • *3-2-1 Code It!*, Chapter 11 • *Instructor's Manual to Accompany 3-2-1 Code It!*, Chapter 11 • *Instructor's Manual to Accompany 3-2-1 Code It!*, Chapter 11 • *3-2-1 Code It!*, Chapter 11
Lab # ___:	• Point out major features of workbook. • Communicate assignments to be accomplished during lab and explain how each is to be completed. • Rotate among students as they complete lab assignments to provide individual assistance. • Consider reviewing rough draft work during lab and allowing students to submit final draft at the beginning of the next lab class. • Assign additional workbook assignments for homework.	• *Workbook to Accompany 3-2-1 Code It!*, Preface • *Workbook to Accompany 3-2-1 Code It!*, Chapter 11
Assessment:	• Homework assignments • Chapter quiz • In-class participation • Lab assignments	

Chapter 12: CPT Surgery II		
Time:	• Instructor preparation (______ hours) • In-class lecture (______ hours) • In-class lab (if laboratory component is included as part of course) (______ hours)	
Topics:	• Musculoskeletal System Subsection • Respiratory System Subsection	
Overview:	This chapter focuses on the CPT Surgery Musculoskeletal System and Respiratory System subsections.	
Objectives:	• Define key terms. • Explain the organization, format, and content of the CPT Surgery Musculoskeletal and Respiratory subsections. • Interpret CPT surgery coding notes for the Musculoskeletal and Respiratory System subsections. • Assign CPT surgery codes from the Musculoskeletal and Respiratory System Integumentary subsections. • Add CPT and/or HCPCS level II modifiers to codes as appropriate.	
	Task	**Resource**
Prior to class:	• Read textbook and prepare lecture notes. • Review answers to chapter review. • Select workbook assignments for homework. • Prepare course syllabus. • Prepare chapter quiz.	• *3-2-1 Code It!*, Chapter 12 • *Instructor's Manual to Accompany 3-2-1 Code It!*, Chapter 12 • *Workbook to Accompany 3-2-1 Code It!*, Chapter 12 • *Instructor's Manual to Accompany 3-2-1 Code It!*, Introduction • *Instructor's Manual to Accompany 3-2-1 Code It!*, Chapter 12
Class # ___:	• Distribute and explain course syllabus. • Point out major features of textbook. • Review WebTutor™ features (if applicable). • Assign Chapter 12 as reading assignment. • Lecture on Chapter 12 content. • Encourage students to create flash cards. • Assign chapter review as homework.	• Prepared course syllabus • *3-2-1 Code It!*, Preface • *3-2-1 Code It!*, Preface • *3-2-1 Code It!*, Chapter 12 • Lecture notes prepared from *3-2-1 Code!*, Chapter 12 • *3-2-1 Code It!*, Chapter 12 • *3-2-1 Code It!*, Chapter 12
Class # ___:	• Review previous class lecture and answer students' questions about chapter content. • Continue lecture on Chapter 12 content. • Collect homework (and grade). • Administer chapter quiz. • Assign Chapter 12 as reading assignment.	• Ask students to identify key topics and issues from previous class lecture. • *3-2-1 Code It!*, Chapter 12 • *Instructor's Manual to Accompany 3-2-1 Code It!*, Chapter 12 • *Instructor's Manual to Accompany 3-2-1 Code It!*, Chapter 12 • *3-2-1 Code It!*, Chapter 12
Lab # ___:	• Point out major features of workbook. • Communicate assignments to be accomplished during lab and explain how each is to be completed. • Rotate among students as they complete lab assignments to provide individual assistance. • Consider reviewing rough draft work during lab and allowing students to submit final draft at the beginning of the next lab class. • Assign additional workbook assignments for homework.	• *Workbook to Accompany 3-2-1 Code It!*, Preface • *Workbook to Accompany 3-2-1 Code It!*, Chapter 12
Assessment:	• Homework assignments • Chapter quiz • In-class participation • Lab assignments	

Chapter 13: CPT Surgery III		
Time:	• Instructor preparation (_____ hours) • In-class lecture (_____ hours) • In-class lab (if laboratory component is included as part of course) (_____ hours)	
Topics:	• Cardiovascular System Subsection • Hemic and Lymphatic Systems Subsection	
Overview:	This chapter focuses on the CPT Surgery Cardiovascular System and Hemic and Lymphatic Systems subsections.	
Objectives:	• Define key terms. • Explain the organization, format, and content of the CPT Surgery Cardiovascular System and Hemic and Lymphatic Systems subsections. • Interpret CPT surgery coding notes for the Cardiovascular System and Hemic and Lymphatic Systems subsections. • Assign CPT surgery codes from the Cardiovascular System and Hemic and Lymphatic Systems subsections. • Add CPT and/or HCPCS level II modifiers to codes as appropriate.	
	Task	**Resource**
Prior to class:	• Read textbook and prepare lecture notes. • Review answers to chapter review. • Select workbook assignments for homework. • Prepare course syllabus. • Prepare chapter quiz.	• *3-2-1 Code It!*, Chapter 13 • *Instructor's Manual to Accompany 3-2-1 Code It!*, Chapter 13 • *Workbook to Accompany 3-2-1 Code It!*, Chapter 13 • *Instructor's Manual to Accompany 3-2-1 Code It!*, Introduction • *Instructor's Manual to Accompany 3-2-1 Code It!*, Chapter 13
Class # ___:	• Distribute and explain course syllabus. • Point out major features of textbook. • Review WebTutor™ features (if applicable). • Assign Chapter 13 as reading assignment. • Lecture on Chapter 13 content. • Encourage students to create flash cards. • Assign chapter review as homework.	• Prepared course syllabus • *3-2-1 Code It!*, Preface • *3-2-1 Code It!*, Preface • *3-2-1 Code It!*, Chapter 13 • Lecture notes prepared from *3-2-1 Code!*, Chapter 13 • *3-2-1 Code It!*, Chapter 13 • *3-2-1 Code It!*, Chapter 13
Class # ___:	• Review previous class lecture and answer students' questions about chapter content. • Continue lecture on Chapter 13 content. • Collect homework (and grade). • Administer chapter quiz. • Assign Chapter 13 as reading assignment.	• Ask students to identify key topics and issues from previous class lecture. • *3-2-1 Code It!*, Chapter 13 • *Instructor's Manual to Accompany 3-2-1 Code It!*, Chapter 13 • *Instructor's Manual to Accompany 3-2-1 Code It!*, Chapter 13 • *3-2-1 Code It!*, Chapter 13
Lab # ___:	• Point out major features of workbook. • Communicate assignments to be accomplished during lab and explain how each is to be completed. • Rotate among students as they complete lab assignments to provide individual assistance. • Consider reviewing rough draft work during lab and allowing students to submit final draft at the beginning of the next lab class. • Assign additional workbook assignments for homework.	• *Workbook to Accompany 3-2-1 Code It!*, Preface • *Workbook to Accompany 3-2-1 Code It!*, Chapter 13
Assessment:	• Homework assignments • Chapter quiz • In-class participation • Lab assignments	

Chapter 14: CPT Surgery IV		
Time:	• Instructor preparation (_____ hours) • In-class lecture (_____ hours) • In-class lab (if laboratory component is included as part of course) (_____ hours)	
Topics:	• Mediastinum and Diaphragm Subsection • Digestive System Subsection • Urinary System Subsection	
Overview:	This chapter focuses on the CPT Surgery Mediastinum and Diaphragm, Digestive System, and Urinary System subsections.	
Objectives:	• Define key terms. • Explain the organization, format, and content of the CPT Mediastinum and Diaphragm, Digestive System, and Urinary System subsections. • Interpret CPT surgery coding notes for the Mediastinum and Diaphragm, Digestive System, and Urinary System subsections. • Assign CPT surgery codes from the Mediastinum and Diaphragm, Digestive System, and Urinary System subsections. • Add CPT and/or HCPCS level II modifiers to codes as appropriate.	
	Task	**Resource**
Prior to class:	• Read textbook and prepare lecture notes. • Review answers to chapter review. • Select workbook assignments for homework. • Prepare course syllabus. • Prepare chapter quiz.	• *3-2-1 Code It!*, Chapter 14 • *Instructor's Manual to Accompany 3-2-1 Code It!*, Chapter 14 • *Workbook to Accompany 3-2-1 Code It!*, Chapter 14 • *Instructor's Manual to Accompany 3-2-1 Code It!*, Introduction • *Instructor's Manual to Accompany 3-2-1 Code It!*, Chapter 14
Class # ___:	• Distribute and explain course syllabus. • Point out major features of textbook. • Review WebTutor™ features (if applicable). • Assign Chapter 14 as reading assignment. • Lecture on Chapter 14 content. • Encourage students to create flash cards. • Assign chapter review as homework.	• Prepared course syllabus • *3-2-1 Code It!*, Preface • *3-2-1 Code It!*, Preface • *3-2-1 Code It!*, Chapter 14 • Lecture notes prepared from *3-2-1 Code!*, Chapter 14 • *3-2-1 Code It!*, Chapter 14 • *3-2-1 Code It!*, Chapter 14
Class # ___:	• Review previous class lecture and answer students' questions about chapter content. • Continue lecture on Chapter 14 content. • Collect homework (and grade). • Administer chapter quiz. • Assign Chapter 14 as reading assignment.	• Ask students to identify key topics and issues from previous class lecture. • *3-2-1 Code It!*, Chapter 14 • *Instructor's Manual to Accompany 3-2-1 Code It!*, Chapter 14 • *Instructor's Manual to Accompany 3-2-1 Code It!*, Chapter 14 • *3-2-1 Code It!*, Chapter 14
Lab # ___:	• Point out major features of workbook. • Communicate assignments to be accomplished during lab and explain how each is to be completed. • Rotate among students as they complete lab assignments to provide individual assistance. • Consider reviewing rough draft work during lab and allowing students to submit final draft at the beginning of the next lab class. • Assign additional workbook assignments for homework.	• *Workbook to Accompany 3-2-1 Code It!*, Preface • *Workbook to Accompany 3-2-1 Code It!*, Chapter 14
Assessment:	• Homework assignments • Chapter quiz • In-class participation • Lab assignments	

Chapter 15: CPT Surgery V		
Time:	• Instructor preparation (_____ hours) • In-class lecture (_____ hours) • In-class lab (if laboratory component is included as part of course) (_____ hours)	
Topics:	• Male Genital System Subsection • Reproductive System Procedures Subsection • Intersex Surgery Subsection • Female Genital System Subsection • Maternity Care and Delivery Subsection • Endocrine System Subsection • Nervous System Subsection • Eye and Ocular Adnexa Subsection • Auditory System Subsection • Operating Microscope Subsection	
Overview:	This chapter focuses on the CPT Surgery Male Genital System, Reproductive System Procedures, Intersex Surgery, Female Genital System, Maternity Care and Delivery, Endocrine System, Nervous System, Eye and Ocular Adnexa, Auditory System, and Operating Microscope subsections.	
Objectives:	• Define key terms. • Explain the organization, format, and content of the CPT Male Genital System, Reproductive System Procedures, Intersex Surgery, Female Genital System, Maternity Care and Delivery, Endocrine System, Nervous System, Eye and Ocular Adnexa, Auditory System, and Operating Microscope subsections. • Interpret CPT surgery coding notes for the Male Genital System, Reproductive System Procedures, Intersex Surgery, Female Genital System, Maternity Care and Delivery, Endocrine System, Nervous System, Eye and Ocular Adnexa, Auditory System, and Operating Microscope subsections. • Assign CPT surgery codes from the Male Genital System, Reproductive System Procedures, Intersex Surgery, Female Genital System, Maternity Care and Delivery, Endocrine System, Nervous System, Eye and Ocular Adnexa, Auditory System, and Operating Microscope subsections. • Add CPT and/or HCPCS level II modifiers to codes as appropriate.	
	Task	**Resource**
Prior to class:	• Read textbook and prepare lecture notes. • Review answers to chapter review. • Select workbook assignments for homework. • Prepare course syllabus. • Prepare chapter quiz.	• *3-2-1 Code It!*, Chapter 15 • *Instructor's Manual to Accompany 3-2-1 Code It!*, Chapter 15 • *Workbook to Accompany 3-2-1 Code It!*, Chapter 15 • *Instructor's Manual to Accompany 3-2-1 Code It!*, Introduction • *Instructor's Manual to Accompany 3-2-1 Code It!*, Chapter 15
Class # ___:	• Distribute and explain course syllabus. • Point out major features of textbook. • Review WebTutor™ features (if applicable). • Assign Chapter 15 as reading assignment. • Lecture on Chapter 15 content. • Encourage students to create flash cards. • Assign chapter review as homework.	• Prepared course syllabus • *3-2-1 Code It!*, Preface • *3-2-1 Code It!*, Preface • *3-2-1 Code It!*, Chapter 15 • Lecture notes prepared from *3-2-1 Code!*, Chapter 15 • *3-2-1 Code It!*, Chapter 15 • *3-2-1 Code It!*, Chapter 15
Class # ___:	• Review previous class lecture and answer students' questions about chapter content. • Continue lecture on Chapter 15 content. • Collect homework (and grade). • Administer chapter quiz. • Assign Chapter 15 as reading assignment.	• Ask students to identify key topics and issues from previous class lecture. • *3-2-1 Code It!*, Chapter 15 • *Instructor's Manual to Accompany 3-2-1 Code It!*, Chapter 15 • *Instructor's Manual to Accompany 3-2-1 Code It!*, Chapter 15 • *3-2-1 Code It!*, Chapter 15
Lab # ___:	• Point out major features of workbook. • Communicate assignments to be accomplished during lab and explain how each is to be completed. • Rotate among students as they complete lab assignments to provide individual assistance. • Consider reviewing rough draft work during lab and allowing students to submit final draft at the beginning of the next lab class. • Assign additional workbook assignments for homework.	• *Workbook to Accompany 3-2-1 Code It!*, Preface • *Workbook to Accompany 3-2-1 Code It!*, Chapter 15
Assessment:	• Homework assignments • Chapter quiz • In-class participation • Lab assignments	

Chapter 16: CPT Radiology		
Time:	• Instructor preparation (_____ hours) • In-class lecture (_____ hours) • In-class lab (if laboratory component is included as part of course) (_____ hours)	
Topics:	• Radiology Terminology • Overview of Radiology Section • Radiology Section Guidelines • Radiology Subsections • Diagnostic Radiology (Diagnostic Imaging) • Diagnostic Ultrasound • Radiologic Guidance • Breast Mammography • Bone/Joint Studies • Radiation Oncology • Nuclear Medicine	
Overview:	This chapter focuses on the CPT Radiology section, which includes diagnostic radiology (diagnostic imaging); diagnostic ultrasound; radiologic guidance; breast, mammography; bone/joint studies; radiation oncology; and nuclear medicine.	
Objectives:	• Define key terms. • Explain the organization, format, and content of the CPT Radiology section. • Interpret CPT radiology coding guidelines and notes. • Assign CPT radiology codes. • Add CPT and/or HCPCS level II modifiers to codes as appropriate.	
	Task	**Resource**
Prior to class:	• Read textbook and prepare lecture notes. • Review answers to chapter review. • Select workbook assignments for homework. • Prepare course syllabus. • Prepare chapter quiz.	• *3-2-1 Code It!*, Chapter 16 • *Instructor's Manual to Accompany 3-2-1 Code It!*, Chapter 16 • *Workbook to Accompany 3-2-1 Code It!*, Chapter 16 • *Instructor's Manual to Accompany 3-2-1 Code It!*, Introduction • *Instructor's Manual to Accompany 3-2-1 Code It!*, Chapter 16
Class # ___:	• Distribute and explain course syllabus. • Point out major features of textbook. • Review WebTutor™ features (if applicable). • Assign Chapter 16 as reading assignment. • Lecture on Chapter 16 content. • Encourage students to create flash cards. • Assign chapter review as homework.	• Prepared course syllabus • *3-2-1 Code It!*, Preface • *3-2-1 Code It!*, Preface • *3-2-1 Code It!*, Chapter 16 • Lecture notes prepared from *3-2-1 Code!*, Chapter 16 • *3-2-1 Code It!*, Chapter 16 • *3-2-1 Code It!*, Chapter 16
Class # ___:	• Review previous class lecture and answer students' questions about chapter content. • Continue lecture on Chapter 16 content. • Collect homework (and grade). • Administer chapter quiz. • Assign Chapter 16 as reading assignment.	• Ask students to identify key topics and issues from previous class lecture. • *3-2-1 Code It!*, Chapter 16 • *Instructor's Manual to Accompany 3-2-1 Code It!*, Chapter 16 • *Instructor's Manual to Accompany 3-2-1 Code It!*, Chapter 16 • *3-2-1 Code It!*, Chapter 16
Lab # ___:	• Point out major features of workbook. • Communicate assignments to be accomplished during lab and explain how each is to be completed. • Rotate among students as they complete lab assignments to provide individual assistance. • Consider reviewing rough draft work during lab and allowing students to submit final draft at the beginning of the next lab class. • Assign additional workbook assignments for homework.	• *Workbook to Accompany 3-2-1 Code It!*, Preface • *Workbook to Accompany 3-2-1 Code It!*, Chapter 16
Assessment:	• Homework assignments • Chapter quiz • In-class participation • Lab assignments	

Chapter 17: CPT Pathology and Laboratory		
Time:	• Instructor preparation (_____ hours) • In-class lecture (_____ hours) • In-class lab (if laboratory component is included as part of course) (_____ hours)	
Topics:	• Overview of Pathology and Laboratory Section • Pathology and Laboratory Section Guidelines • Pathology and Laboratory Subsections	
Overview:	This chapter focuses on the CPT Pathology and Laboratory section.	
Objectives:	• Define key terms. • Explain the organization, format, and content of the CPT Pathology and Laboratory section. • Interpret CPT pathology and laboratory coding guidelines and notes. • Assign CPT pathology and laboratory codes. • Add CPT and/or HCPCS level II modifiers to codes as appropriate.	
	Task	**Resource**
Prior to class:	• Read textbook and prepare lecture notes. • Review answers to chapter review. • Select workbook assignments for homework. • Prepare course syllabus. • Prepare chapter quiz.	• *3-2-1 Code It!*, Chapter 17 • *Instructor's Manual to Accompany 3-2-1 Code It!*, Chapter 17 • *Workbook to Accompany 3-2-1 Code It!*, Chapter 17 • *Instructor's Manual to Accompany 3-2-1 Code It!*, Introduction • *Instructor's Manual to Accompany 3-2-1 Code It!*, Chapter 17
Class # ___:	• Distribute and explain course syllabus. • Point out major features of textbook. • Review WebTutor™ features (if applicable). • Assign Chapter 17 as reading assignment. • Lecture on Chapter 17 content. • Encourage students to create flash cards. • Assign chapter review as homework.	• Prepared course syllabus • *3-2-1 Code It!*, Preface • *3-2-1 Code It!*, Preface • *3-2-1 Code It!*, Chapter 17 • Lecture notes prepared from *3-2-1 Code!*, Chapter 17 • *3-2-1 Code It!*, Chapter 17 • *3-2-1 Code It!*, Chapter 17
Class # ___:	• Review previous class lecture and answer students' questions about chapter content. • Continue lecture on Chapter 17 content. • Collect homework (and grade). • Administer chapter quiz. • Assign Chapter 17 as reading assignment.	• Ask students to identify key topics and issues from previous class lecture. • *3-2-1 Code It!*, Chapter 17 • *Instructor's Manual to Accompany 3-2-1 Code It!*, Chapter 17 • *Instructor's Manual to Accompany 3-2-1 Code It!*, Chapter 17 • *3-2-1 Code It!*, Chapter 17
Lab # ___:	• Point out major features of workbook. • Communicate assignments to be accomplished during lab and explain how each is to be completed. • Rotate among students as they complete lab assignments to provide individual assistance. • Consider reviewing rough draft work during lab and allowing students to submit final draft at the beginning of the next lab class. • Assign additional workbook assignments for homework.	• *Workbook to Accompany 3-2-1 Code It!*, Preface • *Workbook to Accompany 3-2-1 Code It!*, Chapter 17
Assessment:	• Homework assignments • Chapter quiz • In-class participation • Lab assignments	

Chapter 18: CPT Medicine		
Time:	• Instructor preparation (______ hours) • In-class lecture (______ hours) • In-class lab (if laboratory component is included as part of course) (______ hours)	
Topics:	• Overview of Medicine Section • Medicine Section Guidelines • Medicine Subsections	
Overview:	This chapter focuses on the CPT Medicine section.	
Objectives:	• Define key terms. • Explain the organization, format, and content of the CPT Medicine section. • Interpret CPT medicine coding guidelines and notes. • Assign CPT medicine codes. • Add CPT and/or HCPCS level II modifiers to codes as appropriate.	
	Task	**Resource**
Prior to class:	• Read textbook and prepare lecture notes. • Review answers to chapter review. • Select workbook assignments for homework. • Prepare course syllabus. • Prepare chapter quiz.	• *3-2-1 Code It!*, Chapter 18 • *Instructor's Manual to Accompany 3-2-1 Code It!*, Chapter 18 • *Workbook to Accompany 3-2-1 Code It!*, Chapter 18 • *Instructor's Manual to Accompany 3-2-1 Code It!*, Introduction • *Instructor's Manual to Accompany 3-2-1 Code It!*, Chapter 18
Class # ___:	• Distribute and explain course syllabus. • Point out major features of textbook. • Review WebTutor™ features (if applicable). • Assign Chapter 18 as reading assignment. • Lecture on Chapter 18 content. • Encourage students to create flash cards. • Assign chapter review as homework.	• Prepared course syllabus • *3-2-1 Code It!*, Preface • *3-2-1 Code It!*, Preface • *3-2-1 Code It!*, Chapter 18 • Lecture notes prepared from *3-2-1 Code!*, Chapter 18 • *3-2-1 Code It!*, Chapter 18 • *3-2-1 Code It!*, Chapter 18
Class # ___:	• Review previous class lecture and answer students' questions about chapter content. • Continue lecture on Chapter 18 content. • Collect homework (and grade). • Administer chapter quiz. • Assign Chapter 18 as reading assignment.	• Ask students to identify key topics and issues from previous class lecture. • *3-2-1 Code It!*, Chapter 18 • *Instructor's Manual to Accompany 3-2-1 Code It!*, Chapter 18 • *Instructor's Manual to Accompany 3-2-1 Code It!*, Chapter 18 • *3-2-1 Code It!*, Chapter 18
Lab # ___:	• Point out major features of workbook. • Communicate assignments to be accomplished during lab and explain how each is to be completed. • Rotate among students as they complete lab assignments to provide individual assistance. • Consider reviewing rough draft work during lab and allowing students to submit final draft at the beginning of the next lab class. • Assign additional workbook assignments for homework.	• *Workbook to Accompany 3-2-1 Code It!*, Preface • *Workbook to Accompany 3-2-1 Code It!*, Chapter 18
Assessment:	• Homework assignments • Chapter quiz • In-class participation • Lab assignments	

Chapter 19: Insurance and Reimbursement

	Task	Resource
Time:	• Instructor preparation (_____ hours) • In-class lecture (_____ hours) • In-class lab (if laboratory component is included as part of course) (_____ hours)	
Topics:	• Third-Party Payers • Health Care Reimbursement Systems • Impact of HIPAA on Reimbursement	
Overview:	This chapter focuses on health care insurance and reimbursement issues, including third-party payers, health care reimbursement systems, and the impact of the Health Insurance Portability and Accountability Act of 1996 on reimbursement.	
Objectives:	• Define key terms. • Identify and provide examples of third-party payers. • List and define each health care reimbursement system. • Describe the impact of HIPAA on health care reimbursement.	
Prior to class:	• Read textbook and prepare lecture notes. • Review answers to chapter review. • Select workbook assignments for homework. • Prepare course syllabus. • Prepare chapter quiz.	• *3-2-1 Code It!*, Chapter 19 • *Instructor's Manual to Accompany 3-2-1 Code It!*, Chapter 19 • *Workbook to Accompany 3-2-1 Code It!*, Chapter 19 • *Instructor's Manual to Accompany 3-2-1 Code It!*, Introduction • *Instructor's Manual to Accompany 3-2-1 Code It!*, Chapter 19
Class # ___:	• Distribute and explain course syllabus. • Point out major features of textbook. • Review WebTutor™ features (if applicable). • Assign Chapter 19 as reading assignment. • Lecture on Chapter 19 content. • Encourage students to create flash cards. • Assign chapter review as homework.	• Prepared course syllabus • *3-2-1 Code It!*, Preface • *3-2-1 Code It!*, Preface • *3-2-1 Code It!*, Chapter 19 • Lecture notes prepared from *3-2-1 Code!*, Chapter 19 • *3-2-1 Code It!*, Chapter 19 • *3-2-1 Code It!*, Chapter 19
Class # ___:	• Review previous class lecture and answer students' questions about chapter content. • Continue lecture on Chapter 19 content. • Collect homework (and grade). • Administer chapter quiz. • Assign Chapter 19 as reading assignment.	• Ask students to identify key topics and issues from previous class lecture. • *3-2-1 Code It!*, Chapter 19 • *Instructor's Manual to Accompany 3-2-1 Code It!*, Chapter 19 • *Instructor's Manual to Accompany 3-2-1 Code It!*, Chapter 19 • *3-2-1 Code It!*, Chapter 19
Lab # ___:	• Point out major features of workbook. • Communicate assignments to be accomplished during lab and explain how each is to be completed. • Rotate among students as they complete lab assignments to provide individual assistance. • Consider reviewing rough draft work during lab and allowing students to submit final draft at the beginning of the next lab class. • Assign additional workbook assignments for homework.	• *Workbook to Accompany 3-2-1 Code It!*, Preface • *Workbook to Accompany 3-2-1 Code It!*, Chapter 19
Assessment:	• Homework assignments • Chapter quiz • In-class participation • Lab assignments	

SECTION II

Answer Keys to Chapter Exercises and Reviews

Chapter 1
Overview of Coding

EXERCISE 1.1 – CAREER AS A CODER

1. c
2. a
3. b
4. c
5. b
6. c
7. e
8. a
9. b
10. d

EXERCISE 1.2 – PROFESSIONAL ASSOCIATIONS AND DISCUSSION BOARDS

1. c
2. a
3. b
4. a
5. c

EXERCISE 1.3 – OVERVIEW OF CODING

1. b
2. a
3. a
4. a
5. a
6. b
7. b
8. a
9. a
10. b

EXERCISE 1.4 – DOCUMENTATION AS THE BASIS FOR CODING

1. a
2. b
3. b
4. b
5. b
6. medical record
7. demographic data
8. continuity of care
9. medical necessity
10. manual
11. source-oriented
12. integrated
13. electronic medical record (EMR)
14. optical disk imaging (or document imaging)
15. jukebox

EXERCISE 1.5 – HEALTH DATA COLLECTION

1. medical management
2. case abstracting
3. CMS-1500
4. UB-04 (or CMS-1450)
5. medical necessity

REVIEW

Multiple Choice

1. a
2. d
3. c
4. b
5. b
6. c
7. c
8. d
9. a
10. a
11. c
12. a
13. c
14. b
15. b
16. d
17. b
18. a
19. b
20. c

Chapter 2
Introduction to ICD-9-CM and ICD-10-CM/PCS Coding

EXERCISE 2.1 – OVERVIEW OF ICD-9-CM AND ICD-10-CM/PCS

1. 1979, October 1, 2013
2. ICD-10
3. National Center for Health Statistics (NCHS); Centers for Medicare & Medicaid Services (CMS)
4. Medicare Prescription Drug, Improvement, and Modernization Act (MMA)
5. subscription
6. encoder
7. Medicare Catastrophic Coverage Act of 1988, HIPAA
8. medical necessity
9. chest pain
10. multiple lacerations

EXERCISE 2.2 – ICD-9-CM AND ICD-10-CM TABULAR LIST OF DISEASES

1. Tabular List of Diseases
2. Diagnostic and Statistical Manual of Mental Disorders (DSM)
3. V codes
4. E codes
5. Morphology of Neoplasms (M codes)
6. neoplasms
7. benign; malignant
8. Classification of Drugs by AHFS List
9. Classification of Industrial Accidents According to Agency
10. List of Three-Digit Categories

EXERCISE 2.3 – ICD-9-CM AND ICD-10-CM INDEX

1. Index to Diseases
2. Table of Drugs and Chemicals
3. letter-by-letter
4. Launois-Cleret syndrome
5. numerical
6. boldfaced
7. nonessential modifiers

8. essential modifiers
9. Asthmatic
10. History

Note:

The main term is History *in the ICD-9-CM or ICD-10-CM index. The diagnosis "history of affective psychosis" indicates that the patient no longer has the condition. Therefore, do not refer to main term* Psychosis *and subterm* affective, *which would result in an incorrect code assignment.*

	ICD-9-CM	ICD-10-CM
11.	5	6
12.	2	3
13.	6	1
14.	4	5
15.	1	8
16.	9	9
17.	8	8
18.	10	10
19.	7	7
20.	3	4

Note:

In the ICD-9-CM Index to Diseases, "H disease" is sequenced after Hb *because it is interpreted as "Hdisease" according to letter-by-letter alphabetization rules, which means that spaces and hyphens are ignored. However, in the ICD-10-CM Index to Diseases and Injuries, Hb is sequenced* before *"H disease" because spaces are* not *ignored (although hyphens are ignored).*

EXERCISE 2.4 – ICD-9-CM TABULAR LIST OF PROCEDURES AND INDEX TO PROCEDURES

1. Tabular List of Procedures and Index to Procedures
2. *Current Procedural Terminology* (CPT); *Healthcare Financing Administration Common Procedure Coding System, Level II (national)*
3. December 31, 2003
4. two
5. 17

EXERCISE 2.5 - ICD-10-PCS INDEX AND TABLES

1. *International Classification of Diseases, 10th Revision, Procedure Coding System*
2. Hospital inpatient
3. seven-character

4. Each code consists of independent characters, with each individual axis retaining its meaning across broad ranges of codes
5. Imaging section, body system, root type, body part, contrast, qualifier, qualifier
6. Mental health section, body system, root type, type qualifier, qualifier, qualifier, qualifier
7. Medical and surgical section, body system, root operation, body part, approach, device, qualifier
8. The values of characters 2–7 may vary; remain the same
9. Tables, index, list of codes
10. 001U074

EXERCISE 2.6 – OFFICIAL GUIDELINES FOR CODING AND REPORTING

1. cooperating parties for the ICD-9-CM
2. AHA; AHIMA; CMS; NCHS
3. HIPAA
4. encounter
5. provider

REVIEW

Multiple Choice

1. a
2. b
3. a
4. c
5. c
6. a
7. b
8. a
9. c
10. d

Matching

11. b
12. c
13. a
14. d
15. e

Coding Practice

ICD-9-CM and ICD-10-CM Index to Diseases (and Injuries) and Tabular List of Diseases (and Injuries)

ICD-9-CM	ICD-10-CM	
553.20	K46.9	16. Abdominal hernia
790.29	R73.09	17. Abnormal nonfasting glucose tolerance test
382.9	H66.90	18. Acute otitis media
621.30	N85.00	19. Hyperplasia of endometrium
818.0	S42.30-	20. Fracture, right humerus (Fracture, Traumatic in ICD-10-CM index)

Note:

The dash in ICD-10-CM subcategory code S42.30- indicates that a sixth digit is necessary. The ICD-10-CM index includes a dash next to subcategory codes when an additional digit is required.

784.4	E84.9	21. Congenital fibrocystic disease of the lung (Fibrocystic, Disease in ICD-9-CM index) (Fibrosis, Cystic in ICD-10-CM index)
715.90	M19.90	22. Degenerative arthritis (Osteoarthritis in ICD-10-CM index)
610.1	N60.1-	23. Fibrocystic disease of breasts (Fibrocystic disease, then Mastopathy, Cystic in ICD-10-CM index)
448.0	I78.0	24. Hereditary epistaxis
V10.90	Z85.9	25. History of cancer (History, personal (of) in ICD-9-CM and ICD-10-CM indexes)

Note:

Cancer is not listed as a subterm below "History (personal) of." Therefore, refer to subterm "malignant (of) NEC" to assign V10.90 (ICD-9-CM) or Z85.9 (ICD-10-CM). (You also don't know what type of cancer was present.)

ICD-9-CM and ICD-10-CM Index to Diseases (and Injuries) and Tabular List of Diseases and ICD-10-PCS Index and Tables

40.11	07B60ZX	26. Open biopsy, left axillary lymph node (Excision, Diagnostic in ICD-10-PCS)
51.22	0FT40ZZ	27. Cholecystectomy, total (Resection, Gallbladder in ICD-10-PCS index)
57.32	0TJB8ZZ	28. Cystoscopy
54.11	0WJG0ZZ	29. Exploratory laparotomy, open (Inspection, Cavity, Peritoneal in ICD-10-PCS index)
84.73	BT11ZZZ	30. Intravenous right pyelogram (Fluoroscopy, Kidney in ICD-10-PCS index)
47.19	0DTJ0ZZ	31. Incidental appendectomy (Resection, Appendix in ICD-10-PCS index)
22.12	09BT3ZX	32. Open biopsy of left frontal nasal sinus (Excision in ICD-10-PCS index)
60.11	0VB03ZX	33. Percutaneous biopsy of prostate (Excision in ICD-10-PCS index)
01.24	0N81	34. Right frontal craniotomy (Division, Head and Facial Bones in ICD-10-PCS index)
57.33	0TBB	35. Transurethral biopsy of bladder (Excision in ICD-10-PCS index)

Chapter 3
ICD-9-CM and ICD-10-CM/PCS Coding Conventions

EXERCISE 3.1 – FORMAT AND TYPEFACE

ICD-9-CM	ICD-10-CM/PCS	
133.9	B88.0	1. Acariasis infestation
701.1	L44.0	2. Acquired pilaris pityriasis
V52.1	Z44.10	3. Admission for adjustment of artificial leg
309.24	F43.22	4. Adjustment disorder with anxiety
307.1	F50.00	5. Anorexia nervosa
72.9	10D07Z5	6. Forceps delivery
17.69	0H5UXZZ	7. Laser interstitial thermal therapy (LITT) destruction, left breast tissue, with MRI guidance
69.01	10A07ZZ	8. Termination of pregnancy (by) dilation and curettage
37.51	02YA0Z0	9. Heart transplantation, allogenic
88.76	BW40ZZZ	10. Ultrasonography, abdomen

EXERCISE 3.2 – EPONYMS

ICD-9-CM	ICD-10-CM	
524.60	M26.69	1. Costen's complex
755.54	Q74.0	2. Madelung's deformity
362.12	H35.029	3. Coats' disease (In ICD-10-CM, *see* Retinopathy, exudative)
716.00	M12.10	4. Kaschin-Beck disease
386.00	H81.01	5. Meniere disease, right ear
082.1	n/a	6. Mediterranean tick fever
22.39	n/a	7. Caldwell-Luc operation
81.44	n/a	8. Roux-Goldthwait operation
89.42	n/a	9. Masters two-step stress test
59.4	n/a	10. Millin-Read operation

Note:

There are no eponyms or common procedure terms (e.g., appendectomy) in ICD-10-PCS.

EXERCISE 3.3 – ABBREVIATIONS

ICD-9-CM	ICD-10-CM	
287.2	D69.2	1. Purpura
553.00	K41.90	2. Femoral hernia
410.10	I21.09	3. ST elevation myocardial infarction, anterior wall
251.1	E16.1	4. Hyperinsulinism
871.4	S05.31	5. Laceration, right eyeball
67.12	n/a	6. Punch biopsy of cervix
62.41	n/a	7. Bilateral orchidectomy
84.24	n/a	8. Upper arm reattachment
96.56	n/a	9. Irrigation of bronchus
23.19	n/a	10. Surgical removal of tooth

Note:

The NEC and NOS abbreviations do not appear in ICD-10-PCS.

EXERCISE 3.4 – PUNCTUATION

ICD-9-CM	ICD-10-CM	
046.19, 294.10	A81.00, F02.80	1. Creutzfeldt-Jakob syndrome with dementia, without behavioral disturbance
084.9, 573.2	B54, K75.9	2. Malaria with hepatitis
030.3	A30.3	3. Dimorphous leprosy
245.0	E06.0	4. Acute pyogenic thyroiditis
265.0, 357.4	E51.11, G63	5. Neuritis due to beriberi
00.66, 00.40	n/a	6. Percutaneous transluminal coronary angioplasty
01.09	n/a	7. Cranial puncture, subdural tap
68.23	n/a	8. Endometrial ablation
24.5	n/a	9. Alveoloplasty
88.41	n/a	10. Arteriography of basilar artery

Note:

Punctuation is not an ICD-10-PCS coding convention.

EXERCISE 3.5 – BOXED NOTES

Note:

ICD-10-CM/PCS does not use the boxed notes *coding convention; therefore, only ICD-9-CM codes are included in this answer key.*

853.01	1. Traumatic brain hemorrhage with no loss of consciousness
884.0	2. Multiple open wounds to arms
296.21	3. Single episode of mild involutional affective psychosis
730.16	4. Chronic periostitis with osteomyelitis of the lower leg
533.40	5. Recurrent bleeding peptic ulcer
919.3	6. Infected blister
216.7	7. Cellular blue nevus on calf (Neoplasm Table, skin, benign)
91.35	8. Toxicology examination of urine specimen
81.02 81.62	9. Anterior spinal fusion of C4-C6
54.51	10. Laparoscopic lysis of abdominal adhesions

EXERCISE 3.6 – TABLES

ICD-9-CM	ICD-10-CM	
239.1	D49.1	1. Ethmoid tumor (Neoplasm Table)
173.3	C44.39	2. Basal cell carcinoma, skin of external check (Neoplasm Table)
155.2	C22.9	3. Carcinoma of liver (Neoplasm Table)
185	C61	4. Prostate cancer (Neoplasm Table)
987.8, E982.8	T59.894A	5. Poisoning due to inhalation of paint fumes (Table of Drugs and Chemicals) (initial encounter)

Note:

In ICD-10-CM, codes from categories T51–T65 classify toxic effects, which occur when a harmful substance is ingested or comes in contact with a person. Toxic effect codes have an associated intent: accidental, intentional self-harm, assault, and undetermined. If stated, additional code(s) for all manifestations of the toxic effect (e.g., gastroenteritis, respiratory failure, and so on) are assigned and sequenced after the toxic effect code. (In ICD-9-CM, a poisoning code for the toxic effect is assigned from the Table of Drugs and Chemicals in addition to an external cause of injury code, *or E code.)*

785.59, E943.3	R57.9, T47.4x5A	6. Circulatory collapse due to therapeutic use of magnesium sulfate (Table of Drugs and Chemicals) (initial encounter)

Note:

In ICD-10-CM, categories T36–T50 are assigned to classify an adverse effect when the drug was correctly prescribed and properly administered. If stated, additional code(s) for manifestations of adverse effects (e.g., circulatory collapse, tachycardia, delirium, and so on) are assigned and sequenced before the adverse effect *T code.*

969.00, E854.0	T43.201A	7. Accidental overdose of antidepressants (Table of Drugs and Chemicals) (initial encounter)

Note:

ICD-10-CM, category codes T36–T50 are assigned to classify a poisoning or reaction to the improper use of a medication (e.g., overdose, wrong substance given or taken in error, wrong route of administration). (Poisoning codes have an associated intent: accidental, intentional self-harm, assault and undetermined.) If stated, additional code(s) for manifestations of poisonings (e.g., coma, respiratory distress, and so on) are assigned and sequenced after the poisoning T code.

401.0	n/a	8. Malignant idiopathic hypertension (Hypertension Table)
405.99	n/a	9. Secondary hypertension (Hypertension Table)
405.11	n/a	10. Benign hypertension due to renal stenosis (Hypertension Table)

Note:

The hypertension table does not appear in ICD-10-CM; therefore, answers are not entered for items 8–10. Although tables are used in ICD-10-PCS, students will complete those exercises in Chapter 5 of the textbook.

EXERCISE 3.7 – INCLUDES NOTES

ICD-9-CM	ICD-10-CM	
323.9	G04.90	1. Meningoencephalitis
403.90, 585.9	I12.9, N18.9	2. Nephrosclerosis
534.90	K28.9	3. Anastomotic ulcer
401.9	I10	4. Hypertensive vascular degeneration
682.9	L03.91	5. Acute lymphangitis
72.71	10D07Z6, 0W8NXZZ	6. Malstrom's vacuum extraction with episiotomy (Extraction, Products of Conception in ICD-10-PCS) (Episiotomy in ICD-10-PCS)
76.72	n/a	7. Open reduction and fixation of left zygomatic fracture
81.01, 81.62	n/a	8. Open arthrodesis of C1-C2 (cervical spine) anterior column using anterior approach with internal fixation device
88.68	n/a	9. Impedence phlebography with venipuncture for injection of contrast material, chest
14.39	n/a	10. Repair of right retinal defect

Note:

Includes notes do not appear in ICD-10-PCS.

EXERCISE 3.8 – EXCLUDES NOTES

ICD-9-CM	ICD-10-CM	
429.2	I25.10	1. Cardiovascular disease

Note:

The Excludes note below ICD-9-CM code 429.2 excludes that due to hypertension (402.0–402.9). This means if the diagnostic statement was "hypertensive cardiovascular disease," the coder would assign a code from 402.0–402.9 instead of code 429.2.

The Excludes1 note for ICD-10-CM code I51.9 is located below the ***I51 Complications and ill-defined descriptions of heart disease*** *category, and it states any condition in I51.4–I51.9 due to hypertension (I11.-). This means if the diagnostic statement was "hypertensive cardiovascular disease," the Excludes1 note instructs the coder to assign a code from I11.- instead of code I51.9.*

447.6	I77.6	2. Arteritis
626.0	N91.2	3. Absence of menstruation
694.0	L13.0	4. Herpetiformis dermatosis
746.87	Q24.0	5. Dextrocardia
n/a	A17.1, A17.81	6. Meningeal tuberculoma. Tuberculoma of brain and spinal cord.

Note:

The Excludes2 note for ICD-10-CM code A17.1 (meningeal tuberculoma) permits the assignment of code A17.81 when tuberculoma of the brain and spinal cord is also documented.

n/a	C01	7. Malignant neoplasm of dorsal surface of base of tongue. (Neoplasm table).
n/a	E74.31, E73.0	8. Sucrase-isomaltase deficiency. Congenital lactose intolerance
n/a	F28, F20.0	9. Psychotic disorder with hallucinations. Paranoid schizophrenia.
n/a	R04.1, R04.2	10. Hemorrhage from the throat. Hemoptysis.

EXERCISE 3.9 – INCLUSION TERMS

ICD-9-CM	ICD-10-CM	
006.0	A06.0	1. Acute amebic dysentery
116.0	B40.7	2. Disseminated blastomycosis
207.20	C94.20	3. Megakaryocytic (thrombocytic) leukemia, acute
330.1	E75.09	4. GM2 gangliosidosis, juvenile
771.2	P37.1	5. Congenital toxoplasmosis
21.31	n/a	6. Nasal polypectomy
36.39	n/a	7. Intrapericardial poudrage
75.38	n/a	8. Transcervical fetal oxygen saturation monitoring (intrapartum)
92.04	n/a	9. Radio-cobalt B12 Schilling test
68.31	n/a	10. Classic infrafascial SEMM hysterectomy (abdominal)

Note:

Inclusion terms are not used in ICD-10-PCS.

EXERCISE 3.10 – OTHER, OTHER SPECIFIED, AND UNSPECIFIED CODES

ICD-9-CM	ICD-10-CM	
543.9	K38.8	1. Intussusception of appendix
633.90	O00.9	2. Ectopic pregnancy
674.84, 572.4	O90.4	3. Hepatorenal syndrome following delivery (postpartum condition)
445.89	I75.89	4. Arterial atheroembolism
365.9	H40.9	5. Glaucoma
13.19	n/a	6. Cataract extraction, left eye
87.59	n/a	7. Cholecystogram
93.96	n/a	8. Oxygen by nasal cannula
47.09	n/a	9. Abdominal appendectomy
23.19	n/a	10. Removal of impacted tooth

Note:

"Other, other specified, and unspecified codes" is not a coding convention in ICD-10-PCS.

EXERCISE 3.11 – ETIOLOGY AND MANIFESTATION RULES

ICD-9-CM	ICD-10-CM	
252.1, 366.42	E20.9, H28	1. Tetanic cataract in hypoparathyroidism
135, 425.8	D86.89	2. Cardiac sarcoidosis
585.9, 420.0	N18.9, I32	3. Uremic pericarditis
090.0, 567.0	A50.08, K67	4. Congenital syphilitic peritonitis

Note:

ICD-9-CM codes 090.0 and 567.0 are both reported. Code 567.0 in the ICD-9-CM tabular list contains a note that states, "Code first underlying disease." This means code 567.0 is not reported alone and requires a different code to be reported first. In this case, code 090.0 is reported first. Also, code 567.0 contains an excludes code, which directs you elsewhere to assign the first underlying code.

ICD-10-CM codes A50.08 and K67 are also both reported because of the Excludes2 instruction, which indicates that the code and the excluded code can be reported together.

ICD-9-CM	ICD-10-CM	
002.0, 730.80	A01.05	5. Typhoid osteomyelitis

Note:

In ICD-9-CM, typhoid osteomyelitis requires the assignment of two codes. In ICD-10-CM, that condition is assigned a single (combination) code.

EXERCISE 3.12 – AND

ICD-9-CM	ICD-10-CM/PCS	
099.52	A56.3	1. Venereal disease of the rectum due to *Chlamydia*
170.3	C41.3	2. Malignant neoplasm of costal cartilage
253.0	E22.0	3. Acromegaly
516.9	J84.0	4. Parietoalveolar pneumopathy
232.4	D04.4	5. Carcinoma *in situ* of scalp (Neoplasm)
88.71	BH4CZZZ	6. Ultrasonography of head
96.02	0CHY7BZ	7. Insertion of oropharyngeal (mouth and throat) airway
83.19	0K880ZZ	8. Open division of muscle, left upper arm
86.89	0HQFXZZ	9. Repair of skin, right hand
28.11	0CBP0ZX	10. Open biopsy, tonsils (Excision in ICD-10-PCS)

EXERCISE 3.13 – DUE TO

ICD-9-CM	ICD-10-CM	
275.1	E83.01	1. Cirrhosis due to Wilson's disease
099.0	A57	2. Bubo due to *Hemophilus ducreyi*
277.83	E71.43	3. Carnitine deficiency due to hemodialysis
244.1	E89.0	4. Hypothyroidism due to irradiation therapy
478.75	J38.5	5. Airway obstruction due to laryngospasm

Note:

The due to *subterm does not appear in the ICD-9-CM Index to Procedures or ICD-10-PCS Index.*

EXERCISE 3.14 – IN

ICD-9-CM	ICD-10-CM	
696.0	L40.50	1. Arthritis in psoriasis
115.92	B39.9, H32	2. Chorioretinitis in histoplasmosis

Note:

In ICD-9-CM, chorioretinitis in histoplasmosis *is assigned a single (combination) code. In ICD-10-CM, that condition requires the assignment of two (multiple) codes.*

654.13	034.12, D25.9	3. Uterine fibroid tumor in pregnancy (antepartum, second trimester)

Note:

ICD-10-CM tabular list category code 034 states Use additional code for specific condition, *which means code D25.9 is assigned as a secondary code to classify the fibroid tumor. In ICD-9-CM,* uterine fibroid tumor in pregnancy *is assigned a single (combination) code. In ICD-10-CM, that condition requires the assignment of two (multiple) codes.*

057.9, 370.44	B09	4. Keratoconjunctivitis in exanthema

Note:

In ICD-9-CM, keratoconjunctivitis in exanthema *requires the assignment of two codes. In ICD-10-CM, that condition is assigned a single (combination) code.*

078.6	A98.5	5. Nephrosis in epidemic hemorrhagic fever

Note:

ICD-10-PCS does not use the subterm in.

EXERCISE 3.15 – WITH

ICD-9-CM	ICD-10-CM/PCS	
540.0	K35.2	1. Appendicitis with perforation
242.10	E05.10	2. Thyrotoxicosis with uninodular adenomatous goiter
860.4	S27.2	3. Traumatic hemothorax with pneumothorax
309.24	F43.22	4. Adjustment disorder with anxiety
740.0	Q00.0	5. Skull agenesis with anencephalus (or anencephaly)
53.69	OWUF0JZ	6. Open repair of anterior abdominal wall hernia with synthetic substitute
38.34	n/a	7. Correction of coarctation of aorta with anastomosis
66.39	n/a	8. Destruction of fallopian tube with ligation
15.6	n/a	9. Extraocular muscle operation with revision
02.94	n/a	10. Removal of halo traction with synchronous replacement

Note:

There is limited use of subterm with *in the ICD-10-PCS Index.*

EXERCISE 3.16 – CROSS-REFERENCES

ICD-9-CM	ICD-10-CM/PCS	
276.4	E87.4	1. Abnormal acid-base balance
799.89	R68.89	2. Toxicosis
551.8	K46.1	3. Strangulated gangrenous abdominal hernia
752.51	Q53.9	4. Undescended testis
646.23	O12.10	5. Proteinuria complicating pregnancy
86.69	0HX7XZZ	6. Advancement graft, skin of abdomen (split-thickness)
39.59, 00.40	n/a	7. Plasty of peripheral blood vessel
38.10	n/a	8. Removal of thrombus with endarterectomy
79.00, 78.90	n/a	9. Fracture repair with insertion of bone growth stimulator
53.00	n/a	10. Halsted operation

Note:

See is the only cross-reference term used in the ICD-10-PCS Index; thus, there is just one ICD-10-PCS procedure coded above.

REVIEW

Matching I

1. d
2. c
3. e
4. a
5. b

Matching II

6. e
7. c
8. b
9. d
10. a

Matching III

11. d
12. c
13. e
14. a
15. b

Multiple Choice

16. d
17. d
18. b
19. b
20. a
21. c
22. a
23. d
24. c
25. c
26. b
27. c
28. b
29. b
30. c
31. d
32. a
33. b
34. a
35. d
36. b
37. d
38. c
39. a
40. c

Chapter 4
ICD-9-CM and ICD-10-CM Coding Guidelines

EXERCISE 4.1 – ICD-9-CM AND ICD-10-CM OFFICIAL GUIDELINES FOR CODING AND REPORTING

1. cooperating parties for the ICD-9-CM or cooperating parties for the ICD-10-CM
2. encounter
3. provider
4. HIPAA
5. structure and conventions
6. principal diagnosis
7. additional diagnoses
8. comorbidities and complications
9. outpatient coding and reporting
10. present on admission (POA) reporting guidelines

EXERCISE 4.2 – GENERAL ICD-9-CM AND ICD-10-CM DIAGNOSIS CODING GUIDELINES

1. F

Note:

The boxed note below the entry indicates that a fifth-digit subclassification is required for ICD-9-CM category 948 codes.

2. F

Note:

Always verify codes in the tabular list.

3. T
4. T
5. F

Note:

When established diagnoses are coded, do not assign codes to associated signs and symptoms.

6. T
7. F

Note:

When signs and symptoms are integral to the disease process, they are included in the code for the established or definitive disease.

8. T
9. T
10. F

Note:

When possible, assign separate codes for the acute (or subacute) and chronic conditions. (Sometimes there is a combination code for acute and chronic conditions.)

11. F

Note:

Multiple coding involves assigning two or more codes to completely classify the elements of a complex diagnostic statement, which contain words or phrases such as due to, incidental to, secondary to, with, *or other similar terminology.*

12. T
13. T
14. F

Note:

There is no time limit on when a late effect residual code can be reported.

15. F

Note:

Code any condition described at the time of encounter/visit as "impending" or "threatened" as follows: If the condition did occur, code as confirmed diagnosis; if the condition did not occur, reference the disease index to determine if the condition has a subentry term for "impending" or "threatened" and reference main term entries for "Impending" and "Threatened"; if subterms impending *or* threatened *are listed, assign the code; and if subterms* impending *or* threatened *are not listed, code the existing underlying condition(s), not the condition described as "impending" or "threatened."*

ICD-10 ALERT!

ICD-10 ALERT! Beginning with Exercise 4.3, ICD-10-CM codes will be located in parentheses next to the ICD-9-CM codes.

EXERCISE 4.3 – INFECTIOUS AND PARASITIC DISEASES

042 (B20) 1. AIDS

005.1 (A05.1) 2. Botulism

088.81 (A69.20) 3. Lyme disease

055.1 (B05.2) 4. Postmeasles pneumonia

071 (A82.9) 5. Rabies

EXERCISE 4.4 – NEOPLASMS

233.1 (D06.9) 1. Carcinoma *in situ*, cervix uteri (neoplasm)

181 (C58) 2. Choriocarcinoma (female patient)

228.00 (D18.00) 3. Hemangioma

176.9 (C46.9) 4. Kaposi sarcoma

214.1 (D17.39) 5. Lipoma, skin of abdomen

EXERCISE 4.5 – ENDOCRINE, NUTRITIONAL AND METABOLIC DISEASES, AND IMMUNITY DISORDERS

250.03 (E10.8) 1. Diabetes mellitus, type 1 uncontrolled

250.00 (E11.9) 2. Diabetes mellitus, type 2

253.1 (E22.1) 3. Hyperprolactinemia

278.01 (E66.01) 4. Morbid obesity

256.4 (E28.2) 5. Polycystic ovaries

EXERCISE 4.6 – DISEASES OF THE BLOOD AND BLOOD-FORMING ORGANS

289.0 (D75.1) 1. Acquired polycythemia

285.1 (D62) 2. Acute posthemorrhagic anemia

288.09 (D70.9) 3. Agranuloycytosis

281.9 (D53.9) 4. Chronic simple anemia

289.51 (D73.2) 5. Chronic congestive splenomegaly

EXERCISE 4.7 – MENTAL DISORDERS

331.0 (G30.9) 1. Alzheimer's disease

Note:

In ICD-10-CM, code G30.9 contains a Use additional code to identify *note. The conditions listed below the note are not included in the diagnosis statement; therefore, do not assign an additional code.*

295.32 (F20.0) 2. Chronic paranoid schizophrenia

291.0 (F10.231) 3. Alcoholic delirium tremens

305.62 (F14.10) 4. Episodic cocaine abuse

Note:

Code 304.22 (Cocaine dependence, episodic abuse) is incorrect because the diagnostic statement does not include the word "dependence." Refer to ICD index main term "abuse," subterm "drugs (nondependent)," and second modifier "cocaine" for the correct code.

296.30 (F33.9) 5. Major depressive disorder, recurrent episode

EXERCISE 4.8 – DISEASES OF THE NERVOUS SYSTEM AND SENSE ORGANS

380.12 (H60.331) 1. Acute swimmers' ear, right

351.0 (G51.0) 2. Bell palsy

368.2 (H53.2) 3. Diplopia

343.2 (G80.8) 4. Congenital quadriplegia

324.1 (G06.1) 5. Intraspinal abscess

EXERCISE 4.9 – DISEASES OF THE CIRCULATORY SYSTEM

410.21 (I21.19) 1. Acute ST elevation myocardial infarction, inferolateral wall, initial episode of care

391.1 (I01.1) 2. Acute rheumatic endocarditis

438.11 (I69.920) 3. Aphasia, late effect of cerebrovascular disease

401.1 (I10) 4. Benign hypertension

396.3 (I08.0) 5. Mitral and aortic valve insufficiency

EXERCISE 4.10 – DISEASES OF THE RESPIRATORY SYSTEM

461.1 (J01.10) 1. Acute frontal sinusitis

477.0 (J30.1) 2. Allergic rhinitis due to pollen

496 (J44.9) 3. Chronic obstructive pulmonary disease

518.0 (J98.11) 4. Atelectasis

464.4 (J05.0) 5. Croup

EXERCISE 4.11 – DISEASES OF THE DIGESTIVE SYSTEM

555.9 (K50.90) 1. Crohn disease

528.2 (K12.0) 2. Canker sore

534.10 (K28.1) 3. Acute gastrojejunal ulcer, with perforation

530.81 (K21.9) 4. Gastroesophageal reflux

550.90 (K40.90) 5. Inguinal hernia

EXERCISE 4.12 – DISEASES OF THE GENITOURINARY SYSTEM

604.0 (N45.4) 1. Abscess of epididymis

610.1 (N60.11) 2. Chronic cystic mastitis, right breast

601.1 (N41.10) 3. Chronic prostatitis

596.3 (N30.80) 4. Diverticulitis of bladder

626.2 (N92.0) 5. Excessive menstruation

EXERCISE 4.13 – COMPLICATIONS OF PREGNANCY, CHILDBIRTH, AND THE PUERPERIUM

658.40 (041.129) 1. Amnionitis

Note:

In the ICD-10-CM index, main term Amnionitis *states* see Pregnancy, complicated by *where the code for subterm* Amnionitis *is 041.129.*

676.24 (O92.79) 2. Engorgement of breasts (postpartum)
642.33 (O13.3) 3. Gestational hypertension, third trimester (antepartum)

Note:

In the ICD-9-CM Index to Diseases, go to the hypertension table and locate subterm complicating pregnancy *and 2nd qualifier* gestational.

661.41 (O62.4) 4. Incoordinate uterine contractions, delivered

665.34 (O71.3) 5. Laceration of cervix (postpartum complication)

EXERCISE 4.14 – DISEASES OF THE SKIN AND SUBCUTANEOUS TISSUE

704.01 (L63.9) 1. Alopecia areata

680.7 (L02.632) 2. Carbuncle, left foot

707.00, 707.20 (L89.90) 3. Decubitus ulcer

684 (L01.00) 4. Impetigo

701.4 (L91.0) 5. Keloid

EXERCISE 4.15 – DISEASES OF THE MUSCULOSKELETAL AND CONNECTIVE TISSUE

719.49 1. Arthralgia, hand, lower leg, and ankle

Note:

Assign code 719.49 for "multiple sites." Do not assign separate codes 719.44, 719.46, and 719.47 when a combination code for "multiple sites" is available.

736.74 (M21.532) 2. Claw foot, left (acquired)

718.45 (M24.559) 3. Contracture of joint, pelvic region

721.5 (M48.20) 4. Kissing spine

728.85 (M62.838) 5. Muscle spasm

EXERCISE 4.16 – CONGENITAL ANOMALIES

747.21 (Q25.4) 1. Anomalies of aortic arch

746.86 (Q24.6) 2. Congenital heart block

742.3 (Q03.9) 3. Congenital hydrocephalus

743.03 (Q11.0) 4. Cystic eyeball, congenital

750.13 (Q38.3) 5. Fissure of tongue, congenital

EXERCISE 4.17 – CERTAIN CONDITIONS ORIGINATING IN THE PERINATAL PERIOD

770.83 (P28.2) 1. Cyanotic attacks of newborn

766.0 (P08.0) 2. Exceptionally large baby

767.5 (P11.3) — 3. Facial palsy, newborn
779.31 (P92.9) — 4. Feeding problems in newborn
772.0 (P50.9) — 5. Fetal blood loss

EXERCISE 4.18 – SIGNS, SYMPTOMS, AND ILL-DEFINED CONDITIONS

796.1 (R29.2) — 1. Abnormal reflex
781.3 (R27.0) — 2. Ataxia
790.93 (R97.2) — 3. Elevated prostate specific antigen
783.41 (R62.51) — 4. Failure to thrive (child)
796.2 (R03.0) — 5. Elevated blood pressure reading

EXERCISE 4.19 – INJURY AND POISONING

802.22 (S02.60xA) — 1. Closed fracture mandible, subcondylar (initial encounter)
831.04 (S43.109A) — 2. Closed dislocation of clavicle (initial encounter)
850.11 (S06.0x1A) — 3. Concussion with brief loss of consciousness (30 minutes) (initial encounter)
945.22 (T25.229A) — 4. Foot burn, left, blisters, epidermal loss (second-degree) (initial encounter)
861.02 (S26.020A) — 5. Heart laceration without penetration of heart chambers (initial encounter)
708.0, E930.0 (L50.0, T36.0x5A) — 6. Hives resulting from penicillin taken as prescribed (initial encounter)
967.0, 780.01, E950.1 (T42.3x2A, R40.20) — 7. Coma due to overdose of barbiturates (attempted suicide) (initial encounter)
995.29, E948.6 (T50.a15A) — 8. Adverse reaction to pertussis vaccine (initial encounter)

Note:

The specific adverse reaction (e.g., rash, difficulty breathing, fever) is not stated. Therefore, assign ICD-9-CM code 995.29 or ICD-10-CM code T50.a15A.

971.2, 980.0, 427.9, E855.5, E860.0 (T44.991A, T51.91xA, I49.9) — 9. Cardiac arrhythmia due to interaction of prescribed ephedrine and alcohol intoxication (accident) (initial encounter)
963.0, 780.09, E858.1 (T45.0x1A, R40.1) — 10. Stupor due to overdose of Nytol (accident) (initial encounter)

EXERCISE 4.20 – FACTORS INFLUENCING HEALTH STATUS AND CONTACT WITH HEALTH SERVICES

V59.3 (Z52.3) — 1. Bone marrow donor
V58.11 (Z51.11) — 2. Chemotherapy encounter
V70.3 (Z02.89) — 3. Examination for summer camp
V01.3 (Z20.89) — 4. Exposure to smallpox
V17.1 (Z82.3) — 5. Family history of stroke

EXERCISE 4.21 – EXTERNAL CAUSES OF INJURY AND POISONING

Answer	Item
E885.2, E849.4 (V00.131A, Y92.830)	1. Fall from skateboard at public park (Place of occurrence)
E898.0, E05.9, E849.0 (X05.xxA, Y93.g3, Y92.020)	2. Burning bedclothes resulting from cooking in kitchen of mobile home (Place of occurrence)
E837.9 (V93.59xA)	3. Explosion in watercraft
E881.0 (W11.xxxA)	4. Fall from ladder
E849.4 (Y92.320A)	5. Foot injury taking place on baseball field (accident)

REVIEW

Multiple Choice

1. c
2. a
3. b

Note:

There is no stated relationship between the diabetes mellitus and the iritis; therefore, the answer is a.

4. b
5. b
6. b
7. a
8. b
9. d
10. c
11. a
12. a
13. c
14. a
15. b
16. c
17. c
18. c
19. a
20. d
21. c
22. a
23. d
24. c
25. b
26. c
27. d
28. a
29. d
30. a
31. a
32. a
33. c
34. d
35. c
36. d
37. d
38. a
39. a
40. a

Coding Practice: Diseases

Answer	Item
286.0 (D66)	41. Classical hemophilia
V53.31 (Z45.018)	42. Fitting of cardiac pacemaker
779.4, E930.2 (P93.0, T36.2x5A)	43. Gray syndrome from chloramphenicol administration in newborn as prescribed (initial encounter)
959.9, E985.1 (T14.90, Y23.0xx0)	44. Injury by shotgun, undetermined whether accidental or intentional (shooting) (initial encounter)
564.1 (K58.9)	45. Irritable bowel syndrome
174.9 (C50.919)	46. Malignant neoplasm, breast
836.63 (S83.136)	47. Medial dislocation of tibia, proximal end, open (initial encounter)
E814.9 (V03.10xA)	48. Motor vehicle traffic accident involving a collision with a pedestrian (initial encounter)
300.14 (F44.81)	49. Multiple personality
787.01 (R11.2)	50. Nausea with vomiting
V14.0 (Z88.0)	51. Personal history of penicillin allergy
482.32 (J15.3)	52. Pneumonia due to *Streptococcus*, group B
714.31 (M08.09)	53. Polyarticular juvenile rheumatoid arthritis, acute
753.14 (Q61.19)	54. Polycystic kidney, autosomal recessive
244.0 (E89.0)	55. Postsurgical hypothyroidism
416.0 (I27.0)	56. Pulmonary arteriosclerosis
134.1 (B88.1)	57. Sand flea infestation
634.12 (O03.6)	58. Spontaneous abortion, complicated by excessive hemorrhage, complete
651.31, V27.3 (O30.019, Z37.3)	59. Twin pregnancy with loss of one fetus (delivered)
618.1 (N81.2)	60. Uterine prolapse, first degree

Chapter 5
ICD-9-CM and ICD-10-CM/PCS Hospital Inpatient Coding

HOSPITAL INPATIENT CODING ANSWER FORM

Copy and provide the form to students for their use in assigning codes to hospital inpatient case scenarios and records. Using the form will facilitate students' understanding of diagnosis and procedure sequencing.

	Code(s)
Principal Diagnosis:	
Other (Additional) Diagnosis(es): (e.g., comorbidities, complications, and secondary diagnoses)	
Principal Procedure:	
Other Significant Procedure(s):	

EXERCISE 5.1 – ACUTE CARE FACILITIES (HOSPITALS)

1. acute care facility (ACF)
2. ancillary services
3. single hospitals; multihospital systems
4. bed size (or bed count)
5. short-term (or acute)
6. long-term (or long-term acute)
7. four

Note:

The month of May has 31 days. Count the day of admission, May 30, plus the remaining days through June 3 (May 31, June 1, and June 2). Do not count June 3 because it is the day of discharge.

8. nonacute
9. rehabilitation
10. hospitalists

EXERCISE 5.2 – INPATIENT DIAGNOSIS CODING GUIDELINES

Matching

1. b
2. h
3. f
4. a
5. g
6. i
7. d
8. j
9. e
10. c

EXERCISE 5.3 – INPATIENT PROCEDURE CODING GUIDELINES

1. UHDDS definitions
2. ICD-9-CM Volume 3, ICD-10-PCS
3. CPT, HCPCS level II
4. MS-DRGs
5. first
6. performed for definitive treatment rather than for diagnostic or exploratory purposes, necessary to treat a complication, or most closely related to the principal diagnosis.
7. surgical in nature, carrying a procedural (or operative) risk, carrying an anesthetic risk, requiring highly trained personnel, and/or requiring special facilities or equipment.
8. one, five
9. one, 14
10. 24

EXERCISE 5.4 – ICD-9-CM PROCEDURE CODING

1. F
2. F
3. T
4. F
5. T
6. T
7. F
8. F
9. F
10. T

85.50 11. Augmentation mammoplasty

41.32 12. Closed aspiration biopsy of spleen

05.32 13. Injection of neurolytic agent into sympathetic nerve

65.41 14. Laparoscopic unilateral salpingo-oophorectomy

38.59 15. Ligation and stripping of varicose veins, left leg

60.12 16. Open biopsy of prostate

42.21 17. Operative esophagoscopy (by incision)

06.81 18. Parathyroidectomy, complete

72.51 19. Partial breech extraction with forceps to head

81.52 20. Partial hip replacement

55.04 21. Percutaneous nephrostomy with fragmentation

22.01 22. Puncture of nasal sinus for aspiration

00.54 23. Replacement of only cardiac resynchronization defibrillator pulse, generator device

11.31 24. Transposition of pterygium

19.52 25. Type II tympanoplasty

EXERCISE 5.5 – ICD-10-PCS PROCEDURE CODING

1. F
2. F
3. T
4. T
5. F
6. T
7. F
8. T
9. F
10. T

0H0V0JZ 11. Bilateral augmentation mammoplasty using synthetic substitute, open approach (—*see* Alteration, Skin and Breast 0H0)

07BP3ZX 12. Percutaneous biopsy of spleen (—*see* Excision, Diagnostic)

3E0T3CZ 13. Injection of neurolytic agent (nerve block) into peripheral nerve (Block, nerve, anesthetic injection 3E0T3CZ)

0UT10ZZ 14. Laparoscopic oophorectomy, left (—*see* Resection, Female Reproductive System 0UT)

06DS0ZZ 15. Open stripping of varicose veins, left lesser saphenous vein (—*see* Extraction)

0VB00ZX 16. Open biopsy of prostate (—*see* Excision, Diagnostic)

0DJ08ZZ 17. Operative esophagoscopy (by incision)

0GTQ0ZZ 18. Parathyroidectomy, complete (—*see* Resection, Endocrine System 0GT)

10D07Z5 19. Partial breech extraction with high forceps

0SRB0JZ 20. Partial left hip replacement, synthetic substitute

Note:

Do not construct a separate code for resection of the original hip joint.

0TF33ZZ 21. Percutaneous nephrostomy with fragmentation of right kidney pelvis

099U00Z, 099V00Z 22. Puncture of bilateral ethmoid sinuses for aspiration (—*see* Drainage)

Note:

Because there is no bilateral value for the body part, construct codes for the left and right ethmoid sinuses.

02HA0QZ 23. Replacement of cardiac resynchronization defibrillator pulse generator device, heart, open approach (Insertion of device in)

08QTXZZ 24. Repair of pterygium of conjunctiva, left eye

09QE0ZZ 25. Left tympanoplasty (—see Repair, Ear, Nose, Sinus 09Q)

EXERCISE 5.6 – CODING INPATIENT DIAGNOSES AND PROCEDURES

Note:

ICD-10-CM/PCS codes are located in parentheses next to the ICD-9-CM codes.

Note:

Procedure codes are not assigned for ancillary tests (e.g., laboratory tests and x-rays) in the case scenarios because such codes do not impact DRG assignment or the reimbursement amount for an inpatient case. However, because some hospitals do assign codes to ancillary tests (even though codes assigned do not impact the level of reimbursement received), students should be alerted to this practice.

1. 042,136.3,112.0,33.24 (B20, B59, B37.0, 3E1F88X)

Note:

Chapter-specific coding guidelines provide instruction to sequence ICD-9-CM code 042 (or ICD-10-CM code B20) (AIDS) as the principal diagnosis, with AIDS-related conditions sequenced as other additional diagnoses. The bronchoscopy procedure was performed for the purpose of taking cell washings as a type of biopsy. (Do not construct an ICD-10-PCS code for the bronchoscopy. Code only the diagnostic irrigation procedure.)

2. 433.11, 784.59, 342.90 (I63.031, I69.321, I69.359)

Note:

The patient was admitted for treatment of the carotid artery occlusion with cerebral infarction (433.11), which is the principal diagnosis. When codes from categories 430–437 (e.g., 433.11) are assigned, additional codes are assigned to identify any sequelae present, such as dysphasia (784.59) and hemiparesis (342.90). Only after the patient has completed initial treatment or is discharged from care, codes from category 438 are assigned to classify the late effects of cerebrovascular disease codes for dysphasia (438.12) and hemiparesis (438.21). The CT scan (87.03) does not impact the DRG reimbursement rate; therefore, that code is not assigned.

3. 813.42, E882, E849.0, 93.54 (S52.501A, W13.2xxA, Y92.018, 2W3DX1Z)

Note:

The ICD-9-CM Index to Diseases entry for "Fracture" includes subterm radius (alone) (closed) *and 2nd qualifier* lower end or extremity (distal end) (lower epiphysis), *which directs the coder to assign 813.42 (after verifying it in the Tabular List of Diseases). To locate the external cause of injury codes, go to main term* Fall, falling (accidental) *in the Index to External Causes of Injury and Poisonings and subterm* roof (through) *to locate code E882. Then go to main term* Accident (to), *subterm* occurring (at) (in) *and 2nd qualifier* home *to locate code E849.0.*

4. 250.61, 357.2, 707.15, 707.24, 785.4, V58.67, 84.12 (E10.40, E10.622, L97.524, Z79.4, 0Y6N0Z0)

Note:

Chapter-specific ICD-9-CM coding guidelines provide instruction that the diabetes code is to be sequenced as the principal diagnosis for a condition such as "diabetic foot ulcers due to type 1 diabetic peripheral neuropathy" (250.61). The manifestations of the diabetic peripheral neuropathy are reported as other additional diagnosis codes: 357.2 (peripheral neuropathy), 707.15 (toe ulcer), 707.24 (stage of ulcer) and 785.4 (gangrene). To assign the procedure code, go to main term Amputation, forefoot *in the Index to Procedures and assign code 84.12 (after verifying the code in the Tabular List of Procedures).*

5. 345.41 (G40.219)

Note:

To assign the principal diagnosis ICD-9-CM code, go to main term Epilepsy *in the Index to Diseases and locate subterm* localization-related, *2nd qualifier* with, *and 3rd qualifier* complex partial seizures *to assign 345.41 (after verifying the code in the Tabular List of Diseases).*

REVIEW

Multiple Choice

1. a
2. b
3. a
4. b
5. a
6. c
7. b
8. b
9. b
10. b
11. d
12. c

Note:

A pilonidal abscess is located near or on the natal cleft of the buttocks.

13. a
14. d
15. c
16. b
17. c
18. c
19. a

Note:

The Index cross reference for main term Biopsy *included the term* Diagnostic, *which means 7th qualifier value X is assigned instead of Z.*

20. d

Coding Practice: Hospital Inpatient Cases

Note:

- ICD-10-CM and ICD-10-PCS codes are included in parentheses next to ICD-9-CM codes.
- Coding rationales are included for each case to provide direction about how to assign codes.
- Procedure codes are not assigned for ancillary tests (e.g., laboratory tests and x-rays) because they do not impact DRG assignment or the reimbursement amount for an inpatient case. However, because some hospitals do assign codes to ancillary tests (even though codes assigned do not impact the level of reimbursement received), students should be alerted about this practice.

21. 038.42, 276.51, 402.91, 428.0 (A41.51, A40.0, E86.0, III.0, I50.9)

Note:

- A blood culture test was positive for *Escherichia coli*, and the physician documented septicemia as the principal diagnosis.
- Other diagnoses documented in the final diagnosis that are assigned codes include dehydration and hypertensive heart disease, which were treated with "routine medications" during the admission.
- Do not assign a code to the "positive blood culture, *Escherichia coli*" diagnosis because it is included in the septicemia diagnosis.
- To locate the code for acute pulmonary edema due to CHF (congestive heart failure), go the Index to Diseases and locate main term "edema," subterm "lung," second qualifier "acute," third qualifier "with heart disease or failure," and fourth qualifier "congestive."

22. 038.11, 785.52, 584.9, 276.51, 691.0 (A41.0, R65.21, N17.9, E87.0, L22)

Note:

- When septic shock is documented as a discharge diagnosis, report the code for septicemia as the principal diagnosis. (ICD-9-CM category code 038 contains an instructional note that states, "Use additional code for systemic inflammatory response syndrome (SIRS) 995.91-995-92." This means that code 995.91 is reported as an other (additional) diagnosis code.)
- This patient also was diagnosed as having septic shock, to which a separate code is assigned as an other (additional) diagnosis code.
- In addition, make sure you assign a code for any organ dysfunction; in this case, acute renal failure.
- Then assign a code for dehydration and diaper rash.

23. 197.0, 157.0, 244.9, 250.00, 32.39 (C78.02, C25.0, E03.9, E11.9, 0BTJ0ZZ)

Note:

- When a patient is admitted for a primary malignant neoplasm with metastasis and treatment is directed toward the secondary site only, the secondary neoplasm code is assigned as the principal diagnosis. The primary malignant neoplasm code is assigned as an other (additional) diagnosis code.
- In this case, codes for hypothyroidism and diabetes are also assigned.
- A procedure code is assigned for the left lower lobe lung resection procedure.

24. 153.3, 197.0, 496, 414.01, 412 (C18.7, C78.01, C78.02, J44.9, I25.10, I25.2)

Note:

- Assign a code to carcinoma of sigmoid colon as the principal diagnosis. Carcinoma of the sigmoid colon is the primary site of cancer.
- Assign a code to probable metastatic bronchogenic carcinoma, bilaterally, as an other (additional) diagnosis because a suspected condition that receives inpatient treatment is coded as if confirmed. When a primary carcinoma metastasizes from its place of origin, the metastasized site is coded as the secondary site of cancer.
- Assign codes to chronic conditions that were medically managed during the hospitalization: chronic obstructive disease and coronary artery disease. Because documentation indicates that the patient has coronary artery disease with no history of coronary artery bypass surgery, assign a code for CAD of native coronary artery.
- "Previous MI" is a healed or old myocardial infarction, to which a code is also assigned.

25. 250.70, 785.4, 041.7, 041.4, 84.11 (E11.52, B96.5, B96.2, 0Y6Q0Z0)

Note:

- In ICD-9-CM, diabetic gangrene is coded as 250.70, diabetes with peripheral circulatory disorders. Fifth digit 0 is assigned to indicate that the diabetes was not stated as uncontrolled. In ICD-10-CM, code E11.52 is assigned. (Do *not* assign code E08.52 in error, which classifies diabetes mellitus *due* to peripheral angiopathy.)
- In ICD-9-CM, an additional code is assigned to identify the manifestation; and in this case, the manifestation is gangrene (785.4). In ICD-10-CM, an additional code is *not* assigned because the manifestation (gangrene) is included in code E11.52.
- Assign codes to classify *Pseudomonas aeruginosa* and *Escherichia coli* as bacterial agents.
- Assign a procedure code for metatarsal amputation of the left great toe.

26. 244.9, 280.8, 532.30 (E03.9, D63.8, K26.3)

Note:

- Hypothyroidism is the condition established after study to be chiefly responsible for the patient's admission to the hospital. Thus, hypothyroidism is reported as the principal diagnosis.
- The iron deficiency anemia is sequenced as an other (additional) diagnosis; it was due to hypothyroidism.
- A code is assigned for the duodenal ulcer, and a code is assigned for osteoarthritis of the knee because both were treated during this admission.
- The transfusion of packed red blood cells does not impact the DRG reimbursement rate; therefore, do not assign a code for it.

27. 282.62, 517.3 V18.2 (D57.01, Z83.2)

Note:

- In ICD-9-CM, assign code 282.62 for sickle cell disease in crisis as the principal diagnosis. In ICD-10-CM, combination code D57.01 is assigned.
- In ICD-9-CM, assign an other (additional) code for acute chest syndrome (517.3) to identify the type of crisis.
- Assign a code for the family history of sickle cell anemia.

28. 285.22, 174.9, 198.5, 197.7, V58.69 (C50.911 , D63.0, C79.51, C78.7, Z79.3)

Note:

- In ICD-9-CM, when an admission is for treatment of anemia due to a malignancy and only the anemia is treated, assign the code for anemia as the principal diagnosis. Anemia in neoplastic disease is coded as 285.22 and sequenced as principal diagnosis because it is the condition responsible for admission. In ICD-10-CM, the index directs you to report code C50.911 first, followed by code D63.0.
- The underlying chronic conditions are coded as other (additional) diagnoses: carcinoma of breast with metastases to bone and liver. These chronic conditions are underlying causes of the anemia. Also, assign a code for long-term current use of other medications (e.g., chemotherapy).
- The transfusion of packed red blood cells does not impact the DRG reimbursement rate.

29. 965.61, 427.1, 311, V62.0, V62.81, E950.0, E849.0 (T39.312A, I47.2, F32.9, Z56.0, Z65.8, T39.012A, Y92.00)

Note:

- If an overdose of a drug was intentionally taken, it is coded as a poisoning. Sequence the poisoning code first, followed by a code for the manifestation (paroxysmal ventricular tachycardia).
- Codes for unemployment and relationship problems provide additional information about the patient's status.
- External cause codes are also assigned in this case to indicate that the poisoning was a suicide attempt and that the incident occurred at home.
- A code for depression is also assigned as an other (additional) diagnosis.

30. 296.32 (F32.1)

Note:

- Involutional psychotic reaction is assigned as the principal diagnosis. In ICD-9-CM, fifth digit 2 is assigned because the physician stated that the reaction was moderate.)
- An other (additional) code for the depression is *not* assigned because it is implicit in the involutional psychotic reaction diagnosis.
- The electroconvulsive therapy does not impact the DRG reimbursement rate; thus, do not assign a code.

31. 331.0, 294.11, 492.8, 250.00 (G30.9, F02.81, J43.9, E11.9)

Note:

- When coding Alzheimer's disease, assign an additional code for associated behavioral disturbances. (In ICD-9-CM, "dementia in conditions classified elsewhere" has been expanded to identify the presence or absence of behavioral disturbances. In this case, code 294.11 is assigned to identify that the patient was having behavioral disturbances (e.g., aggressive behavior and wandering). When assigning code 294.11, first code the underlying physical condition (331.0).)
- Then assign other (additional) codes for emphysema and type 2 diabetes mellitus, controlled.

32. 435.9, 182.0, 599.0, 041.3 (G45.9, C54.1, N39.0, B96.1)

Note:

- The patient was admitted with dizziness, weakness, and nystagmus, which are symptoms of the transient ischemic attack diagnosed by the physician. The transient ischemic attack (TIA) is sequenced as the principal diagnosis. The symptoms are not coded because they are associated with the principal diagnosis of TIA.
- The patient is currently being treated for the endometrial carcinoma; therefore, an other (additional) diagnosis is assigned for the endometrial carcinoma.
- Assign a code for the urinary tract infection, with an additional code to identify the organism, *Klebsiella pneumoniae.*
- The gait training physical therapy code does not impact the DRG reimbursement rate; therefore, that code is not assigned.

33. 401.9, 444.81, 438.22, 438.11, 427.31 (I10, I74.5, I69.953, I69.920, I48.0)

Note:

- Hypertension is reported as the principal diagnosis. In ICD-9-CM, assign hypertension to category 401 with the appropriate fourth digit to indicate malignant (.1), benign (.0), or unspecified (.9). Do not assign fourth digit .0 or .1 unless "malignant" or "benign" is documented in the patient record. (There is no documented cause-and-effect relationship between the hypertension and possible iliofemoral emboli; therefore, combination code 405.99 is *not* assigned.)
- Assign a code to possible iliofemoral emboli as an other (additional) diagnosis. For inpatient hospitalizations, conditions stated as "possible" are coded as established diagnoses. To assign an other (additional) diagnosis code for "possible femoral and popliteal artery embolism," the coder would query the physician because that diagnosis was not included in the list of final diagnoses.
- In ICD-9-CM, codes from category 438 are assigned to indicate conditions classifiable to categories 430–437 as the cause of late effects. These include neurological deficits that persist after initial onset of the condition.
- Assign an additional diagnosis code for atrial fibrillation.

34. 410.11, 401.9, 272.0, 278.01 (I21.09, I10, E78.0, E66.01)

Note:

- Assign a code to acute ST elevation anterior wall myocardial infarction as the principal diagnosis. In ICD-9-CM, fifth digit 1 designates the first episode of care for a newly diagnosed myocardial infarction.
- Additional diagnosis codes for chest pain and diaphoresis are *not* assigned because they are considered components of the myocardial infarction. Such symptoms integral to a myocardial infarction are *not* coded.
- Assign a code to hypertension as an other (additional) diagnosis.
- Other (additional) diagnosis codes are also assigned for hypercholesterolemia and morbid obesity.

35. 466.0, 280.1, 787.01 (J20.6, D50.8, R11.2)

Note:

- Acute bronchitis due to RSV is the principal diagnosis because pneumonia was ruled out.
- Do not code the cough because it is a sign of the bronchitis.
- The meningitis also is not coded because it is no longer being medically managed.
- Assign additional diagnosis codes for the nutritional anemia due to poor dietary iron intake and nausea and vomiting because they were treated during the hospitalization.

36. 491.22, 429.2, 440.9, 411.1, 424.0 (J44.0, I51.9, I25.119, I34.0)

Note:

- The patient was admitted with shortness of breath and chest pain. The increasing chest pain was due to the chronic obstructive pulmonary disease with acute bronchitis; and when acute bronchitis is documented with chronic obstructive pulmonary disease, code 491.22 (or J44.0) is assigned and sequenced as the principal diagnosis.
- Do *not* assign an other (additional) diagnosis code for acute bronchitis. Do *not* assign a code for the respiratory distress because it is included in the principal diagnosis code.
- When the cause of the angina is clearly documented, sequence the cause before the appropriate angina code. In ICD-9-CM, progressive angina (411.1) is sequenced as an other (additional) code after the underlying cause of arteriosclerotic cardiovascular disease (429.2 and 440.9). In ICD-10-CM, a combination code (I25.119) classifies ASCVD of native artery with angina.
- Also assign a code for mitral insufficiency as an other (additional) diagnosis.

37. 153.3, 560.89, 332.0, 46.03 (C18.7, G20, 0D1L3J4)

Note:

- In ICD-9-CM, when a patient is admitted with a bowel obstruction due to sigmoid carcinoma, assign 153.3 as the principal diagnosis and sequence code 560.89, other intestinal obstruction, as an other (additional) diagnosis. In ICD-10-CM, the intestinal obstruction code contains an Excludes1 note that states, "intestinal obstruction due to specified condition–code to condition." Thus, just code C18.7 is assigned.
- Do *not* assign a code for the abdominal distention because it is a symptom of the bowel obstruction.
- Assign an other (additional) diagnosis code to Parkinson's disease.
- Assign a procedure codes to the loop colostomy. Do not assign a code to insertion of the nasogastric tube because it does not impact DRG reimbursement.

38. 532.30, 532.70, 553.3, 575.6, 733.00, 724.03 (K26.3, K26.7, K44.9, K82.4, M81.0, M48.06)

Note:

- If the same condition is described as both acute and chronic, code both the acute and chronic condition, sequencing the acute condition first. (In ICD-9-CM, assign fifth digit 0 for the acute and chronic ulcer to identify the ulcer as being without obstruction.)
- Do *not* assign a code for the abdominal pain because it is a symptom of the ulcer. Assign additional diagnosis codes for the hiatal hernia, gallbladder polyps, osteoporosis, and lumbar spinal stenosis because all conditions were medically managed during the inpatient stay.

39. 584.9, 276.51, 285.21, 585.6 (N17.9, E86.0, N18.6, D63.1)

Note:

- When a patient is diagnosed with acute renal failure and dehydration and the only treatment is intravenous hydration, it is appropriate to assign the code for acute renal failure as the principal diagnosis. In most cases, intravenous hydration corrects the acute renal failure. The fact that the renal function was not investigated does not affect the code assignment.
- Assign an other (additional) diagnosis, code for the dehydration.
- Assign an other (additional) diagnosis, code for the anemia due to end-stage renal disease.
- The transfusion of packed red blood cells code does not impact the DRG reimbursement rate; therefore, that code is not assigned.

40. 600.90, 724.79, 401.9, 60.29 (N40.0, M53.3, I10, 0VT07ZZ)

Note:

- Assign benign prostatic hyperplasia as the principal diagnosis. (In ICD-9-CM, fifth digit 0 is assigned to indicate the absence of urinary obstruction.)
- Assign an other (additional) diagnosis code for coccygodynia, which was evaluated and treated during the patient's stay.
- Assign a diagnosis code for the hypertension that was under medical management.
- Do not assign a code for "straining on urination" because it was not included in the list of discharge diagnoses; a physician query would be generated to ask if a code should be assigned.
- Assign a procedure code for the transurethral resection of the prostate.

41. 620.2, 218.9, 617.9 (N83.20, D25.9, N80.9)

Note:

- When two or more interrelated conditions meet the definition of principal diagnosis, either condition may be sequenced first as long as official coding guidelines do not indicate otherwise. Because it was determined that both the ovarian cyst and the uterine fibroid resulted in the patient's admission, either condition may be sequenced as the principal diagnosis.
- Assign an other (additional) diagnosis code for the possible endometriosis. If a diagnosis at the time of hospital discharge is qualified as "possible," code the condition as if it were an established diagnosis.

42. 634.11, 69.02 (O03.1, 0UB97ZZ)

Note:

- The principal diagnosis is spontaneous abortion with excessive bleeding. (In ICD-9-CM, a fifth digit is required for abortion category 634. Fifth digit 1, incomplete, indicates that not all of the products of conception were expelled from the uterus.)
- A procedure code is assigned for dilatation and curettage following an abortion.

43. 660.11, 653.41, 661.21, V27.0, 74.1 (O65.0, O33.4xx0, O62.2, Z37.0, 10D00Z1)

Note:

- When a patient undergoes a cesarean delivery, the reason for the cesarean delivery is sequenced as the principal diagnosis. In this case, the cause is "obstructed labor." Two codes are reported for an obstructed labor. First code the obstructed labor, followed by the code for the cause of the obstruction. In this case, the cause is borderline cephalopelvic disproportion. (In ICD-9-CM, to assist you in proper sequencing of the codes, category code 653 contains an instructional note that states, "Code first any obstructed labor" and category code 660.1 contains an instructional note that states, "Use additional code from 653.0–653.9." Fifth digit 1 is assigned to indicate "delivered, with or without mention of antepartum (before birth) condition.")
- A code is assigned for failure to progress as an other (additional) diagnosis.
- A code for outcome of delivery is always reported on maternal delivery records. It is always sequenced as an other (additional) diagnosis. In this case, the code indicates that the outcome of delivery was a single liveborn.
- Assign a procedure code for the low cervical cesarean section.

44. 727.41, V25.2, 706.2, 82.21, 63.73, 21.32 (M67.411, Z30.2, L72.0, 0LB73ZZ, 0V5Q0ZZ, 0HB1XZZ)

Note:

- Ganglion cyst of joint is the principal diagnosis because it is the condition after study that occasioned the admission to the hospital.
- Assign a code for the other (additional) diagnosis of sterilization.
- Assign a code for the other (additional) diagnosis of cyst, skin of the nose.
- Assign procedure codes for excision of ganglion cyst, bilateral vasectomy, and excision, lesion, skin of nose. A ganglion cyst is a swelling that often appears on or around joints and tendons in the hand (or foot); thus, for ICD-10-PCS, Table 0LB is used to construct the procedure code for "excision of ganglion cyst, right wrist." Also, ICD-10-PCS Table 0LB does not include a value for "right wrist" because it is considered part of the "right hand.")

45. 707.07, 707.24, 785.4, 041.11, 84.15 (L89.624, I96, B95.6, 0Y6G0ZZ)

Note:

- Decubitus ulcer of the heel is the principal diagnosis. It is a Stage IV decubitus ulcer.
- A code is assigned to gangrene as an additional diagnosis to identify its presence.
- Assign an additional diagnosis code to identify the *Staphylococcus aureus* infection.
- Assign a procedure code for the below-the-knee amputation as the principal procedure.
- The whirlpool physical therapy treatment does not impact the DRG reimbursement rate; therefore, that code is not assigned.

46. 996.78, 338.18, 458.29, 998.59, 041.4, E878.1, 78.65 (T84.84xA, I95.81, T81.4xxA, B96.2, Y83.1, 0QW604Z)

Note:

- Diagnosis "painful Gouffon pins" is coded as a complication due to presence of other internal fixation device. (In ICD-9-CM, subcategory code 996.7 classifies the pain, and fifth digit 8 indicates that the pain is due to presence of the pin.)
- In ICD-9-CM, you can assign an other (additional) code for "pain" (338.18). However, do *not* assign ICD-10-CM code G89.18 for "pain" because its Excludes1 note lists code T84.84.
- Assign an external cause code as an other (additional) diagnosis code to indicate that this complication was due to the surgical procedure, implant of an internal orthopedic device.
- Assign an other (additional) diagnosis code for postoperative hypotension.
- Assign other (additional) diagnosis code for the postoperative wound infection and assign a code for *Escherichia coli* as an other (additional) diagnosis to indicate the organism.
- Assign an external cause code as an other (additional) diagnosis to classify the complications due to surgical operation for the removal of the pin.
- Assign the principal procedure code for removal of the pin. (The proximal end of the femur, near the hip joint).
- The gait training with a walker code does not impact the DRG reimbursement amount; therefore, that code is not assigned.

47. 715.16, 81.54 (M17.11, 0SRC07Z)

Note:

- Degenerative arthritis is coded to category 715.9, with fifth digit 6 assigned to indicate that the knee is the site of the arthritis (715.96).
- Assign a code for total knee replacement as the principal procedure.
- The gait training with a walker code does not impact the DRG reimbursement amount; therefore, that code is not assigned.

48. V30.00, 758.1, 764.08, 765.29, 749.23, 755.01, 752.61, 756.3, 756.14, 753.3 (Z38.00, Q91.4, P05.18, Q37.0, Q69.0, Q54.1, Q76.6, Q76.49, Q63.2)

Note:

- The appropriate ICD-9-CM code from the V30–V39 categories (or ICD-10-CM Z38 category) is sequenced as the principal diagnosis. In this case, the principal diagnosis code is V30.00 (or Z38.00) for single liveborn, baby born in the hospital, and no cesarean section.
- When congenital condition(s) are diagnosed during the hospital episode in which an infant is born, appropriate code(s) from the Congenital Malformations . . . chapter of the coding manual are assigned as other (additional) diagnoses. The following other (additional) diagnoses are assigned codes:
  - Trisomy 13
  - Small for dates
  - Cleft lip and palate, complete
  - Accessory finger, left hand
  - Hypospadias
  - Extra rib
  - Hemivertebra
  - Dextroversion malrotation, left kidney

49. 745.0, 780.2 (Q20.0, R55)

Note:

- Persistent truncus arteriosus is the principal diagnosis.
- Assign a code to syncope as an other (additional) diagnosis.
- Do not assign codes for the shortness of breath, fatigue, and vague chest pain because they are symptoms of (and included in) the principal diagnosis code.

50. V30.00, 765.17, 765.26, 779.5 (Z38.00, P07.17, P07.32, P96.1)

Note:

- The principal diagnosis is single liveborn, born in the hospital spontaneous vaginal delivery.
- Assign a diagnosis code for "premature infant."
- Assign an additional code for the weeks of gestation."
- Assign an other (additional) diagnosis code for withdrawal symptoms due to the mother's drug addiction.

51. V30.01,774.6 (Z38.01, P59.9)

Note:

- The principal diagnosis is single liveborn, born in hospital via cesarean section.
- Assign a code to hyperbilirubinemia as an other (additional) diagnosis.
- The phototherapy treatment of a newborn does not impact the DRG reimbursement amount; therefore, that code is not assigned.

52. 780.31, 381.01 (R56.00, H65.01)

Note:

- Assign febrile seizure as the principal diagnosis because it is the condition that occasioned the admission to the hospital.
- Do *not* assign a code to the fever because it is included in the febrile seizure code.
- Assign a code for the acute serous otitis media, right ear, as an other (additional) diagnosis.

53. 789.03 (R10.31)

Note:

The patient was admitted to the hospital due to her abdominal pain, and a definitive diagnosis was never made for the cause of the abdominal pain. Therefore, the principal diagnosis is right lower quadrant abdominal pain.

54. 943.21, 942.25, 945.26, 948.00, E924.0, E849.0 (T22.211A, T21.27xA, T24.211A, T31.0, X10.0xxA, Y92.00)

Note:

- The principal diagnosis code reflects the highest degree of burn when a patient is admitted with more than one burn. Because the patient's burns were all second-degree, sequence the second-degree burn of the forearm second-degree burn of the vulva, or second-degree burn of the thigh as the principal diagnosis.
- Then assign a code classify "burns according to extent of body surface involved." This code is assigned when it is necessary to provide data for evaluating burn mortality.
- Assign an external cause code to indicate that the burn was due to a hot liquid and another external cause code to indicate that the accident occurred at home.
- The nonexcisional debridement of burns does not impact the DRG reimbursement amount; therefore, that code is not assigned.
- Do *not* assign a code for the placement of dressings.

55. 823.32, 813.42, 873.64, E812.2, E849.8, 79.36, 25.51 (S82.255C, S82.455C, S52.531A, S01.512A, V21.4xxA, Y92.481, 0QSG04Z, 0QSJ04Z, 0CQ7XZZ)

Note:

- Codes for multiple fractures are sequenced according to severity, and the code for an open fracture is sequenced before a closed fracture. For this case, sequence the open fracture as the principal diagnosis.
- Assign an other (additional) diagnosis code for closed fracture of the distal radius.
- Assign an other (additional) diagnosis code for tongue laceration. (In ICD-9-CM, the laceration of the tongue is coded "without mention of complication" because there was no mention of delayed healing, delayed treatment, foreign body, or infection. ICD-10-CM does not classify such complications with laceration codes.)
- Assign an external cause code to indicate that the patient was the driver of a motorcycle that collided with a parked vehicle. Then, assign an external cause code to indicate that the place of occurrence was a parking lot.
- Assign open reduction, internal fixation of tibia/fibula as the principal procedure code(s). (In ICD-9-CM, a combination code is assigned. ICD-10-PCS, two codes are assigned.)
- Assign a code for the suture repair of the tongue laceration. In ICD-10-CM, assign an *external* approach value for the 5th character because the tongue is located in the oral cavity, which is an orifice visible and does not require an incision or use of instrumentation (e.g., endoscope).
- The casting does not impact the DRG reimbursement rate; therefore, that code is not assigned.

Chapter 6
ICD-9-CM and ICD-10-CM Outpatient and Physician Office Coding

EXERCISE 6.1 – OUTPATIENT CARE

1. outpatient (or ambulatory)
2. primary
3. primary care provider
4. ambulatory patients (or outpatients)
5. ambulatory surgery patients
6. emergency department patients (or emergency care patients)
7. observation patients
8. triage
9. clinic
10. referred

EXERCISE 6.2 – DIAGNOSTIC CODING AND REPORTING GUIDELINES FOR OUTPATIENT SERVICES – HOSPITAL-BASED AND PHYSICIAN OFFICE

1. skin lesion
2. shortness of breath
3. fractured humerus
4. gastroenteritis
5. urinary frequency
6. acute bronchitis
7. back pain
8. diabetes mellitus
9. outpatient chemotherapy
10. acute cholecystitis with cholelithiasis

EXERCISE 6.3 – ICD-9-CM CODING GUIDELINES FOR OUTPATIENT DIAGNOSTIC TESTS

1. intra-abdominal abscess
2. pulmonary nodule
3. wheezing
4. degenerative joint disease at L1 and L2
5. pneumonia due to *Streptococcus,* Group B

REVIEW

Multiple Choice

1. d
2. a
3. c
4. d
5. a
6. a
7. c
8. d
9. c
10. c
11. c
12. d
13. d
14. c
15. d
16. c
17. c
18. d
19. a
20. b

Coding Practice

Note:

- ICD-10-CM codes are included in parentheses next to ICD-9-CM codes.
- Coding rationales are included for each case to provide direction about assigning codes.
- ICD-9-CM and ICD-10-PCS codes are *not* assigned to procedures or services because HCPCS level II and CPT codes are assigned to outpatient procedures and services. (ICD-9-CM and ICD-10-PCS procedure codes are assigned to inpatient cases, as discussed in textbook Chapter 5.)
- ICD-10-CM codes are located in parentheses next to ICD-9-CM codes for each case.

Ambulatory Surgery Center (ASC)

21. 244.9 (E03.9)

Note:

Do not assign a code for asthma because that condition was not medically managed during this outpatient encounter. Providers medically manage conditions when they evaluate the condition, prescribe medications, order tests, and so on.

22. 211.1, V18.59 (D13.1, Z83.79)

Note:

Assign the benign neoplasm of stomach *code even though the diagnosis documents "multiple" gastric polyps.*

23. V25.2 (Z30.2)

24. 550.90 (K40.90)

Note:

Do not assign a procedure code for the right inguinal herniorrhaphy because CPT (not ICD-9-CM or ICD-10-PCS) codes are assigned to outpatient surgery cases.

25. V25.2, V61.5 (Z30.2, Z64.1)

Note:

This case scenario documents the patient complaint of multiparity, which is assigned as a secondary diagnosis code.

Chiropractic Office

26. 722.71, E927.0, E016.2, E849.9 (M50.00, Y93.h9, Y93.h3, Y92.9)
27. 847.0, E007.6, E917.0, E849.4 (S13.4xxA, Y93.67, W51.xxA, Y92.310)

Note:

Do not assign codes for the neck pain and stiffness because those are symptoms of the definitive diagnosis, acute cervical sprain.

28. 847.0, E011.0, E849.3 (S13.4xxA, M54.9, Y93.c1, Y92.69)

Note:

The numbness and tingling in her left arm is due to the cervical neck strain; therefore, do not assign codes for these symptoms.

29. 721.0 (M47.812)

Note:

Index main term Osteoarthritis *and subterm* Spine *contains a* see also *Spondylosis cross reference, which directs you to the appropriate code.*

30. 847.0, E819.9 (S13.9xxA, V89.2xxA)

Note:

Assign a code for the neck sprain *only. To assign additional codes, you would generate a physician query to ask the chiropractor to document additional conditions.*

Hospital Emergency Department

31. 784.0 (R51)

Note:

Assigning a code for the headache *only is appropriate even though physical examination indicated abnormalities of the eyes. The patient's current symptoms in light of his past history may have prompted the ED visit.*

32. 719.41, E927.0, E029.9, E849.9 (M25.511, Y93.h9, Y93.89, Y92.9)

Note:

The shoulder is a joint. Therefore, in the Index to Diseases, go to main term Pain, *subterm* joint, *and 2nd qualifier* shoulder *to assign the code.* Probable strain, deltoid muscle, and possibly the deeper muscles of the anterior shoulder area, *because is a qualified diagnosis, which is not coded for outpatient (e.g., ED) care.*

33. 490, 481 (J40, J18.1)

Note:

- Because the chest x-ray documents "slight increased density at right lower lobe," assign the code for "pneumonia, lobar." The radiologist who documents the x-ray report findings is a physician; so even though the attending physician did not document "lobar pneumonia" in the diagnosis statement, the x-ray report supports the code assignment for "lobar pneumonia."
- There is no documentation of the infectious organism; therefore, do not assign a code for the type of infection. (If performed, sputum culture results would document the infectious organism.)
- Do not assign a code to the "chest pain" symptom because a definitive diagnosis of "pneumonia" was documented.

34. 845.00 E007.3, E927.0, E849.4 (S93.402A, Y93.64, Y92.328)

35. 883.0, E920.3, E849.9 (S61.235xA, W26.0xxA, Y92.9)

Hospital Outpatient Department

36. V81.2, V17.49 (Z13.6, Z82.49)

Note:

- The patient's EKG was negative, which means she was not diagnosed as having cardiovascular disease. The nonspecific T-wave changes were explained as probably due to anxiety and positional changes during the procedure. Therefore, go to main term *Screening* and subterm *cardiovascular disease* (ICD-9-CM) or *cardiovascular disorder* (ICD-10-CM).
- Assign code V17.49 for *family history of cardiovascular disease.*
- Do not assign code V71.7 (ICD-9-CM) or Z03.89 (ICD-10-CM) because the patient did not present with cardiovascular symptoms. This patient underwent a screening EKG because of a family history of cardiovascular disease.

37. 710.0 (M32.9)

38. 414.01 (I25.10)

Note:

- There is no past history of coronary artery bypass graft surgery; therefore, assign the ASHD code that describes "native coronary artery" as the type of vessel.

39. 428.0, V65.3, V65.42 (I50.9, Z71.3)

Note:

In addition to a code for CHF, assign ICD-9-CM codes for dietary counseling and substance use and abuse counseling, which includes tobacco use. Before assigning ICD-10-CM codes for alcohol abuse counseling and tobacco abuse counseling, query the physician to determine if the codes are appropriate. In ICD-9-CM, the code descriptions include the word "use" in reference to alcohol and tobacco, respectively; however, in ICD-10-CM, the word "abuse" is included in the code description.

40. V56.0, 996.81,753.0, E878.0 (T86.12, Q60.0, Z76.82, Y83.0)

Note:

- In ICD-9-CM, assign codes for *hemodialysis* (reason for encounter) (V56.0), *failure of transplanted kidney* (996.81), *congenital absence of kidney* (753.0), and *external cause of surgical complication* (E878.0). In ICD-10-CM, assign codes for *failure of kidney transplant* (T86.12), *unilateral renal agenesis* (Q60.0), *awaiting organ transplant status* (Z76.82), and *external cause of surgical complication* (Y83.0).
- Also, query the physician to request documentation of *chronic kidney disease* and its severity (e.g., Stages I–V) and/or end-stage renal disease (ESRD), which are not documented in the case study.

Hospital Same-Day Surgery

41. 474.10 (J35.3)

Note:

Do not report ICD-9-CM code 474.9 (or ICD-10-CM code J35.9) because hypertrophied tonsils and adenoids *results in a more specific code.*

42. 600.00, 585.9, 599.0, 041.04 (N40.0, N18.9, N39.0, B95.2)

Note:

- Anemia, *ischemia*, and *pre-pyloric gastric ulcer* were not medically managed during this encounter; therefore, do not assign codes to these conditions.

43. 565.0, 455.6 (K60.2, I84.20)

Note:

- Although *obesity* is likely a contributing factor to the development of the anal fissure and hemorrhoids, there is no documentation that this condition was medically managed. Therefore, do not assign a code for obesity.

44. 241.9, 226 (N04.9, D34)

Note:

- There is no documentation as to type of *nodular colloid goiter*, which means the unspecified code is assigned.
- *Degenerating follicular adenoma, right lobe of thyroid* is a benign neoplasm of the thyroid gland.

45. 634.91 (O03.4)

Note:

An incomplete abortion *is a* miscarriage.

Physician Office

46. 871.4, E917.9, E849.6 (S05.32, W22.8xxA, Y92.214)

Note:

In ICD-9-CM, main term Laceration *and subterm* cornea *contains an instruction to* see Laceration, eyeball *to assign code 871.4. In ICD-10-CM, main term* Laceration *and subterm* eye(ball) *lists code S05.3-.*

47. 891.0, E917.9, E849.9 (S81.032xA, W22.8xxA, Y92.9)

Note:

Go to main term Wound *and subterm* knee *to assign the code. There is no documentation of a complication, such as a wound infection.*

48. 603.9 (N43.3)

49. 883.0, E920.1, E849.9 (S61.112A, W29.8xxA, Y92.9)

Note:

- In ICD-9-CM, main term *Laceration* contains the instruction to *see also Wound*, open, by site. Go to main term *Wound* and subterm *thumb* (the word *nail* is a nonessential modifier) to assign code 883.0.
- In ICD-10-CM, main term *Laceration*, subterm *thumb*, 2nd qualifier left, 3rd qualifier *with*, and 4th qualifier *damage* to *nail* lists code S61.112A.

50. 729.81, 729.5 E917.9, E849.0 (M79.89, M79.641, W22.8xxA, Y92.010)

Note:

- Main term *Swollen* contains the instruction to "*see also Swelling.*" Therefore, go to main term *Swelling* and subterm *hand* in to assign the code.
- Go to main term *Pain* and subterm *hand* to assign the code 729.5 for "hand . . . painful to touch."

Stand-Alone Radiology Center

51. 585.9, 996.74 (N18.9, T82.398A)

Note:

- An *occluded dialysis access graft* is a complication of the access graft, which needs surgical repair (to clear the occlusion). In ICD-9-CM, go to main term *Complication*, subterm *blood vessel graft,* and 2nd qualifier *occlusion* to assign code 996.74. In ICD-10-CM, go to main term *Complication*, subterm *graft*, 2nd qualifier *vascular*, and 3rd qualifier *specified complication NEC* to assign code T82.898A.
- An occluded graft is *not* a mechanical complication of the blood vessel graft, which would be assigned a different code to describe the mechanical complication (e.g., torn graft or twisting of graft).

52. 575.8 (K82.8)

Note:

Do not assign a code to moderate hypertrophic change of lumbar spine *because the purpose of the outpatient encounter was for a cholecystogram, which resulted in a related diagnosis.*

53. 577.1 (K86.1)

Note:

Do not *assign a code to* stomach pain *because that is a symptom of recurrent pancreatitis.*

54. 788.30 (R32)

Note:

The first-listed diagnosis is urinary incontinence, *and there are no secondary diagnoses.*

55. 719.06, 836.0 (M25.461, S83.241A)

Note:

- Go to main term *Effusion*, subterm *joint,* and 2nd qualifier *knee to* assign the first-listed code.
- In ICD-9-CM, go to main term *Tear,* subterm *meniscus,* 2nd qualifier *medial,* and 3rd qualifier *posterior horn* in the Index to Diseases to assign the secondary code. In ICD-10-CM, go to main term *Tear*, subterm *meniscus*, 2nd qualifier *medial*, 3rd qualifer *specified* type *NEC* to assign the secondary code.

Stand-Alone Urgent Care Center

56. 913.0, 916.0, 881.01, 844.9, 845.00, E819.9, E849.9 (S50.811A, S50.812A, S80.811A, S80.812A, S51.012A, S93.401A, S83.91xA, W50.0xxA, Y92.9)

Note:

- In ICD-9-CM, main term *Abrasion* contains an instruction to "see also *Injury, superficial, by site.*" Therefore, go to main term *Injury,* subterm *superficial,* and 2nd qualifier *arm* to assign code 913.0 (after selecting the fourth digit 0 from the Tabular List of Diseases).
- Return to main term *Injury,* and subterm *superficial;* locate 2nd qualifier leg to assign code 916.0 (after selecting the fourth digit 0 from the Tabular List of Diseases).
- In ICD-9-CM, main term *Laceration* contains an instruction to "see also *Wound, open, by site.*" Therefore, go to main term *Wound* and subterm *elbow to* assign the code (881.01).
- In ICD-10-CM, the *see also* cross reference instruction for main terms *Abrasion* and *Laceration* were removed, which makes it easier to locate the appropriate codes.
- In ICD-9-CM, the condition "sprain, right knee, lower leg" is assigned combination code 844.9 (for knee and leg). A separate code (845.00) is assigned for "sprain, ankle." In ICD-10-CM, there is no *lower leg* 2nd qualifier for main term *Sprain* and subterm *knee.* However, separate codes are assigned for the ankle sprain and the knee sprain.

57. 682.4, 796.2, E917.9, E849.9, V12.3 (L03.113, W50.0xxA, Y92.9, Z86.2)

Note:

Code 796.2 is assigned to "elevated blood pressure reading" because the provider discussed the sign with the patient and made plans for follow-up treatment.

58. 720.2 (M46.1)

Note:

Go to main term Inflammation, *subterm* joint, *and 2nd qualifier* sacroiliac to *assign the code.*

59. 706.2 (L72.1)

Note:

Go to main term Cyst *and subterm* sebaceous *to assign the code. There is no 2nd qualifier for "infected" or "right cheek."*

60. 784.7 E917.9, E849.9 (R04.0, W50.0, Y92.9)

Chapter 7
HCPCS Level II National Coding System

EXERCISE 7.1 – OVERVIEW OF HCPCS

1. national
2. durable medical equipment, prosthetics, orthotics, supplies (DMEPOS)
3. level I
4. five
5. A–V

EXERCISE 7.2 – HCPCS LEVEL II CODES

1. HCPCS National Panel
2. Medicare Carriers Manual (MCM)
3. Medicare National Coverage Determinations Manual
4. HCPCS National Panel
5. American Dental Association (ADA)
6. DMEPOS dealer
7. annual
8. -AE
9. -50
10. modifiers

EXERCISE 7.3 – ASSIGNING HCPCS LEVEL II CODES

1. injection, medication
2. twice
3. once
4. supplies
5. Medicare
6. medications
7. table of contents
8. alphabetical first character
9. commercial payers
10. CPT

EXERCISE 7.4 - DETERMINING PAYER RESPONSIBILITY

1. c
2. b
3. a
4. b
5. c
6. b
7. b
8. a
9. c
10. c

REVIEW

Multiple Choice

1. c
2. d
3. b
4. a
5. a
6. d
7. c
8. d
9. a
10. d
11. d
12. c
13. a
14. c
15. c
16. c
17. a
18. b
19. d
20. c

Coding Practice I

Transportation Services Including Ambulance (A0000–A0999)

> **Note:**
>
> *The main term* Ambulance *requires review of codes A0021–A0999 to locate the appropriate five-character HCPCS level II code and two-character modifier.*

21. A0433-PH
22. A0225-HH
23. A0429-RH
24. A0422-NH
25. A0130-EP

Medical and Surgical Supplies (A4000–A8999)

26. A4208-AG
27. A4246-TD
28. A4261

> **Note:**
>
> *According to Encoder Pro Expert, code A4261 is exempt from adding a modifier to identify the type of practitioner who performed the procedure.*

29. A4282-NU
30. A6410

Administrative, Miscellaneous and Investigational (A9000–A9999)

31. A9526
32. A9300-RR

33. A9528 × 2
34. A9700
35. A9152

Enteral and Parenteral Therapy (B4000–B9999)

36. B4224, B4224
37. B4155
38. B9002-NU
39. B4036-NU
40. B4224 × 2

Outpatient PPS (C1300–C9899)

41. C1717-AF
42. C1764-SC
43. C1789
44. C8905-LT
45. C1752-RT

Dental Procedures (D0000–D9999)

46. D3410
47. D1120
48. D5912
49. D2722
50. D7510

Durable Medical Equipment (E0100–E9999)

51. E0910
52. E0455
53. E0202
54. E0570
55. E0135-NU

Procedures/Professional Services (Temporary) (G0000–G9999)

56. G0307
57. G0127
58. G9016, G9016 × 2
59. G0104
60. G0252

Alcohol and/or Drug Abuse Treatment Services (H0001–H2037)

61. H0004-HJ × 2
62. H0035
63. H2013
64. H0045 × 3
65. H2032-GP × 2

Drugs Administered Other Than Oral Method (J0000–J9999)

66. J0706
67. J1460 × 10
68. J2501
69. J3265
70. J9000

Temporary Codes (K0000–K9999)

71. K0072-RB × 2
72. K0105
73. K0038 × 2
74. K0012-RR
75. K0603

Orthotic Procedures (L0000–L4999)

76. L0160
77. L0220
78. L0830
79. L3310 × 2
80. L1960-AV

Prosthetic Procedures (L5000–L9999)

81. L5150
82. L7007
83. L5000
84. L6708, L6895
85. L8030

Medical Services (M0000–M0301)

86. M0064
87. M0075
88. M0300
89. M0301
90. M0076

Pathology and Laboratory Services (P0000–P9999)

91. P9612
92. P3000
93. P9045
94. P9019 × 2
95. P9010 × 2

Q Codes: Temporary Codes (Q0035–Q9968)

96. Q0083
97. Q3031
98. Q2017

99. Q4023
100. Q0112

Diagnostic Radiology Services (R0000–R5999)

> **Note:**
> *HCPCS level II diagnostic radiology services codes are reported in addition to CPT radiology codes.*

101. R0075-US
102. R0076-UR
103. R0075-UN

Temporary National Codes (Non-Medicare) (S0000–S9999)

104. S2142
105. S2202
106. S3708
107. S0400
108. S2055

National T Codes Established for State Medicaid Agencies (T1000–T9999)

109. T1027
110. T2101
111. T1502-TE
112. T1000-TD × 2
113. T2035

Vision Services (V0000–V2999)

114. V2208 × 2
115. V2025
116. V2744 × 2
117. V2785
118. V2626

Hearing Services (V5000–V5999)

119. V5010
120. V5140
121. V5245
122. V5240
123. V5268

Coding Practice II

124. J0456 Zithromax (azythromycin) 500-mg injection
R0070 Chest x-ray by mobile service; one patient seen

> **Note:**
> *Code R0070 is reported by the mobile x-ray service.*

125. J1670 Injection, tetanus immune globulin, human, up to 250 mg
E0112 Wooden crutches

Note:

Do not assign HCPCS level II code to the pHisoHex solution, sterile gauze, or paper tape. Those supplies are included in the provision of the evaluation and management service, which would be assigned a separate CPT code for this case.

Do not assign HCPCS code J2001 for Xylocaine. Although lidocaine HCL is the generic name for Xylocaine, code J2001 is assigned only when lidocaine HCL is injected for intravenous infusion.

Chapter 8
Introduction to CPT Coding

EXERCISE 8.1 – HISTORY OF CPT

1. b
2. e
3. a
4. d
5. c

EXERCISE 8.2 – OVERVIEW OF CPT

1. clinical providers
2. third-party payer
3. medical necessity
4. II
5. III

EXERCISE 8.3 – ORGANIZATION OF CPT

1. six
2. these codes are reported by all specialties
3. Anesthesia
4. vesiculotomy; complicated
5. Code 47560 is assigned for a surgical laparoscopy with guided transhepatic cholangiography, without biopsy. Code 47562 is assigned for a laparoscopic cholecystectomy.

EXERCISE 8.4 – CPT INDEX

1. T
2. F
3. F
4. T
5. F

EXERCISE 8.5 – CPT APPENDICES

1. d
2. a
3. f
4. l
5. g
6. b
7. b
8. h
9. j
10. c
11. k
12. e
13. i
14. n
15. m

EXERCISE 8.6 – CPT SYMBOLS

1. a
2. d
3. e
4. f
5. c
6. b
7. i
8. g
9. h
10. f

EXERCISE 8.7 – CPT SECTIONS, SUBSECTIONS, CATEGORIES, AND SUBCATEGORIES

1. F
2. F
3. T
4. T
5. F

EXERCISE 8.8 – CPT MODIFIERS

1. -80
2. -79
3. -25
4. -57
5. -56
6. -55
7. -76
8. -51
9. -50
10. -32

EXERCISE 8.9 – NATIONAL CORRECT CODING INITIATIVE

1. Medicare Part B claims
2. Outpatient Code Editor (OCE)
3. comprehensive/component; mutually exclusive
4. Advanced Beneficiary Notice (ABN); Notice of Exclusions from Medicare Benefits (NEMB)
5. unbundling

REVIEW

Multiple Choice

1. d
2. c
3. a
4. b
5. c
6. b
7. c
8. d
9. d
10. b
11. b
12. c
13. d
14. d
15. b
16. b
17. a
18. a
19. d
20. b

Note:

Modifier -26 is added to the code because "interpretation only" was performed. Without modifier -26, reimbursement from the payer would be higher than allowed.

Coding Practice

CPT Index

21. Main term Debridement
    Subterm Skin
    2nd qualifier Subcutaneous tissue
    3rd qualifier Infected
    Code range 11004–11006

22. Main term — Arthrodesis
    Subterm — Elbow
    Code range — 24800–24802
    - or -
    Main term — Elbow
    Subterm — Arthrodesis
    Code range — 24800–24802

Note:

When the CPT index contains more than one main term for a procedure, look up either the name of the procedure (e.g., arthrodesis) or the organ or anatomic part (e.g., elbow).

23. Main term — Kocher pylorectomy
    Cross-reference — *See* Gastrectomy; partial

    Main term — Gastrectomy
    Subterm — Partial
    Code range — 43631–43635, 43845
24. Main term — Hysterectomy
    Subterm — Abdominal
    2nd qualifier — Resection of Ovarian Malignancy
    Code range — 58951,58953–58956
25. Main term — PET
    Cross-reference — *See* Positron Emission Tomography
    Main term — Positron Emission Tomography (PET)
    Subterm — Brain
    Code range — 78608–78609

CPT Appendices

26. 1007F— Assessment for use of anti-inflammatory or analgesic OTC (over-the-counter) medications.
27. Category — Dysmorphology
    Modifier — 9N
28. three

Note:

The patient underwent two nerve conduction studies, and the maximum number allowed is three. This means that the patient can return for an additional nerve conduction study.

29. The gastroduodenal and proper hepatic arteries are third-order branches that branch from the celiac trunk, a first-order artery.
30. Code 43228 is included in the list of CPT codes that includes moderate (conscious) sedation, which means that a code from range 99143–99145 is *not* reported.

CPT Symbols

31. The flash (⁄⁄) symbol precedes code 90736, which means it is pending FDA approval.
32. The plus (✚) symbol precedes code 59525, which means it is an add-on code and modifier -51 is not added to the code.
33. The bull's-eye (◉) symbol precedes code 45380, which means that conscious sedation is included. Conscious sedation is not coded and reported separately.

34. The forbidden (⃠) symbol precedes code 31500, which means that modifier -51 is not added to the code.
35. The semicolon (;) symbol is included in the description of code 21480 to save space in CPT. The description of code 21480 is "closed treatment of temporomandibular dislocation; initial or subsequent." The description of code 21485 is "closed treatment of temporomandibular dislocation; complicated (e.g., recurrent requiring intermaxillary fixation or splinting), initial or subsequent. Thus, code 21480 must be referred back to as the common portion of the code description.

CPT Modifiers

36. Modifier -51 is added to code 12002 to indicate that multiple procedures were performed during the same operative session on the same day of service.
37. Modifier -50 is added to 30905 to indicate that a bilateral procedure was performed during the same operative session on the same day of service.
38. Modifier -26 (Professional Component) is added to the CPT code for the MRI.
39. Modifier -76 (Repeat Procedure by Same Physician) is added to code 56420.
40. Modifier -77 should be assigned to report a repeat procedure by another physician.

Chapter 9
CPT Evaluation and Management

EXERCISE 9.1 – OVERVIEW OF EVALUATION AND MANAGEMENT SECTION

1. Preventive Medicine Services
2. Emergency Department Services
3. history and examination
4. 5
5. place of service (POS)
6. type of service (TOS)
7. office visit
8. physician's office
9. Office or Other Outpatient Services
10. Established Patient

EXERCISE 9.2 – EVALUATION AND MANAGEMENT SECTION GUIDELINES

1. established patient
2. new
3. established
4. fractured pelvis
5. numbness, left foot

EXERCISE 9.3 – LEVELS OF EVALUATION AND MANAGEMENT SERVICES

1. a. 99204
   b. 99211
   c. 99222
   d. 99345
   e. 99283
2. a. yes
   b. 99284-25

Note:

Modifier -25 was added to facilitate reimbursement of both the E/M service and procedure performed (reduction of fracture). Students will learn to code procedures starting with Chapter 11 of 3-2-1 Code It!

3. a. no
   b. no code
4. extent of history, extent of examination, and complexity of medical decision making
5. three
6. two out of three
7. counseling, coordination of care, nature of presenting problem, and time
8. a. Office or Other Outpatient Services, Established Patient
   b. 99213
9. To assign the E/M code, the following is determined:
   a. established (The patient was seen in the office for "routine three-month follow-up.")
   b. expanded problem focused

Note:

Chief complaint is "follow-up for evaluation and management type 2 diabetes mellitus and hypertension." According to the 1997 E/M documentation guidelines, two elements of the history of present illness (HPI) were documented: quality (stable) and severity (home monitoring), which means that a brief HPI was performed. Documentation of the review of system (ROS) included five body areas/systems (chest pain—cardiovascular; headache—neurologic; extremities—musculoskeletal; shortness of breath—respiratory; and visual changes—eyes), making this an extended ROS. Since there is no documentation of past, family, or social history, the highest extent of history that can be selected is expanded problem focused.

   c. detailed

Note:

According to the 1997 E/M documentation guidelines, general multisystem exam elements are counted as follows: constitutional (1) (blood pressure, weight, and pulse count as one element); eyes (1) (pupils equal, round, and reactive to light and accommodation); ears, nose, and throat (2) (external auditory canals/tympanic membranes negative; oropharynx benign); neck (2) (supple; no bruits, jugular venous distention, or thyromegaly) (maximum of two elements can be identified for neck); respiratory (2) (breath sounds clear to auscultation and percussion; auscultation, or listening to the lungs, revealed no rubs, rales, rhonchi, or wheezing) (maximum of four elements can be identified for respiratory); cardiovascular (3) (no click, gallop, irregularity, murmur, or rub; distal pulses intact; no edema); musculoskeletal (1) (no cyanosis, clubbing); and neurological (2) (deep tendon reflexes within normal limits and symmetrical; no decreased lower extremity sensation noted). A total of 14 elements in this general multisystem exam were documented, which means that a detailed examination was performed.

   d. moderate complexity

Note:

The number of diagnoses and management options documented is multiple because two diagnoses and management options must be considered. The amount and complexity of data to be reviewed are minimal because just lab tests are considered. The risk of complications and/or morbidity or mortality is moderate because of the documented prescription drug therapy for two stable chronic illnesses. Since the complexity of medical decision making is determined by the two highest of the three options, the level for this encounter is moderate complexity.

e. The E/M code is 99214.

Note:

An expanded problem-focused history, a detailed examination, and moderate complexity of medical decision making were documented. Because two of three key components determine the E/M level for an established patient visit, assign 99213. Code selection is based on extent of examination and complexity of medical decision making. (No contributory components, such as counseling or coordination of care, were documented.)

10. 99344

EXERCISE 9.4 – EVALUATION AND MANAGEMENT CATEGORIES AND SUBCATEGORIES

1. F
2. F
3. T
4. F
5. T
6. F
7. F
8. T
9. T
10. F
11. T
12. T
13. F
14. T
15. F
16. T
17. F
18. T
19. F
20. T
21. F
22. T
23. F
24. T
25. T
26. T
27. F
28. F
29. F
30. T

REVIEW

Multiple Choice

1. a
2. b
3. a
4. c
5. c
6. b
7. a
8. c
9. b
10. c
11. c
12. d
13. d
14. c
15. c
16. a

Note:

The nursing facility patient is "recovering," which means that code 99307 is reported.

17. a
18. b
19. a
20. b

Coding Practice

Office or Other Outpatient Services

21. 99213

Note:

An established patient requires two out of three key components be met or exceeded for a particular level of E/M service to be assigned. In this case, a problem-focused history was performed. (It is part of code 99212.) The examination and medical decision making are level 3 (code 99213). Since just two key components need to be met, the level 3 E/M code is assigned.

22. 99202

Note:

For a new patient, three out of three key components must be met or exceeded to assign an E/M code. Code 99202 requires an expanded problem-focused history and examination and straightforward medical decision making.

Hospital Observation Services

23. 99219

Note:

For initial hospital observation care, three out of three key components must be met or exceeded for a level to be assigned. In this case, documentation warrants assignment of a level 2 initial observation code.

24. 99218 (5/7), 99217 (5/8)

Note:

Two codes are assigned to this case: one for initial observation care and one for observation care discharge. For the initial observation care, three out of three key components must be met or exceeded to assign a level. For the discharge care, the physician must document a final exam, patient instructions, and discussion of the hospital stay.

Hospital Inpatient Services

25. 99222 (10/10), 99232 (10/11), 99232 (10/12), 99238 (10/13)

Note:

Four codes are required for this case. 99222 is the E/M code for initial hospital care level 2, 99232 reflects subsequent hospital care level 2, and 99238 reflects discharge day management 30 minutes or less.

26. 99233

Note:

For an established patient, two out of three key components are required. For this case, the coder can use the detailed physical examination and the MDM of a high level. The detailed history does not have to be used to assign a subsequent hospital care E/M code.

Consultations

27. 99242

Note:

For office consultations with new patients, three out of three key components must be met or exceeded for a level to be assigned. For 99242, an expanded problem-focused history, expanded problem-focused exam, and medical decision making of a straightforward nature are the requirements.

28. 99255

Note:

Initial inpatient consultation codes require three out of three key components be met in order to assign a specific level. A comprehensive history, comprehensive exam, and MDM of high level would code to 99255.

Emergency Department Services

29. 99285

Note:

The presenting problem in this patient warrants a high E/M level. The diagnoses of shortness of breath and chest pain are critical medical issues. Since no time was documented by the physician, critical care service code 99291 or 99292 could not be used.

30. 99288

Critical Care Services

31. 99291

Note:

ED is the abbreviation for emergency department, and MDM is the abbreviation for medical decision making. The presenting problem of this patient and the fact that critical services were provided for 70 minutes requires the coding of 99291. The patient is unable to provide history due to his medical condition; however, time is the component used to assign a critical care code and the fact that the patient's medical problem is of a critical nature. The lack of history documentation does not prevent the use of code 99291 in this case.

32. 99291, 99292, 99292, 99292, 99292

Note:

Three hours of critical care support equals 180 minutes, which is coded to 99291 and 99292 × 4. The criteria for critical care code assignment are the documentation of time by the physician and the patient's medical illness/condition being of a critical nature.

Nursing Facility Services

33. 99304

Note:

For initial nursing facility care, all three key components must be met for a specific level to be assigned. Based on the history, exam, and MDM levels in this case, 99304 is the only E/M code that can be assigned. The physician exceeds the MDM requirement for this level but does not meet the comprehensive examination requirement to be able to assign the next highest level, 99305.

34. 99308

Note:

For the subcategory of subsequent nursing facility care, two out of three key components must be met to assign a specific level. The exam noted in this case meets the requirement of 99308. The MDM meets the requirement of 99309. However, the case does not document that either the history or exam requirement for 99309 are met. Therefore, E/M code 99308 is assigned.

Domiciliary, Rest Home, or Custodial Care Services

35. 99324

Note:

The code range for domiciliary, rest home, or custodial care services is 99324 to 99328 for new patients. As with other new patient codes, three out of three key components must be met for a specific level to be assigned.

36. 99335

Note:

Only two out of three key components must be met for this established patient. A problem-focused history is part of level 1, an expanded problem-focused exam is part of level 2, and an MDM of moderate complexity is part of level 3. The only level where two key components were met or exceeded was level 2. The physician met the exam requirement and exceeded the MDM requirement.

Home Services

37. 99347

> **Note:**
>
> *For the subcategory of established patient, home services, two out of three key components must be met or exceeded to assign a specific level. An MDM of a moderate level is under E/M code 99349; however, based on the level of exam and history provided, the code assigned to this case is 99347. For that code, the physician met the examination required and exceeded the MDM required. The physician also documented a problem-focused history, which is the minimal requirement for 99347. The history level and the exam level can be used to assign this code; but if the coder uses the exam and the MDM level, the E/M code is still 99347. 99348 or 99349 cannot be assigned because the documentation does not met or exceed two out of three key components. Only one (MDM) is met for either of these levels.*

38. 99343

> **Note:**
>
> *For a new patient in the category of home services, all three key components must be met or exceeded for a specific level to be assigned. For 99343, the requirements are a detailed history, a detailed examination, and MDM of moderate complexity.*

Prolonged Physician Service

39. 99214, 99354, 99355

> **Note:**
>
> *First, you have to determine the established patient office visit level based on the documentation. Then given the information of two hours of service, prolonged physician service codes are added. Based on information in CPT, 99214 has a typical time of 25 minutes. (120 minutes minus 25 minutes equals 95 minutes.) 99354 covers 74 of the 95 minutes, which leaves 21 minutes unaccounted for. 99355 is assigned for the remaining 21 minutes. Both 99354 and 99355 are add-on codes; therefore, no modifier is needed.*

Physician Standby Services

40. 99360

> **Note:**
>
> *99360 is assigned for standby (non-face-to-face) service. This code is assigned based on full units of 30 minutes.*

Case Management Services

41. 99367

> **Note:**
>
> *Code 99367 is assigned for a medical team conference of 30 minutes' duration or more with participation by the physician. Team conferences are typically face-to-face meetings of health professionals from the same discipline or from various medical specialties.*

42. 99213

Note:

The patient received E/M services on the same day as the telephone service, which means the telephone is considered part of the E/M service provided. Report E/M code 99213 only.

Care Plan Oversight Services

43. 99375

44. 99378

Preventive Medicine

45. 99384

Note:

A preventive medicine service E/M code should be assigned in this case. These codes are assigned by age of the patient.

46. 99397

Note:

BPH is the abbreviation for benign prostate hypertrophy, HTN is the abbreviation for hypertension, and NIDDM is the abbreviation for non-insulin dependent diabetes mellitus. The fact that the patient is counseled on treatment options for his BPH does not preclude the assignment of a preventive medicine code. The patient came in for a check-up, which would warrant a code from this category.

Non-Face-to-Face Physician Services

47. 99441
48. 99444

Special Evaluation and Management Services

49. 99455

Note:

Work-related or medical disability evaluation services is the subcategory of E/M codes that should be used in this case. The requirements for the assignment of an E/M from this category are the completion of a history, exam, the forming of a diagnosis, the development of a treatment plan, and the completion of a report. No special level of key components is required.

Newborn Care

50. 99460 (7/8), 99462 (7/9)

Chapter 10
CPT Anesthesia

EXERCISE 10.1 – ANESTHESIA TERMINOLOGY

1. b
2. e
3. c
4. d
5. a
6. d
7. c
8. a
9. e
10. b

EXERCISE 10.2 – OVERVIEW OF ANESTHESIA SECTION

1. Students should include five from the following list of services:
   - Draping, positioning, prepping, and transporting the patient
   - Inserting nasogastric or orogastric tubes
   - Inserting peripheral intravenous lines for fluid and medication administration
   - Interpreting laboratory results
   - Interpreting monitored functions
   - Placing airway tubes, including laryngoscopy for airway management
   - Positioning external devices for capnography, cardiac monitoring, CNS evoked responses, Doppler flow, pulse oximetry, and temperature
   - Stimulating nerves to determine level of paralysis or localization of nerve(s)
2. -59
3. False
4. Students should include three from the following list of services:
   - Monitors vital signs and maintains patient's airway and continual evaluation of vital functions
   - Diagnoses and treats clinical problems that occur during the procedure
   - Administers analgesics, anesthetic agents, hypnotics, sedatives, or other medications as necessary to ensure patient safety and comfort
   - Provides other medical services as needed for the safe completion of the procedure
5. -QS (monitored anesthesia care)

EXERCISE 10.3 – ANESTHESIA SECTION GUIDELINES

1. c
2. e
3. a
4. d
5. b
6. a
7. b
8. a
9. a
10. b
11. T
12. T
13. T
14. F
15. F
16. T
17. T
18. T
19. T
20. F

Note:

The anesthesia time unit is 4 because 60 ÷ 15 = 4. The anesthesia code's base unit value is 5, and the physical status modifier's relative value is 0; thus, (5 + 4 + 0) × $17.45 = 9 × $17.45 = $157.05.

21. b
22. c
23. a
24. d
25. e

EXERCISE 10.4 – ANESTHESIA SUBSECTIONS

1. add-on
2. -59
3. False

Note:

The code description for 00326 includes the phrase, ". . . in children younger than 1 year of age." Therefore, code 99100 is not reported in addition to code 00326.

4. 00406
5. -QS
6. 01935–01936
7. 00796
8. 01990
9. 01922–23
10. 01953

REVIEW

Multiple Choice

1. d
2. a
3. d
4. a
5. b
6. b
7. a
8. d
9. d
10. a
11. a
12. a
13. b
14. b
15. c
16. b
17. b
18. b
19. c
20. b

Coding Practice I—Modifiers

21. 01961-P1-AA, 99140, 62318-59

Note:

Modifier -P1 is assigned for a healthy patient. Modifier -AA is a HCPCS modifier that is assigned to reflect anesthesia performed by an anesthesiologist. Modifier -59 is assigned to indicate that a distinct procedural service was provided in addition to anesthesia services.

22. 01832-P2-QX, 62318-59

Note:

CRNA is the abbreviation for certified registered nurse anesthetist. The physical status anesthesia modifier -P2 is assigned due to the patient being a diabetic. Modifier -QX is assigned to reflect CRNA service under medical direction of a physician. Modifier -59 is assigned to indicate that a distinct procedural service was provided in addition to anesthesia services.

Do not report code 01996-P2-QX for monitoring on the day after surgery. That code applies to "daily hospital management of epidural or subarachnoid continuous drug administration performed after insertion of an epidural or subarachnoid catheter placed primarily for anesthesia administration during an operative session, but retained for postoperative pain management."

23. 01402-P1-AA

Note:

P1 is the anesthesia modifier assigned to a healthy patient, and -AA is the HCPCS modifier assigned when services are provided by an anesthesiologist.

24. 01400-P1-AA, 64447-59

Note:

Modifier -59 is assigned to indicate that a distinct procedural service was provided in addition to anesthesia services.

25. 00540-P2-QZ, 62318-59

Note:

The physical status anesthesia modifier of P2 is assigned due to this patient's chronic asthma condition. The HCPCS modifier QZ is assigned for CRNA services not under the direction of a physician. Modifier -59 is assigned to indicate that a distinct procedural service was provided in addition to anesthesia services.

Coding Practice II—Anesthesia

Head

26. 00142-P2-AA, 99100

Note:

The physical status anesthesia modifier of P2 is assigned due to the fact that this patient has controlled diabetes mellitus. Qualifying circumstances code 99100 is reported because the patient is over age 70.

27. 00120-P1-AA

Neck

28. 00326-P4-AA, 99140

> **Note:**
>
> *The physical status anesthesia modifier of P4 is assigned to reflect the severity of the patient's cardiopulmonary state. Code 99140 is reported to indicate emergency conditions of treatment. Qualifying circumstance code 99100 is not assigned, per the note located below code 00326 in the CPT coding manual.*

29. 00320-P2-AA

> **Note:**
>
> *The physical status anesthesia modifier of P2 is assigned in this case due to the nature of the patient's condition, thyroid tumor.*

Thorax (Chest Wall and Shoulder Girdle)

30. 00400-P1-AA
31. 00474-P2-AA

> **Note:**
>
> *The patient's chest pain, shortness of breath, and possible lordosis are symptoms of pectus excavatum. While most patients with pectus excavatum are asymptomatic, this patient exhibited symptoms that interfered with physiologic functioning. Therefore, the physical status modifier is -P2. (If the patient had remained untreated and his symptoms had worsened, resulting in heart and/or respiratory disease, physical status modifier -P3 would have been assigned.)*

Intrathoracic

32. 00524-P3-AA, 99100

> **Note:**
>
> *The qualifying circumstance code of 99100 is assigned due to the patient's age being over 70. The physical status anesthesia modifier -P3 is assigned for the systemic disease of pneumonia and the severity that caused the patient to have drainage of fluid (pneumocentesis).*

33. 00530-P2-AA

Spine and Spinal Cord

34. 00600-P2-AA
35. 00635-P2-AA

Upper Abdomen

36. 00756-P2-AA
37. 00702-P1-AA

Lower Abdomen

38. 00802-P1-AA

Note:

This patient has no medical history or chronic conditions; therefore, the physical status anesthesia modifier -P1 is assigned.

39. 00851-P1-AA

Perineum

40. 00952-P2-AA
41. 00921-P1-AA

Pelvis

42. 01112-P1-AA
43. 01170-P1-AA

Upper Leg

44. 01230-P2-AA

Note:

Type 2 diabetes mellitus is a systemic disease that is under control in this patient. Therefore, the physical status modifier -P2 is assigned.

45. 01214-P3-AA, 99100

Note:

The physical status modifier -P3 is assigned due to the admitted condition of the patient.

Knee and Popliteal Area

46. 01392-P1-AA
47. 01400-P1-AA

Lower Leg

48. 01462-P2-AA

Note:

The physical status modifier -P2 is assigned in this case due to the patient's preexisting condition of Down syndrome.

49. 01462-P1-AA

Note:

The fact that this patient is a smoker does not warrant a higher-level physical status modifier. There is no documentation of any disease process or condition; therefore, modifier -P1 is assigned.

Shoulder and Axilla

50. 01620-P1-AA
51. 01636-P1-AA

Upper Arm and Elbow

52. 01710-P1-AA
53. 01716-P1-AA

Forearm, Wrist, and Hand

54. 01810-P1-AA
55. 01830-P1-AA

Radiologic Procedures

56. 01920-P2-AA
57. 01922-P3-AA

Burn Excisions or Debridement

58. 01952-P3-AA, 01953, 01953, 01953

Note:

01952 covers 9 percent of this patient's 35 percent total body burn. Thirty-five percent minus 9 percent equals 26 percent (35 − 9 = 26). 01953 is added × 3 to reflect the remaining 26 percent. 01953 is an add-on code; therefore, no -51 modifier is required. In CPT, the 9% described in code 01953 is interpreted as "up to 9%," which is why code 01953 is reported × 3.

59. 01952-P2-AA

Obstetric

60. 01960-P1-AA
61. 01961-P2-AA

Other Procedures

62. 01996-P1-AA
63. 01990-P6-AA
64. 96365

Note:

Do not report Modifiers -P1 or -AA with code 96365.

65. 00172-P2-AA, 99100

Note:

Modifier -P2 is added due to the diagnosis of cleft palate. Qualifying code of 99100 is assigned because the child is under the age of 1 year.

Chapter 11
CPT Surgery I

EXERCISE 11.1 – OVERVIEW OF SURGERY SECTION

1. body area or organ system
2. diagnostic
3. therapeutic
4. a. urinary system
   b. urinary bladder
   c. endoscopic
   d. biopsy
   e. cystourethroscopy with biopsy
   f. 52204

Note:

Combination code 52204 includes cystourethroscopy with biopsy. No incision is made to access the urinary bladder because the cystourethroscope is inserted through the urethra into the urinary bladder.

5. a. digestive system
   b. large intestine (colon)
   c. laparotomy (incision)
   d. excision
   e. partial colon resection (colectomy) with anastomosis
   f. 44140

Note:

Do not code the lysis of adhesions or exploratory laparotomy. The lysis of adhesions is incidental to the colon resection procedure, and the exploratory laparotomy is the surgical approach. To find the code, refer to the CPT index and locate main term Colon, *subterm* Excision, *and 2nd qualifier* Partial. *Review the range of codes to select 44140 (Colectomy, partial; with anastomosis). (Since there is no mention of laparoscopic approach in the case study, do not report code 44204.)*

EXERCISE 11.2 – SURGERY GUIDELINES

1. F
2. T
3. T
4. F
5. F
6. T
7. T

Note:

When a diagnostic procedure (e.g., diagnostic esophagogastroduodenoscopy) is performed and the provider performs follow-up evaluation and management (E/M) services, the E/M service(s) are separately coded and reported. (If the patient had undergone a therapeutic procedure, such as a partial gastrectomy to remove that part of the stomach that had ulcers, and the physician provided follow-up E/M services, a separate code would not be reported. Such follow-up E/M services are part of the global period and, therefore, included in the procedure code that was initially reported.)

8. F
9. T
10. T
11. July 30
12. March 15
13. October 14
14. -24
15. Although code 29870 contains "(separate procedure)" in its description, that procedure was performed separately and independently of the related and more comprehensive procedure performed the next day. In addition, the first procedure was diagnostic and the second procedure was performed to repair the knee.
16. -50
17. Typically a biopsy of the vulva or perineum is not performed during the same operative session as an inguinal hernia repair. The biopsy is unrelated to the repair of the inguinal hernia. Therefore, modifier -59 is added to code 56605 to indicate that the biopsy was unrelated to the repair of the inguinal hernia.
18. 29999 (Unlisted procedure, arthroscopy)
19. Ablation of benign, premalignant, or malignant tissues by any method, with or without curettement, including local anesthesia, and not usually requiring closure
20. Once because the description states "15 or more lesions." (Also, do *not* report modifier -51 with code 17004.)

EXERCISE 11.3 – GENERAL SUBSECTION

1. 10021
2. 10022
   76942

EXERCISE 11.4 – INCISION AND DRAINAGE

1. 10180
2. 10140
3. 10120
4. 10040
5. 10061

EXERCISE 11.5 – LESION REMOVAL

1. 11401

Note:

Do not report modifier -LT with CPT integumentary system codes because the skin is not a paired organ. The procedure in #1, above, was performed on the "skin" of the left forearm.

2. 11100, 11101
3. 11643, 11602–51, 11602–51
4. 11056
5. 11442

EXERCISE 11.6 – NAILS

1. 11719-TA, 11719-T1, 11719-T2, 11719-T3, 11719-T4, 11719-T5, 11719-T6, 11719-T7, 11719-T8, 11719-T9

Note:

- *Do not add modifier -50 to the code because the code description includes the phrase* any number.
- *Report code 11719 × 10, with the appropriate modifier attached to each (to indicate that all ten toes were treated).*

2. 11762-T1
3. 11730-T5, 11732-T6, 11732-T7, 11732-T8, 11732-T9
4. 11740-F1
5. 11765-T7

EXERCISE 11.7 – PILONIDAL CYST

1. 11772
2. 11770
3. 11771
4. 10080
5. 10081

EXERCISE 11.8 – INTRODUCTION

1. 11980
2. 11900
3. 11954
4. 11976
5. 11901

EXERCISE 11.9 – REPAIR (CLOSURE)

1. 12002
2. Report an appropriate E/M code because there is no CPT surgery code for a wound closure with adhesive strips.
3. 16020
4. 15200, 15002
5. 15780

EXERCISE 11.10 – DESTRUCTION

1. 17000, 17003 x 2

Note:

Report code 17003 twice because of the word each in the CPT code description.

2. 11200, 11201

Note:

Report code 11201 in addition to 11200 because a total of 17 skin tags were removed. Code 11200 is reported for the first 15 skin tags removed, and code 11201 is reported for up to the next 10 skin tags removed.

3. 17110
4. 17000, 17003
5. 11200
6. 17274
7. 17262
8. 17276
9. 17280
10. 17263-LT

EXERCISE 11.11 - BREAST

1. 19125-RT, 19126-RT
2. 19367-RT
3. 19301-LT
4. 19302-RT
5. 19102-LT, 19295-LT, 77032

REVIEW

Multiple Choice

1. d
2. b
3. a
4. d
5. c
6. b
7. b
8. c
9. c
10. a
11. c
12. c
13. c
14. b
15. b
16. d
17. b

Note:

Modifier -LT is not added to any codes in this question because the surgery was performed on skin, which is not considered a paired organ.

18. d
19. a
20. b

Coding Practice

General

21. 10021
22. 10022, 77012

Integumentary System

23. 11404
24. 11771

Note:

Code 11771 is reported for extensive excision of a pilonidal cyst, which is one that is over 2 cm in size, is recurrent, and/or requires subcutaneous or layer closure. For this case, a 5.0-cm pilonidal subcutaneous cyst was removed and layered closure was required.

25. 10060
26. 15100, 11606

Note:

Do not report modifier -LT for general skin procedures because the skin is not considered a paired organ.

27. 13132-F1

Note:

For this case, surgical debridement and depth of the repair indicates the complex closure of a traumatic laceration.

28. 16020
29. 11730-T5, 11732-TA

Note:

Code 11730 is assigned for removal (or avulsion) of one nail plate, and code 11732 is assigned for removal of the second nail plate of the left great toe. HCPCS level II modifiers are added to the codes to indicate the digits on which the procedures were performed. (-T5 is added to indicate surgery on the right foot, great toe. -TA is added to indicate surgery on the left foot, great toe.)

30. 12002

Note:

Per CPT notes, wound repairs of the same anatomical group and *same level of repair have lengths added together to determine the code assignment. In this case, the lengths of the neck and scalp wounds are totaled. (3.0 + 2.0 = 5.0 cm.) Both repairs are simple, and the correct code is 12002. (Do* not *assign codes 12002 and 12001.)*

31. 15740
32. 15840

Note:

Obtaining the fascial graft is included in code 15840. Do not *report a separate code for obtaining the graft.*

33. 17273

Note:

Surgical curettement is a type of destruction, and a code from range 17000–17286 is assigned.

34. 19301-LT
35. 19000-RT

Chapter 12
CPT Surgery II

EXERCISE 12.1 – MUSCULOSKELETAL SYSTEM NOTES

1. body area
2. open or closed fractures and joint injuries
3. treatment
4. normal, uncomplicated follow-up care
5. manipulation

EXERCISE 12.2 – GENERAL

1. 20000
2. 20005
3. 20101

Note:

Surgical exploration and enlargement of the wound, debridement removal of a foreign body, and ligation of subcutaneous tissue is included in 20101; do not *report separate codes.*

4. 20240

Note:

Even though this procedure was performed on the left femur, do not *add modifier -LT to code 20240. Its code description does not represent a procedure performed on paired organs because the sternum and spinous process is listed as an example. They are not paired organs.*

5. 20612-RT
6. 20692-RT
7. 20816-F6

Note:

Do not report modifier -RT. Modifier -F6 specifies the right second (index) finger. MCP is the abbreviation for metacarpophalangeal (joint).

8. 20920
9. 22950, 20931
10. 20975

EXERCISE 12.3 – HEAD

1. 21010-50
2. 21026

Note:

Report code 21026 just once because the code description includes the term bone(s).

3. 21084
4. 21121
5. 21150
6. 21198
7. 21270
8. 21401

Note:

There is no mention of the term blowout; *therefore, do not report a code from 21385–21395.*

9. 21440
10. 21465

EXERCISE 12.4 – NECK (SOFT TISSUES), THORAX, BACK, AND FLANK

1. 21510
2. 21685
3. 21820
4. 21600
5. 21627
6. 20206

Note:

The parenthetical note below code 21550 provides instruction to report code 20206 for a needle *biopsy of (any) soft tissue.*

7. 21930
8. 21935

Note:

A radical resection includes excision of the tumor; therefore, do not report code 21930 in addition to code 21935.

9. 21920
10. 21925

EXERCISE 12.5 – SPINE (VERTEBRAL COLUMN)

1. 22630

Note:

Just one interspace was fused; therefore, report code 22630. Also, code 22630 includes laminectomy and diskectomy when performed to prepare the vertebral interspace for fusion.

2. 22505

Note:

Report code 22505 just once even though three spinal regions were manipulated under anesthesia.

3. 22220
4. 22595, 22841
5. 22800, 20937

EXERCISE 12.6 – ABDOMEN, SHOULDER, HUMERUS (UPPER ARM) AND ELBOW, FOREARM AND WRIST, AND HAND AND FINGERS

1. 22900
2. 23000-LT
3. 23900-RT

Note:

An interthoracoscapular amputation (forequarter) *is the surgical amputation of the arm, including disarticulation (separation at the joint) of the humerus and removal of the scapula and outer part of the clavicle (collarbone).*

4. 23331-LT
5. 24075-RT
6. 24357-RT
7. 24300-LT
8. 25606-LT
9. 25246-RT
10. 26121-LT

EXERCISE 12.7 – PELVIS AND HIP JOINT, FEMUR (THIGH REGION) AND KNEE JOINT, LEG (TIBIA AND FIBULA) AND ANKLE JOINT, AND FOOT AND TOES

1. 27097
2. 27125-RT

Note:

If the patient returns in the future for replacement of the prosthetic device (e.g., broken device), report code 27236.

3. 27372-LT
4. 27323-LT
5. 27357-LT

Note:

Code 27357 includes obtaining (harvesting) graft, such as femur tissue, when performed during the same operative episode.

6. 27498-RT
7. 27650-RT
8. 27604-LT
9. 28296-RT
10. 28110-RT

EXERCISE 12.8 – APPLICATION OF CASTS AND STRAPPING AND ENDOSCOPY/ARTHROSCOPY

1. 29830-LT
2. 29065-LT

Note:

Do not report code 29705-LT because the same physician who applied the first cast removed the wet cast and applied the new cast.

3. 29086-F9

Note:

The proximal interphalangeal (PIP) joint is part of the finger. Therefore, add modifier -F9 (not -RT) to the code.

4. 29445-LT
5. 29125-LT
6. 29892-RT
7. 29901-RT
8. 29824-LT
9. 29807-RT
10. 29881-LT

EXERCISE 12.9 – NOSE

1. 30200

Note:

Do not add modifier -50 to code 30200 because its description indicates turbinate(s), indicating surgery performed on multiple and bilateral turbinates.

2. 30110-LT

Note:

Do not report a code for single-layer closure, which is a simple closure that is included with code 30110.

3. 30100-LT
4. 30118-LT

Note:

The CPT index entry for "Rhinotomy, lateral" lists code 30118 and 30320. No foreign body was removed; therefore, report code 30118 with the appropriate directional modifier.

5. 30462

EXERCISE 12.10 – ACCESSORY SINUSES

1. 31200
2. 31238
3. 31255-LT, 31256-51-LT
4. 31237
5. 31276-LT

Note:

Do not report a code for diagnostic endoscopy (31231) because it is included in the surgical endoscopy code.

EXERCISE 12.11 – LARYNX

1. 31500
2. 31365
3. 31587
4. 31502
5. 31365, 38720-59

Note:

- For a total laryngectomy with bilateral radical neck dissection (31365), do not add modifier -50 to the code. The larynx is a single midline organ, and it is not appropriate to add modifier -50 to code 31365. (A laryngectomy cannot be performed bilaterally.)
- Instead, report code 31365 for the total laryngectomy and radical neck dissection on one side. Then, report code 38720-59 for the radical neck dissection on the other side (even though the description of code 38720 is "Cervical lymphadenectomy (complete)."
- Add modifier -59 to indicate a distinct procedural service.

EXERCISE 12.12 – TRACHEA AND BRONCHI

1. 31603
2. 31717
3. 31635-LT
4. 31624
5. 31623, 31625, 31635

Note:

Codes 31623, 31625, and 31635 are distinct surgical procedures, and they are not considered integral components of one another. Therefore, report each code separately and do not add modifier -51 to any of the codes.

EXERCISE 12.13 – LUNGS AND PLEURA

1. 32551
2. 32997
3. 32405, 10021
4. 32663

Note:

Do not report code 32601 because diagnostic thoracoscopy is included in the code for surgical thoracoscopy.

5. 32851, 32850, 35216, 32855

REVIEW

Multiple Choice

1. b
2. a
3. b
4. c
5. d
6. d
7. a
8. c

Note:

C3-C4 contains just one interspace; therefore, report code 22554 just once (with modifier -62 added to indicate that two surgeons were required to perform the procedure).

9. d
10. c
11. c
12. c
13. b
14. a
15. d
16. c
17. c
18. a
19. b
20. d

Coding Practice

Musculoskeletal System

21. 20100

Note:

Codes 20100–20103 are reported for wound exploration resulting from penetrating trauma (e.g., penetrating gunshot or stab wound). These codes include surgical exploration, extension of dissection, debridement, removal of foreign bodies, and ligation/coagulation of minor subcutaneous/muscular blood vessels (not requiring thoracotomy or laparotomy). Do not report simple, intermediate, or complex repair (closure) codes from the Integumentary subsection with a wound exploration (trauma) code.

22. 21179

Note:

Do not report a separate code for the bone allograft.

23. 27506-RT

Note:

Do not report a separate code for placement of the cast. The cast application is included in the code for the open fracture treatment.

24. 27301-RT
25. 27570-LT
26. 29345-LT

Note:

For cast reapplication, assign a code from 29000–29799. Do not code the cast removal. Cast removal is coded only when performed by a different physician.

27. 29730-LT
28. 29830-LT
29. 26080-F6

Note:

The incision was made between the first and second bones of the right index finger, which is an interphalangeal joint. Code 26080 is assigned. (Do not mistakenly assign code 26075, which involves surgery on the metacarpophalangeal joint, which is located between the first bone of the finger and bones of the wrist.)

30. 25600-RT

Note:

Do not report a separate code for application of the cast. The cast application is included in the code for the open fracture treatment.

Respiratory System

31. 31231

Note:

Do not add modifier -50 to the code. The code descriptor states that this code is applied to unilateral or bilateral procedures. There is no need to apply the -50 modifier.

32. 31510

Note:

An indirect laryngoscopy uses a mirror to visualize the larynx.

33. 31576
34. 32656

Note:

The insertion of a chest tube is a common component of this procedure and is not separately coded.

35. 31628
36. 31561

Note:

Do not report a separate code for use of the operating microscope (69990).

37. 30520
38. 30100
39. 30300
40. 30460

Chapter 13
CPT Surgery III

EXERCISE 13.1 – HEART AND PERICARDIUM

1. 33410
2. 33824
3. 33533, 33517

Note:

Do not report modifier -51 with code 33517.

4. 33920
5. 33207, 33225

Note:

Do not report modifier -51 with code 33225.

6. 33031
7. 33282 (May 1), 93285 (May 16)
8. 33702
9. 33261
10. 33922
11. 33010, 76930
12. 33215
13. 33250
14. 33510, 33508
15. 33690
16. 33464
17. 33496
18. 33512
19. 33533, 33572
20. 33606
21. 33641

Note:

Do not report separate codes for the cardiopulmonary bypass or patch. Code 33641 includes repair of the defect, cardiopulmonary bypass, and placement of the patch.

22. 33852
23. 33780
24. 33641
25. 33860

EXERCISE 13.2 – ARTERIES AND VEINS

1. 37202

Note:

NCCI edits allow the reporting of code 37202 with the cardiac catheterization code.

2. 75710-RT, 36120-RT
3. 36200, 75605, 75625
4. 36555
5. 36011-LT, 36012-LT, 75831-LT

EXERCISE 13.3 – HEMIC AND LYMPHATIC SYSTEMS SUBSECTION

1. 38572
2. 38204
3. 38242
4. 38208
5. 38221
6. 38207
7. 38100
8. 38115
9. 38200, 75810
10. 38100
11. 38120
12. 38700
13. 41155, 38724-59

> **Note:**
>
> *When a cervical lymphadenectomy (38720–38724) is performed during the same operative session as a bilateral neck resection or dissection, report code 41155 for the cervical lymphadenectomy and resection on side. Report code 38724 with the appropriate modifier for the modified neck dissection performed on the other side. (Do not report directional modifiers -LT and -RT because each side of the neck is not considered a paired organ.)*

14. 31365, 38720-59

> **Note:**
>
> *When a total laryngectomy with* bilateral *radical neck dissection (31365) is performed, code 31365 is reported for the total laryngectomy and radical neck dissection on one side. (There is just one larynx, which means that modifier -50* cannot *be added to code 31365.) Code 38720-59 is reported for the radical neck dissection on the other side. (Modifier -59 is added to indicate a distinct procedural service.) (Do not report directional modifiers -LT and -RT because each side of the neck is not considered a paired organ.) (A radical neck dissection removes all lymphatic tissue along with the spinal accessory nerve, (SAN), sternocleidomastoid muscle (SCM), and internal jugular vein (IJV). Thus, modifier -50 cannot be added to code 38720 (cervical lymphadenectomy, complete) because that code does not completely describe the procedure is performed.)*

15. 38792, 78195

REVIEW

Multiple Choice

1. d
2. a
3. c
4. d
5. d
6. b
7. b
8. d
9. c
10. d
11. c
12. d
13. b
14. b
15. c
16. b
17. d
18. d
19. c
20. c

Coding Practice

Cardiovascular System

21. 37722-50, 37718-51-LT

> **Note:**
>
> *The patient had bilateral long saphenous vein stripping, which is reflected with CPT code 37722; modifier -50 identifies this as a bilateral procedure. The patient had short veins stripped of the left leg. Modifier -51 is added to code 37718 to reflect multiple procedures reported on the same date of service. HCPCS modifier -LT is added to reflect that the procedure of stripping short veins was done on the left side of the patient's body.*

22. 33430
23. 33208

> **Note:**
>
> *33208 includes insertion of the pulse generator and electrodes into the atrial and ventricular areas.*

24. 33820
25. 36425
26. 36830
27. 35301-LT

> **Note:**
>
> *EEG is the abbreviation for electroencephalogram. The EEG done during the operation is a common component of this procedure and is not separately coded or reported. To do so would be unbundling.*

28. 33241, 33240-78

> **Note:**
>
> *This case documents the insertion of a new pulse generator only. The leads were not replaced.*

29. 32140
30. 33510

Hemic and Lymphatic Systems

31. 38221
32. 38100
33. 38555
34. 38770
35. 38520
36. 38120
37. 38790, 75805

> **Note:**
>
> *Code 38790 is reported for the injection, and code 75805 is reported for the radiologic procedure.*

38. 38382

> **Note:**
>
> *Chyle in the pleural cavity is a condition called* chylothorax.

39. 38204
40. 38300

Chapter 14
CPT Surgery IV

EXERCISE 14.1 – MEDIASTINUM AND DIAPHRAGM SUBSECTION

1. 39561
2. 39010
3. 39501
4. 39400
5. 39540

EXERCISE 14.2 – ORAL CAVITY

1. 41874
2. 40500
3. 40810
4. 41010

Note:

Do not report code 40819, which classifies an excision of the frenum.

5. 42330

Note:

Do not report code 42405, which classifies an incisional biopsy.

6. 42953
7. 42700
8. 42820
9. 42960
10. 42826

Note:

Do not report code 42821, which classifies a tonsillectomy and adenoidectomy. This patient underwent tonsillectomy only.

EXERCISE 14.3 – ESOPHAGUS AND STOMACH

1. 43217
2. 43045

Note:

Do not report code 43101, which classifies excision of a lesion from the esophagus. This patient underwent foreign body removal from the esophagus through an incision in the chest wall and esophagus (esophagotomy).

3. 43460
4. 43116-52-62 (Dr. Smith), 43496-62 (Dr. Jones)
5. 43250, 43251-59

6. 43520
7. 43848
8. 43761, 76000

Note:

Do not report code 43752, which classifies the original placement of a nasogastric or orogastric tube. Because fluoroscopic guidance is not included in code 43761, report code 76000.

9. 43644

Note:

Do not report code 43645, which classifies small intestine reconstruction to limit absorption in addition to *the gastric bypass procedure.*

10. 49440

EXERCISE 14.4 – INTESTINES (EXCEPT RECTUM), MECKEL'S DIVERTICULUM AND THE MESENTERY, APPENDIX, RECTUM, AND ANUS

1. 44955 (in addition to cesarean section code)
2. 44005
3. 44120, 44121

Note:

Two segments of small intestine were resected and anastomosed. Therefore, report primary code 44120 and add-on code 44121. Do not *report code 44625, which classifies the* closure of an enterostomy *with resection and anastomosis.*

4. 44850
5. 44206
6. 45000
7. 45114

Note:

Do not *report code 45135, which classifies an excision of rectal* procidentia, *with anastomosis, abdominal and* perineal *approach.*

8. 45300
9. 45333
10. 45384

EXERCISE 14.5 – LIVER; BILIARY TRACT; PANCREAS; AND ABDOMEN, PERITONEUM, AND OMENTUM

1. 47011
2. 47141
3. 47380

Note:

Do not *report code 47370, which is performed via laparoscopy. The procedure for this case was performed via open* laparotomy.

4. 47564

Note:

Do not report code 47610, which is performed via open incision (not laparoscopy).

5. 47480
6. 49081
7. 49002
8. 49650

Note:

Do not report a code for use of the mesh. (A code for the use of mesh is reported for incisional or ventral hernia repair only.)

9. 49560, 49568
10. 49495

Note:

Do not report code 49496, which classifies an incarcerated or strangulated hernia.

EXERCISE 14.6 – URINARY SYSTEM SUBSECTION

1. 50020
2. 50590-LT
3. 50060-RT
4. 50392-RT, 74475-RT
5. 50542-LT
6. 50600-LT
7. 50953-50
8. 50727-RT
9. 50684-LT, 74425-LT
10. 50605-LT
11. 52500

Note:

Do not report code 52640, which is performed for a postoperative bladder neck contracture.

12. 52325
13. 52700
14. 51102

Note:

Do not report code 51045, which classifies a cystotomy (incision made into the urinary bladder) with insertion of ureteral catheter or stent.

15. 52214, 52320-51
16. 53440
17. 53600
18. 53400
19. 53850
20. 53200

REVIEW

Multiple Choice

1. b
2. b
3. a
4. d
5. c
6. d
7. b
8. a
9. a
10. c
11. b
12. d

13. c
14. b
15. a
16. b
17. c
18. a
19. b
20. c

Coding Practice

Mediastinum and Diaphragm

21. 39200

> **Note:**
>
> *MRI is the abbreviation for magnetic resonance imaging.*

22. 39540
23. 39545

> **Note:**
>
> *Imbrication is the overlapping of diaphragm tissue.*

24. 39501
25. 39400

Digestive System

26. 43840
27. 40510
28. 43611
29. 42821
30. 49553
31. 47562
32. 45331
33. 47100
34. 41015
35. 42410

> **Note:**
>
> *Do* not *report code 42415 because there is no documentation of "nerve dissection." The mass was dissected free; however, the facial nerve was not dissected.*

Urinary System

36. 52214
37. 52310
38. 52235
39. 50021
40. 50590-RT
41. 52332-RT

> **Note:**
>
> *Do not report code 52000-LT in addition to 52332-RT even though the cystourethroscope was also passed into the left ureter to visualize it. Because the cystourethroscope had already been passed through the urethra to visualize the right ureter (and to facilitate inserting the double-J stent), third-party payers will not consider passing the cystourethroscope into the left ureter a separate procedure. (After using the cystourethroscope to insert the double-J stent), the surgeon withdraws the instrument from the right ureter and inserts it into the left ureter. The instrument did not have to be completely withdrawn from the urethra and reinserted through the urethral to then visualize the left ureter.)*

42. 51535
43. 50200-RT
44. 50060-LT
45. 53400

Chapter 15
CPT Surgery V

EXERCISE 15.1 – MALE GENITAL SYSTEM SUBSECTION

1. 55150
2. 55520-LT
3. 54550-RT

Note:

Do not report code 55110, which classifies scrotal exploration.

4. 55812
5. 54050

EXERCISE 15.2 – REPRODUCTIVE SYSTEM PROCEDURES AND INTERSEX SURGERY SUBSECTIONS

1. 55920
2. 55970
3. 55980

EXERCISE 15.3 – FEMALE GENITAL SYSTEM SUBSECTION

1. 58605 (in addition to vaginal delivery code)
2. 57020

Note:

Colpocentesis involves making an incision in the vaginal wall to drain peritoneal fluid from the area behind the vagina. This case did not mention the presence of a peritoneal abscess; therefore, do not report code 57010.

3. 58970
4. 58300
5. 58662

EXERCISE 15.4 – MATERNITY CARE AND DELIVERY SUBSECTION

1. 59120
2. 59000, 76946
3. 59012, 76941
4. 59025
5. 59426, 59430

EXERCISE 15.5 – ENDOCRINE SYSTEM SUBSECTION

1. 60300
2. 60225

Note:

- The total thyroid lobectomy was performed on the right, which means it's a unilateral total thyroid lobectomy. A contralateral subtotal lobectomy including isthmusectomy was also performed during the same operative episode, which means it was performed on the left side. Thus, code 60225 is assigned because it states, "Total thyroid lobectomy, unilateral; with contralateral subtotal lobectomy, including isthmusectomy."
- Do *not* assign modifiers to code 60225.
- Do *not* assign code 60220 in addition to code 60225 because that would be considered overcoding. Code 60225 includes all elements of the procedure performed.

3. 60260
4. 60100
5. 60000
6. 60650
7. 60500, 60512

Note:

The parenthetical note below code 60512 instructs the coder to report that code with 60500, 60502, 60505, 60212, 60225, 60240, 60252, 60254, 60260, 60270, and 60271.

8. 60540
9. 60500
10. 60600

EXERCISE 15.6 – NERVOUS SYSTEM SUBSECTION

1. 61305

Note:

Per the parenthetical note below code 61253 in CPT, do not report code 61253 with code 61305 when burr holes are drilled into the infratentorial area prior to craniectomy during the same operative session.

2. 61210
3. 61215
4. 62252
5. 61070
6. 63012
7. 62270
8. 63740
9. 62361
10. 63064

Note:

T-1 represents one thoracic vertebral segment. Therefore, code 63064 is reported. If more than one thoracic vertebral segment was decompressed, code 63066 would be reported for each additional segment.

11. 64410
12. 64493-50, 64494-50
13. 64420
14. 64786
15. 64550

EXERCISE 15.7 – EYE AND OCULAR ADNEXA SUBSECTION

1. 65222-RT
2. 65275-LT
3. 65125
4. 65265-RT
5. 65205-E3
6. 65450-LT
7. 65820-RT, 66990-RT

Note:

Report add-on code 66990 as an additional code to indicate the use of an ophthalmic endoscope during the goniotomy procedure.

8. 66985-58-RT

Note:

Modifier -58 indicates that a staged or related procedure was performed.

9. 65400-LT
10. 66984-LT
11. 67015-RT
12. 67220-RT, 92235-RT
13. 67227-50

Note:

Do not *report code 67101, which classifies repair of retinal detachment.*

14. 67255-LT
15. 67141-LT
16. 67415-RT
17. 67312-50
18. 67805-E1–E3
19. 67311-RT, 67318-LT
20. 67312-RT, 67320-RT

Note:

Report code 67320 just once because its description does not *specify "each" muscle.*

21. 68200-LT
22. 68761, 68761, 68761, 68761

Note:

- *There are four puncta, two associated with each eye. Reporting code 68761 four times classifies surgery performed on the puncta of both eyes.*

23. 68810-50
24. 68705-LT, 68705-LT

Note:

Two puncta are associated with each eye. Therefore, report code 68705-LT twice to classify surgery performed on two puncta of one eye.

25. 68020-RT

EXERCISE 15.8 – AUDITORY SYSTEM SUBSECTION

1. 69000-LT
2. 69200-LT
3. 69300-RT
4. 69220-RT
5. 69090-50
6. 69424-50
7. 69436-50
8. 69405-50
9. 69710-LT
10. 69650-LT
11. 69720
12. 69930-50
13. 69610-RT
14. 69642-LT
15. 69676-LT
16. 69970-LT
17. 69955
18. 69960-RT
19. 69970
20. 69950

EXERCISE 15.9 – OPERATING MICROSCOPE SUBSECTION

1. 69610

Note:

Operating Microscope notes state that code 69990 are not reported for visualization with magnifying loupe or corrected vision.

2. 31526

Note:

The description for code 31526 states "with operating microscope," which means that code 69990 is not *reported separately.*

3. 19301-RT, 69990
4. 54901, 69990
5. 61548

Note:

Do not add code 69990 because below code 61548 is a parenthetical note that states, "(Do not report code 69990 in addition to code 61548.)"

REVIEW

Multiple Choice

1. d
2. b
3. b
4. c
5. a
6. a
7. d
8. b
9. d
10. c
11. c
12. d
13. a
14. b
15. b
16. d
17. d
18. c
19. b
20. b

Coding Practice

Male Genital System

21. 55700
22. 55041

Note:

The code description for 55041 states that it is a bilateral code. Do not add modifier -50 to the code.

23. 54057
24. 54150-24
25. 54520-50
26. 55250
27. 55815
28. 54600-LT
29. 54840
30. 54300

Female Genital System

31. 58240

Note:

Due to this patient's diagnosis of gynecologic malignancy, the code assignment is different than that of a non-gynecologic abdominal hysterectomy (58150). Also, this patient had a pelvic exenteration, or removal, of the contents of the cavity.

32. 58558
33. 58671
34. 57454
35. 57135
36. 56740
37. 57513
38. 58770-RT
39. 58974
40. 58925

Intersex Surgery

41. 55980
42. 55970

Maternity Care and Delivery

43. 59050

Note:

Fetal monitoring during labor by the attending obstetrician is not a separately billable or reportable service. The service done in this case is performed by a specialist, or neonatologist, which is billable and reportable per CPT guidelines.

44. 59618

Note:

This patient requested a VBAC (vaginal birth after cesarean). However, due to fetal distress, this request could not be granted; and the mother had a repeat c-section. Attempted VBAC that is unsuccessful is reported with 59618, not 59610. 59610 is the code used to report a successful VBAC.

45. 59866
46. 59812
47. 59414
48. 59120
49. 59400

Note:

Per CPT guidelines, the performing of an episiotomy during a delivery is not a separately billable or reportable procedure. To do so is unbundling. This code also reflects antepartum and postpartum care.

50. 59425
51. 59400, 59412

Note:

CPT code 59400 reflects normal antepartum care, vaginal delivery, and routine postpartum care. CPT code 59412 reflects the turning of the fetus from a breech presentation to a cephalic presentation. Modifier -51 is added to reflect multiple procedure codes being reported.

Endocrine System

52. 60100
53. 60220
54. 60540-50
55. 60281
56. 60500
57. 60650-LT
58. 60220
59. 60254

Note:

The patient has a thyroid malignancy, which requires the assignment of code 60254 for a total excision, not code 60240.

60. 60260
61. 60545-LT

Nervous System

62. 62360
63. 64402

Note:

A nerve block is the terminology used to identify the injection of an anesthetic agent into a nerve.

64. 64831-LT
65. 64553
66. 63700
67. 62270
68. 61150
69. 61680

Note:

AV is the abbreviation for arteriovenous.

70. 64712
71. 63744

Eye and Ocular Adnexa System

72. 65222-LT
73. 67312-LT

Note:

Each eye has four extraocular muscles: superior rectus, inferior rectus, lateral rectus, and medial rectus. In this case, two muscles were surgically treated.

74. 67800-E1
75. 68520-RT
76. 65400-RT
77. 66761-LT
78. 67145-RT
79. 67938-E4
80. 68550-LT
81. 66984-LT

Note:

- *IOL* is the abbreviation for intraocular lens.
- The use of the operating microscope is included in the code because it is an integral part of cataract surgery. Assigning a separate code for use of an operating microscope (69990) in addition to the code for the eye surgery is unbundling.
- The injection of an antibiotic is considered an integral part of the procedure, and a separate code is *not assigned.*

Auditory System

82. 69210

Note:

Modifier -50 is not added to the code for this case. The description of code 69210 indicates that this code is reportable for unilateral or bilateral procedures.

83. 69300-LT
84. 69200-LT
85. 69105-RT
86. 69641-LT

Note:

The removal of the cholesteatoma is an incidental part of this procedure, and it is not separately coded.

87. 69540-LT
88. 69020-RT
89. 69400-RT
90. 69552-LT

Note:

The tegmen is part of the mastoid bone; it is the roof the mastoid sinuses.

91. 69220-LT

Operating Microscope

Note:

Code 69990 for use of the operating microscope is an add-on code. Do not add modifier -51 to the code.

92. 69801-RT, 69990
93. 42600-LT, 69990
94. 39503, 69990
95. 34501-LT, 69990
96. 26548-F4, 69990
97. 35207-F3, 69990
98. 64865, 69990
99. 42808, 69990
100. 31420, 69990
101. 26415-LT, 69990
102. 69424-50, 69990

Note:

Modifier -50 is added to the procedure code to reflect that it is a bilateral procedure.

103. 51500, 69990
104. 26850-F6, 69990
105. 24495-RT, 69990

Chapter 16
CPT Radiology

EXERCISE 16.1 – RADIOLOGY TERMINOLOGY

1. d
2. a
3. c
4. b
5. b
6. d
7. a
8. c
9. g
10. c
11. d
12. e
13. f
14. a
15. b

EXERCISE 16.2 – OVERVIEW OF RADIOLOGY CODING

1. type of service; anatomic site; use of contrast material
2. technical
3. professional
4. global service
5. report (or results)

EXERCISE 16.3 – RADIOLOGY SECTION GUIDELINES

1. invasive
2. noninvasive
3. Surgical component: 36200
   Radiological component: 75625
4. intravascularly, intra-articularly, or intrathecally
5. False

EXERCISE 16.4 – DIAGNOSTIC RADIOLOGY (DIAGNOSTIC IMAGING)

1. 19102-RT, 77012
2. 70373
3. 75710-LT

Note:

- Do not assign code 75658-LT (instead of code 75710-LT) because there is no mention of a "retrograde" approach in the case. "Retrograde" means the contrast medium was injected "against the flow" of blood in the artery.
- The surgeon would report the catheterization code (e.g., 36140-LT).

4. 72220
5. 76390

EXERCISE 16.5 – DIAGNOSTIC UTRASOUND

1. 76700
2. 76801
3. 76818
4. 76705
5. 76514
6. 47000, 77002
7. 61751, 77011
8. 20982-LT, 77022
9. 19102-LT, 77031
10. 77056

EXERCISE 16.6 – RADIATION ONCOLOGY

1. 77321
2. 77620
3. 77280
4. 77401
5. 77789

EXERCISE 16.7 – NUCLEAR MEDICINE

1. 79101
2. 78195
3. 79403
4. 78587

Note:

- Anterior, posterior, and lateral views are considered multiple views.
- Do not report code 78588 (Pulmonary perfusion imaging, particulate, with ventilation imaging, aerosol, one or multiple projections). This case did not include documentation of "pulmonary perfusion imaging, particulate."

5. 78428

REVIEW

Multiple Choice

1. a
2. d
3. c
4. a
5. c
6. a
7. c
8. d
9. b
10. b
11. d
12. d
13. b
14. a
15. b
16. c
17. c
18. d
19. a
20. a

Coding Practice

21. 74000

Note:

AP is the abbreviation for anteroposterior.

22. 74270
23. 74290
24. 74245
25. 74250
26. 71020
27. 71100
28. 70250
29. 73120-LT
30. 71010
31. 74410, 50394
32. 70240
33. 72040
34. 73080-LT

Note:

A complete elbow x-ray includes a minimum of three views.

35. 73562-50 (or 73562, 73562)

Note:

Modifier -50 is approved for use with code 73562. However, it is also acceptable to report code 73562 two times on a claim.

36. 73100-LT
37. 74010
38. 78635
39. 70120
40. 78215
41. 76805
42. 77402
43. 76870
44. 70491

Note:

CT is the abbreviation for computed tomography.

45. 72131
46. 73030-RT
47. 78811

Note:

PET is the abbreviation for positron emission tomography.

48. 73610-LT
49. 75557

Note:

MRI is the abbreviation for magnetic resonance imaging.

50. 78306

Chapter 17
CPT Pathology and Laboratory

EXERCISE 17.1 – OVERVIEW OF PATHOLOGY AND LABORATORY SECTION

1. professional
2. methods
3. chargemaster
4. specimen
5. phlebotomy
6. 36415
7. 36400–36410
8. -26
9. -90
10. Clinical Laboratory Improvement Act of 1988 (CLIA)

EXERCISE 17.2 – PATHOLOGY AND LABORATORY SECTION GUIDELINES

1. specimen
2. twice

Note:

When multiple specimens are received for pathological examination, each specimen is considered a single unit of service and each is reported with a separate code. Thus, code 88302 is reported twice.

3. date of service
4. unlisted service or procedure; special report
5. -91; -51

EXERCISE 17.3 – PATHOLOGY AND LABORATORY SUBSECTIONS

1. 81000
2. 36415, 80162
3. 80051
4. 88331, 88331-59, 88332, 88305, 88305-59

Note:

- The frozen section of the first specimen is reported with code 88331.
- The first frozen section on the second specimen is reported with code 88331-59, and the second frozen section for this specimen is reported with code 88332.
- Code 88305 is reported twice to classify the two separately identified basal cell carcinomas for surgical pathology (definitive examination). Modifier -59 is added to the second code (88305-59).

5. 81025
6. 36600, 82800
7. 82310, 82374, 82435, 82565, 84295, 84520

Note:

Do not report code 80048 (Basic metabolic panel) because potassium and glucose levels were not performed. A code for each laboratory test performed is reported separately: calcium (82310), carbon dioxide (82374), chloride (82435), creatinine (82565), sodium (84295), and urea nitrogen (BUN) (84520).

8. 88331, 88309
9. 85730
10. 36416, 82948
11. 88331, 88305

Note:

- The frozen section of this specimen is reported with code 88331.
- Surgical pathology evaluation of the breast biopsy is reported with code 88305.

12. 80061, 82947

Note:

- Code 80061 is reported for the lipid panel.
- Code 82947 is reported for the quantitative glucose test.

13. 80050

Note:

Code 80050 includes a hemogram. Therefore, a separate code is not reported for the hemogram.

14. 82374, 82435, 82565, 82947, 84132, 84295, 84520

Note:

- Do not report code 80053 (Comprehensive Metabolic Panel) because albumin, bilirubin (total), calcium, phosphatase (alkaline), protein (total), and transferase (alanine and aspartate amino) tests were not performed.
- Instead, each test is reported separately: carbon dioxide (82374), chloride (82435), creatinine (82565), glucose (82947), potassium (84132), sodium (84295), and urea nitrogen (BUN) (84520).

15. 86021
16. 87172
17. 88304

Note:

Although surgical pathology evaluation of appendix tissue is also included below code 88302, that code is for an incidental appendectomy (e.g., appendix removed incidentally during another procedure). For this case, the appendix was abnormal (due to acute appendicitis), which means that code 88304 is reported.

18. 87181
19. 89230
20. 88331, 88332, 88331-59, 88332-59, 88332-59, 88307, 88307-59, 88309

Note:

- The frozen section of two blocks from the right specimen are reported with codes 88331 and 88332.
- The frozen section of three blocks from the left specimen are reported with codes 88331-59, 88332-59, and 88332-59.
- Surgical pathology evaluation of right and left obturator lymph node resections are reported with codes 88307 and 88307-59.
- Surgical pathology evaluation of prostate tissue (as the result of radical prostatectomy) is reported with code 88309.

REVIEW

Multiple Choice

1. a
2. b
3. c
4. c
5. d
6. a
7. c
8. b
9. b
10. b
11. a
12. a
13. b
14. c
15. d
16. c
17. d

Note:

ABO, Rh, and MN blood typing are just 3 of 27 blood typing systems used to describe the absence or presence of antigens. (Many are named after the patients in whom they were initially encountered.)

- ABO testing results in the determination of four principal blood group types: A, B, AB, and O.
- Blood tested for the presence or absence of a Rhesis (Rh) blood protein results in Rh positive (Rh+) or Rh negative (Rh-) status.
- The MN system tests for blood types M, N, or MN, which is useful in maternity and paternity testing.

18. d
19. d
20. a

Coding Practice

21. 80055

Note:

- The combination of these eight blood laboratory testing constitutes an obstetric panel. Assigning a separate code to each test is incorrect.
- Rh(D) is the terminology used to identify a group of antigens on the surface of red blood cells.
- ABO is the medical terminology used to classify blood types; A, B, AB, and O.
- CBC is the abbreviation for complete blood count.
- WBC is the abbreviation for white blood count.

22. 80069, 85027

Note:

- The ten tests—albumin, carbon dioxide, calcium, sodium, glucose, chloride, creatinine, urea nitrogen, potassium, and phosphorus inorganic—constitute a renal function panel.
- Because a CBC is not a part of a renal function panel, a separate code (85027) is assigned.

23. 81001
24. 89260

Note:

Code 89260 is reported for the sperm isolation procedure and semen analysis.

25. 80418

Note:

- These seven tests are done for suppression testing, and they are coded as a pituitary evaluation panel code.
- ACTH is the abbreviation for adrenocorticotropic hormone.
- HGH is the abbreviation for human growth hormone.
- TSH is the abbreviation for thyroid-stimulating hormone.
- LH is the abbreviation for luteinizing hormone.
- FSH is the abbreviation for follicle-stimulating hormone.

26. 87265
27. 83009
28. 85014
29. 82810
30. 88331
31. 87220

Note:

KOH is the abbreviation used to identify the method of using potassium hydroxide prep.

32. 84443, 84479
33. 80100
34. 86038

Note:

- ANA is the abbreviation for antinuclear antibodies.
- SLE is the abbreviation for systemic lupus erythematosus.

35. 88309

Note:

- The gross and microscopic exam of radically resected prostate tissue is coded to level VI under the Surgical Pathology subsection.
- TURP is the abbreviation for transurethral resection of the prostate.

36. 86771
37. 84478
38. 86631

39. 88305

Note:

The gross and microscopic exam of this type of tissue is classified as level IV below the Surgical Pathology subsection.

40. 86485

41. 86901

42. 84153

Note:

PSA is the abbreviation for prostate-specific antigen.

43. 86359

44. 88304

Note:

The examination of this type of tissue is classified as level III below the Surgical Pathology subsection.

45. 86200

Note:

CCP is the abbreviation for cyclic citrullinated peptide.

46. 88029

47. 88142

48. 89050

49. 88230-5C

Note:

- Freidreich ataxia is a non-neoplastic disorder.
- Modifier -5C is added to the code to identify the disorder (Freidreich ataxia in this case) that is being investigated via tissue analysis. Genetic testing modifiers are located in Appendix I of the CPT coding manual. They identify CPT codes that are reported for procedures performed for genetic testing purposes.

50. 88037

Chapter 18
CPT Medicine

EXERCISE 18.1 – INTRODUCTION AND OVERVIEW OF MEDICINE SECTION

1. noninvasive
2. minimally invasive
3. can
4. diagnostic and therapeutic
5. procedure-oriented

EXERCISE 18.2 – MEDICINE SECTION GUIDELINES

1. notes
2. separate
3. plus
4. separate procedure
5. HCPCS level II

EXERCISE 18.3 – MEDICINE SUBSECTIONS

1. 90473
2. 90822

Note:

Code 90822 includes individual psychotherapy (to modify the patient's obsessive-compulsive behavior) with medical evaluation and management services (performed to check the lithium blood levels).

3. 92980, 92981

Note:

Do not report codes 92982–92984 for coronary angioplasty or codes 92995–92996 for atherectomy. When performed in the same artery as the stent procedure, these procedures are included in the stent procedure codes (92980–92981).

4. 90968 × 10

Note:

Code is reported for each day when less than a full month (e.g., 30 days) of ESRD services are provided to a patient between age 2 and 11 years.

5. 96374

Note:

Neither of the IV flush procedures is coded and reported because an IV flush is integral to the infusion/injection service provided. HCPCS level II code J0696 is reported for each 250-mg dosage.

REVIEW

Multiple Choice

1. b
2. d
3. d
4. a
5. c
6. a
7. b
8. c
9. d
10. a
11. d
12. d
13. d
14. c
15. a
16. b
17. b
18. a
19. b
20. b

Coding Practice

21. 92341
22. 96120
23. 92002
24. 91030
25. 93875
26. 92579
27. 94667
28. 93797
29. 90911
30. 93288
31. 93303
32. 98941
33. 90636, 90471
34. 97535, 97535
35. 95813
36. 91132
37. 92516
38. 90718, 90471
39. 90816
40. 93000
41. 92982, 92984

Note:

The procedure described in this note is a percutaneous transluminal coronary angioplasty (PTCA). Two vessels were treated, requiring assignment of codes 92982 and 92984. CPT code 92984 is an add-on code; therefore, do not add modifier -51.

42. 93015
43. 91034
44. 99503
45. 97001
46. 95125
47. 96920
48. 90375, 96372
49. 90960
50. 96413, 96415

Chapter 19
Insurance and Reimbursement

EXERCISE 19.1 – THIRD-PARTY PAYERS

1. Medicare administrative contractors (MAC)
2. Centers for Medicare & Medicaid Services (CMS)
3. CMS-1500; UB-92 or CMS-1450 (UB-04 in 2007)
4. clearinghouse
5. hold harmless clause
6. CHAMPVA
7. Medicaid
8. Medicare
9. managed care
10. fee-for-service

EXERCISE 19.2 – HEALTH CARE REIMBURSEMENT SYSTEMS

1. $1,200 ($1,500 × 80%); $300 ($1,500 × 20%).
2. $4,480 ([$1,400 × 4] × 80% = $4,480); $4,500, which is the DRG prospective payment amount
3. chargemaster review
4. Tax Equity and Fiscal Responsibility Act of 1983 (TEFRA)
5. ambulatory payment classifications (APCs)
6. a
7. a
8. b
9. b
10. a

EXERCISE 19.3 – IMPACT OF HIPAA ON REIMBURSEMENT

1. a
2. b
3. b
4. a
5. a
6. national health plan identifier (PlanID)
7. national standard employer identifier number (EIN)
8. national provider identifier (NPI)
9. electronic data interchange (EDI)
10. security

REVIEW

Multiple Choice

1. c
2. a
3. b
4. d
5. c
6. b
7. b
8. b
9. a
10. d
11. d
12. c
13. b
14. c
15. b
16. b
17. b
18. d
19. c
20. c
21. b
22. b
23. a
24. d
25. c

SECTION III

Chapter Exams and Answer Keys to Chapter Exams

Chapter 1
Overview of Coding

1. An at-home coding specialist enters manifestation codes into the computer. Which type of HIPAA code set is being used?
   a. ASP
   b. CPT
   c. large
   d. SNOMED CT
2. A facility enters into a contract with a billing service to convert health information and claims from a nonstandard to a standard format. The billing service is considered a:
   a. health care clearinghouse.
   b. health care plan.
   c. third-party administrator.
   d. third-party payer.
3. A claims examiner reviews a patient's chart to locate documentation of a diagnosis to justify treatment provided. What is the examiner trying to establish?
   a. medical coding
   b. medical necessity
   c. medical nomenclature
   d. medical record
4. Which coding system is currently used in the United States?
   a. CPT
   b. HCPCS level III
   c. ICD-9
   d. ICD-10
5. The medical record is considered a _______ for a patient encounter.
   a. business record
   b. financial record
   c. medical nomenclature
   d. registration report
6. Secondary purposes of the medical record:
   a. do not relate directly to patient care.
   b. have as an option, medicolegal purposes.
   c. include the planning of individual patient care.
   d. usually do not require accurate documentation.
7. Which of the following statements about a student internship is true?
   a. Because students are not considered employees, they do not have to adhere to a dress code.
   b. Breach of confidentiality can result in termination from the internship site.
   c. Sometimes students receive monetary compensation for their work.
   d. Students must submit a professional resume to the facility supervisor.
8. A student is preparing to sit for a credentialing exam offered through the American Health Information Management Association. Which is the student pursuing?
   a. Certified Coding Specialist
   b. Certified Medical Billing Specialist
   c. Certified Professional Coder
   d. Registered Medical Assistant
9. Students join their professional organizations:
   a. after they graduate.
   b. only if they are sponsored by a member.
   c. to receive all of the benefits provided to active members.
   d. usually for a reduced fee.
10. A health care professional would like to network with other professionals via the Internet. Which would be most helpful for this purpose?
    a. ASP
    b. hyperlink
    c. listerv
    d. WAN

11. Which nomenclature is in use today?
    a. CMIT
    b. SNDO
    c. SNOMED CT
    d. SNOP
12. Which coding system would a physician's office most likely use?
    a. CDT
    b. CPT
    c. DSM
    d. NDC
13. Susan just attended a lecture on new procedures and techniques used in cardiac care, and she received continuing education (CE) credits for her participation. How will CE credits professionally benefit Susan?
    a. Susan can apply the CE credits towards maintenance of her professional credential.
    b. Susan can use CE credits to earn a degree in the coding profession.
    c. Susan can use CE credits to earn a professional credential.
    d. Susan's CE credits are required to maintain her professional degree.
14. A coding specialist is more likely to be credentialed by:
    a. AHIMA.
    b. AMT.
    c. MAB.
    d. NEBA.
15. Which problem-oriented record SOAP note is documented for the statement "Patient's diagnosis is acute bronchitis"?
    a. subjective
    b. objective
    c. assessment
    d. plan
16. Which problem-oriented record SOAP note is documented for the statement "Chest X-ray reveals areas of lung consolidation"?
    a. subjective
    b. objective
    c. assessment
    d. plan
17. Which problem-oriented record SOAP note is documented for the statement "Patient complains of headache"?
    a. subjective
    b. objective
    c. assessment
    d. plan
18. Which problem-oriented record SOAP note is documented for the statement "Patient is scheduled for brain scan on Tuesday?"
    a. subjective
    b. objective
    c. assessment
    d. plan
19. The physician documents "acute and chronic asthma" on the patient's record. Which coding system is used to assign codes for claims submission?
    a. CPT
    b. HCPCS level I
    c. HCPCS level II
    d. ICD-9-CM (or ICD-10-CM)
20. Which credentialing exam is offered by the American Academy of Professional Coders?
    a. CCA
    b. CCS
    c. CMRS
    d. CPC

Chapter 2
Introduction to ICD-9-CM and ICD-10-CM/PCS Coding

1. The Medicare Prescription Drug, Improvement, and Modernization Act (MMA) requires ICD-9-CM codes to be updated:
   a. after a 90-day grace period so computer systems can be updated.
   b. annually; and updated codes must be implemented immediately.
   c. as the cooperating parties for the ICD-9-CM make monthly changes.
   d. each April 1 and October 1; and they must be implemented immediately.
2. Which originally mandated the reporting of ICD-9-CM diagnosis codes on Medicare claims?
   a. cooperating parties for the ICD-9-CM (or ICD-10-CM/PCS)
   b. Medicare Catastrophic Coverage Act of 1988
   c. Medicare Prescription Drug, Improvement, and Modernization Act
   d. third-party payers, including commercial insurance companies
3. Which automates the coding process using computerized or web-based software?
   a. encoder
   b. grouper
   c. maximizer
   d. optimizer
4. Which ICD-9-CM supplementary classification would be referenced to code a homicide attempt?
   a. Contact with health services
   b. External cause of injury
   c. Factors influencing health status
   d. Morphology of neoplasms
5. Subterms, which are indented two spaces below main terms, are also called _______ modifiers.
   a. essential
   b. necessary
   c. nonessential
   d. secondary
6. To initially locate an external cause of injury code, go to the:
   a. Alphabetic Index to External Causes of Injury and Poisoning.
   b. Index to Diseases (and Injuries).
   c. Index to Procedures.
   d. Table of Drugs and Chemicals.
7. ICD-9-CM Volume 3 includes a(n):
   a. alphabetical index of all outpatient procedures and services.
   b. alphanumeric anatomic listing of inpatient procedures and services.
   c. tabular list of 17 chapters.
   d. Tabular List of Procedures and Index to Procedures.
8. The ICD-9-CM Tabular List of Procedures chapters are arranged:
   a. according to anatomic site.
   b. alphabetically.
   c. by service or procedure.
   d. numerically.
9. The cooperating parties for the ICD-9-CM (or ICD-10-CM/PCS) approve guidelines that have been prepared for coding and reporting using the ICD-9-CM (or ICD-10-CM/PCS) and consist of which organizations?
   a. AHA, AHIMA, CMS, and NCHS
   b. APA, AHIMA, DHHS, and AHA
   c. MMA, CMS, APA, and NCHS
   d. WHO, DHHS, AHIMA, CMS, and NCHS
10. The guidelines prepared by the cooperating parties for the ICD-9-CM (or ICD-10-CM/PCS):
    a. are required by the Medicare Prescription Drug, Improvement, and Modernization Act (MMA).
    b. contain rules for the Tabular List of Diseases only.
    c. had been developed to override the official conventions in ICD-9-CM (or ICD-10-CM).
    d. include coding and sequencing instructions for ICD-9-CM (or ICD-10-CM).

11. ICD-9-CM (or ICD-10-CM) index subterms are indented _______ spaces with respect to main terms.
    a. two
    b. four
    c. five
    d. six
12. Within the ICD-9-CM (or ICD-10-CM) tabular list, which contain groups of three-character categories?
    a. categories
    b. sections
    c. subcategories
    d. subclassifications
13. "Persons with health hazards related to communicable diseases" is an example of a(n):
    a. chapter in the ICD-9-CM (or ICD-10-CM) tabular list.
    b. chapter in the ICD-9-CM Tabular List of Procedures.
    c. ICD-9-CM (or ICD-10-CM) grouping of external cause of injury codes.
    d. ICD-9-CM grouping of V codes (or ICD-10-CM grouping of Z codes).
14. "Place of occurrence" is an example of a:
    a. chapter in the ICD-9-CM (or ICD-10-CM) tabular list.
    b. chapter in the ICD-9-CM Tabular List of Procedures.
    c. grouping of ICD-9-CM (or ICD-10-CM) external cause of injury codes.
    d. grouping of ICD-9-CM V codes (or ICD-10-CM Z codes).
15. To properly assign a code from the neoplasm table when a diagnosis is documented as "neoplasm of the pyloric antrum," the coder should:
    a. assign a code from the Unspecified column.
    b. contact the state cancer registry for clarification.
    c. refer to the morphology entry in the index.
    d. review the pathology report to determine the type of neoplasm.
16. The ICD-9-CM Table of Drugs and Chemicals contains a main entry for "Drug," which:
    a. can be referenced when the AHFS list number has not been provided.
    b. contains a list of drugs that are not listed elsewhere in the Table of Drugs and Chemicals.
    c. directs the coder to Appendix C of the ICD-9-CM coding manual.
    d. lists drugs according to the American Hospital Formulary Services (AHFS) list number.
17. The ICD-9-CM (or ICD-10-CM) Tabular List of Diseases (and Injuries) should be referenced:
    a. for verification of external cause of injury codes only.
    b. if the phrase *omit code* is included in the index.
    c. to verify codes selected and to review instructions.
    d. when a procedure code is listed as unspecified.
18. Which connecting term(s) immediately follow the main term to which they refer in the ICD-9-CM Index to Procedures?
    a. by
    b. for
    c. to
    d. with and without
19. The phrase *omit code* located after a main term or subterm in the ICD-9-CM Index to Procedures indicates that the operative approach is:
    a. considered an integral part of the procedure, and it is coded.
    b. considered an integral part of the procedure, and it is not coded.
    c. not considered an integral part of the procedure, and it is coded.
    d. not considered an integral part of the procedure, and it is not coded.
20. After locating a code in the ICD-9-CM Index to Procedures, the coder's next step is to:
    a. link the procedure code to a diagnosis code.
    b. locate that code in the Tabular List of Procedures to review instructions and verify the code.
    c. locate the main term in the Index to Procedures.
    d. review the code description in the Tabular List of Procedures to determine if the "omit code" instruction applies.

Chapter 3
ICD-9-CM and ICD-10-CM/PCS Coding Conventions

1. ICD-9-CM (or ICD-10-CM) index subterms are indented _______ spaces below main terms.
   a. two
   b. four
   c. five
   d. six
2. Where would the abbreviation NEC (not elsewhere classifiable) be found in ICD-9-CM?
   a. Index to Diseases and Index to Procedures
   b. Index to Diseases and Tabular List of Diseases
   c. Index to Procedures and Tabular List of Procedures
   d. Tabular List of Diseases and Tabular List of Procedures
3. Where would the abbreviation NOS (not otherwise specified) be found in ICD-9-CM?
   a. Index to Diseases and Index to Procedures
   b. Tabular List of Diseases and Index to Diseases
   c. Tabular List of Diseases and Tabular List of Procedures
   d. Tabular List of Procedures and Index to Procedures
4. Which are used in the ICD-10-CM Index to Diseases and Injuries to identify manifestation codes?
   a. colons
   b. parentheses
   c. slanted brackets
   d. square brackets
5. The ICD-9-CM (or ICD-10-CM) _______ contains "includes" notes.
   a. index (diseases)
   b. index (procedures)
   c. table of drugs and chemicals
   d. tabular list (diseases)
6. The appearance of an "excludes" note beneath an ICD-9-CM code indicates that codes for:
   a. excluded conditions are always to be reported with the code from which the condition is excluded.
   b. excluded conditions are never to be reported with the code from which the condition is excluded.
   c. excluded conditions may or may not be reported with the code from which the condition is excluded.
   d. unspecified conditions must be assigned as a code number to the condition.
7. Inclusion terms are:
   a. antonyms of the code title or for "unspecified" codes, are a list of conditions assigned to that code.
   b. exhaustive; so if the correct term is not listed below the code, that code cannot be assigned.
   c. listed below certain four- and five-character ICD-9-CM codes in the indexes.
   d. listed below certain four- and five-character ICD-9-CM (or ICD-10-CM) codes in the tabular list.
8. An ICD-9-CM "other specified" code:
   a. generally contains a fourth digit of 9 and/or a fifth digit of 0.
   b. is sufficient to assign a more specific code.
   c. requires the reporting of multiple codes for a case.
   d. usually contains a fourth and/or fifth digit of 8 and/or 9.
9. The relationship between etiology and manifestation codes results in the ICD-9-CM (or ICD-10-CM):
   a. manifestation code being sequenced first, followed by the etiology code.
   b. etiology code being printed in slanted (or square) brackets in the index.
   c. etiology code being reported first, followed by the manifestation code.
   d. manifestation code defining the underlying condition or disease.

10. The "see also" instruction in ICD-9-CM (or ICD-10-CM):
    a. appears in the tabular list and is an optional guideline.
    b. does not have to be followed if the original main term provides the correct code.
    c. is considered a mandatory optional guideline in the index.
    d. must always be followed for disease codes to be assigned properly.
11. Which must be included in the diagnostic statement to classify a condition or procedure?
    a. inclusion terms
    b. modifier included after the colon
    c. nonessential modifiers enclosed in parentheses
    d. synonyms enclosed in square brackets
12. A patient is diagnosed with phlyctenulosis due to tuberculosis. Codes 017.3 and *[370.31]* are located in the Index to Diseases. Upon verification in the Tabular List of Diseases, report code(s):
    a. 017.3 with an appropriate fifth digit only.
    b. 017.3 with an appropriate fifth digit and 370.31 in that order.
    c. 370.31 only.
    d. 370.31 and 017.3 with an appropriate fifth digit in that order.
13. The description for code J00 in the ICD-10-CM Tabular List of Diseases and Injuries is "acute nasopharyngitis [common cold]." How is this code description interpreted?
    a. acute nasopharyngitis and common cold are synonymous.
    b. acute nasopharyngitis due to common cold
    c. acute nasopharyngitis with common cold
    d. common cold due to acute nasopharyngitis
14. The ICD-9-CM (or ICD-10-CM) index contains nonessential modifiers that may be present or absent in the provider's diagnostic statement, and the modifiers are surrounded by _____.
    a. parentheses
    b. slanted brackets
    c. square brackets
    d. tildes
15. ICD-9-CM (or ICD-10-CM) disease coding conventions are:
    a. based on official coding guidelines.
    b. chapter-specific rules used to code diagnoses.
    c. general coding rules that are independent of coding guidelines.
    d. used only in the Tabular List of Diseases (or Tabular List of Diseases and Injuries).
16. The concept "trust the index" in the ICD-9-CM (or ICD-10-CM disease index) means that:
    a. if a term has been used to correctly locate a code in the disease index but that term is not described in the disease tabular list code entry, trust that the index directed you to the correct code.
    b. all terms that apply to a particular code will be listed in the disease tabular list code description; thus, if there is no inclusion term for that condition, the code cannot be assigned.
    c. inclusion terms located in the disease index are not meant to be exhaustive, and additional terms found in the disease tabular list may also be associated with a code.
    d. if a term has been used to correctly locate a code in the disease index and the code listed in the index contains a fifth digit, it is not necessary to verify the code in the disease tabular list.
17. The concept of "moving up the ladder" of codes in the disease tabular list means:
    a. assigning the proper codes to ensure that maximum reimbursement is obtained for the facility.
    b. ensuring that the most specific code is always assigned using the disease tabular list.
    c. querying the physician about documentation to determine whether a more specific code can be assigned.
    d. sequencing codes so the first-listed code reflects the reason for the encounter and secondary codes list additional diagnoses, complications, and comorbidities.

18. Which instruction is optional in ICD-9-CM (or ICD-10-CM) when a secondary condition is not documented?
    a. code first underlying condition
    b. code, if applicable, any causal condition first
    c. in diseases classified elsewhere
    d. use additional code
19. Which is listed alphabetically according to main term in the ICD-9-CM Index to Diseases?
    a. External Causes of Injury and Poisoning
    b. Index to Procedures
    c. Neoplasm Table
    d. Table of Drugs and Chemicals
20. Boxed notes provide information or instruction in the ICD-9-CM Index to Diseases and Index to Procedures. Which functions of boxed notes are associated with the ICD-9-CM Index to Diseases but *not* with the ICD-9-CM Index to Procedures? Boxed notes:
    a. identify manifestation codes.
    b. include nonessential modifiers.
    c. list fifth-digit subclassifications.
    d. provide coding instruction.

Chapter 4
ICD-9-CM and ICD-10-CM Coding Guidelines

ICD-9-CM Coding

1. Which procedure requires the assignment of an ICD-9-CM code for the surgical approach?
   a. Surgeon performed exploratory laparotomy to remove mass; surgery halted prior to removal of mass.
   b. Neurosurgeon performed a craniotomy and removed a brain lesion.
   c. Surgeon made a laparotomy incision and performed a laparoscopic appendectomy.
   d. Surgeon made a skin incision and performed a vein stripping procedure.

2. A symptomatic HIV-positive patient is admitted to the hospital following a motor vehicle accident. The patient is diagnosed as having an open fracture of the femoral shaft and undergoes open reduction with internal fixation. The patient receives HIV antiviral medication while in the hospital.
   a. 042, E919.9, 79.35
   b. 042, 821.11, E919.9, 79.35
   c. 821.11, E919.9, 79.35
   d. 821.11, 042, E919.9, 79.35

3. A patient with chronic choroiditis presents with complaints of decreased vision. The patient is diagnosed with cataract due to choroiditis. Which is the proper assignment (and sequencing if more than one code is assigned) of ICD-9-CM disease code(s)?
   a. 363.20
   b. 366.32
   c. 363.20, 366.32
   d. 366.32, 363.20

4. A patient was admitted after an accidental industrial explosion occurred at his workplace, resulting in a fire. The patient sustained second-degree burns of the right ear, second- and third-degree burns of the shoulder, and first- and second-degree burns of the hand. Thirty-five percent of the body sustained burns, with 10% third-degree burns, 20% second-degree burns, and 5% first-degree burns.
   a. 941.21, 943.25, 943.35, 944.10, 944.20, 948.21, E891.3
   b. 941.21, 943.35, 944.20, 948.21, E891.3
   c. 943.35, 941.21, 944.20, 948.21, E891.3
   d. 943.35, 943.25, 944.20, 941.21, 943.13, 948.21, E891.3

5. A patient had an encounter with his family doctor to receive a preemployment physical examination and was diagnosed with an external ear infection. Which is the proper assignment (and sequencing if more than one code is assigned) of ICD-9-CM disease code(s)?
   a. 380.10
   b. 380.10, V70.5
   c. V70.5
   d. V70.5, 380.10

6. A woman was admitted to the hospital in labor, and she delivered. The final diagnoses included uterine pregnancy, delivery of oversized infant with low forceps and episiotomy; and postdelivery hematoma of episiotomy. Which is the proper assignment and sequencing of ICD-9-CM disease and procedure codes?
   a. 653.51, 674.31, V27.0, 72.1
   b. 653.51, 674.32, V27.0, 72.1
   c. 653.51, 674.32, V27.0, 72.9
   d. 674.32, 653.51, V27.0, 72.1

7. A patient recently underwent a mastectomy for treatment of an upper/inner quadrant adenocarcinoma of the breast. Today the patient has an outpatient encounter for radiation therapy. Which is the proper coding (and sequencing if more than one is assigned) of ICD-9-CM disease code(s)?
   a. 174.2
   b. 174.2, V58.0
   c. V58.0
   d. V58.0, 174.2

8. A patient presents with complaint of pain and stiffness in the left ankle. The diagnosis is documented as traumatic arthritis of the ankle. Which is the proper coding and sequencing of ICD-9-CM disease codes?
   a. 716.17, 908.9
   b. 716.17, 959.7
   c. 908.9, 716.17
   d. 959.7, 716.17
9. A patient is admitted with complaints of chest pain and shortness of breath. During the exam, the patient revealed that he had recently come into contact with a white powdery substance in his duties as a postal employee and that a coworker had contracted anthrax. After examination, the physician diagnosed the patient with pneumonia due to pulmonary anthrax. Which is the proper coding and sequencing of ICD-9-CM disease codes?
   a. 022.1, 484.5, E915
   b. 022.1, 484.5, E979.6
   c. 484.5, 022.1, E915
   d. 484.5, 022.1, E979.6
10. Which of the following is classified by assigning an adverse effect code from the ICD-9-CM Table of Drugs and Chemicals?
    a. A patient was admitted in a comatose state. The patient's brother said that an empty bottle of Tylenol with Codeine, which had just been filled that morning, was found on the table beside the patient. The patient had threatened to hurt herself the day before.
    b. A patient was prescribed Percocet for back pain due to a muscle injury and was admitted after a motor vehicle accident. The patient claimed that he wasn't getting enough relief from the pain, so he took an "extra dose" that morning and must have fallen asleep at the wheel.
    c. A patient who takes prescribed doses of diclofenac for arthritis frequently takes aspirin for headaches. She is admitted to the hospital with gastrointestinal bleeding.
    d. A patient with back pain due to a displaced disk was prescribed Darvocet. While taking prescribed doses, the patient experienced extreme fatigue and bradycardia.
11. A patient is diagnosed as having renal and heart disease due to hypertension. Which is the proper coding (and sequencing if more than one code is assigned) of ICD-9-CM disease code(s)?
    a. 402.90, 403.90
    b. 404.90
    c. 404.90, 401.9
    d. 404.90, 402.90, 403.90
12. A pregnant woman underwent outpatient termination of a pregnancy. The diagnosis was elective abortion due to maternal rubella. Aspiration curettage was performed. Which is the proper coding and sequencing of ICD-9-CM disease and procedure codes?
    a. 635.92, 647.53, 655.33, 69.51
    b. 635.92, 655.30, 69.51
    c. 635.92, 655.33, 69.52
    d. 655.33, 635.90, 69.51
13. A patient had an encounter for the fitting and adjustment of his artificial arm. Which is the proper coding (and sequencing if more than one code is assigned) of ICD-9-CM disease code(s)?
    a. 682.3, V52.0
    b. V52.0
    c. V52.0, 682.3
    d. V52.0, 887.4
14. The patient is a toddler who was traveling, unrestrained, in a motor vehicle driven by the patient's mother. A bee flew through the open window of the vehicle and stung the driver, causing her to veer off the road and hit a tree. The patient sustained multiple contusions and abrasions and a facial laceration. Which is the proper sequencing of E code(s) for this encounter?
    a. E905.3, E816.1
    b. E816.1, E905.3
    c. E816.1, E967.2
    d. E967.2, E816.1
15. A 5-hour-old infant, premature at 30 weeks, spontaneous birth, is transferred to the hospital's neonatal intensive care unit. Final diagnoses include male newborn; suspected respiratory distress syndrome due to prematurity.
    a. V30.00, 765.10, 769
    b. 765.10, 765.25, V71.89
    c. V30.00, 765.10, 765.25
    d. V30.00, 765.25, 769

16. Which procedure requires the assignment of an ICD-9-CM screening code?
    a. A seemingly well 52-year-old woman has an encounter for an occult blood test.
    b. A woman has an encounter for a routine postpartum examination.
    c. During an encounter, a patient states that he had poliomyelitis when he was young.
    d. Patient is admitted for observation for suspected tuberculosis.

17. A patient was admitted for the repair of a hiatal hernia by abdominal approach. The patient, who suffers from chronic paranoid schizophrenia, became agitated and, after consultation, received treatment for acute exacerbation of the condition. Which is the proper coding and sequencing of ICD-9-CM disease and procedure codes?
    a. 553.3, 295.30, 53.75
    b. 553.3, 295.34, 53.75
    c. 553.3, 53.75
    d. 750.6, 295.34, 53.75

18. A patient is admitted for breathing treatments due to acute exacerbation of chronic obstructive pulmonary disease (COPD) with asthma. Which is the proper coding (and sequencing if more than one code is assigned) of ICD-9-CM disease code(s)?
    a. 493.22
    b. 493.82
    c. 493.92, 496
    d. 496, 493.92

19. The patient was admitted for open biopsy of the frontal nasal sinus. Open biopsy was performed, and frozen section results from pathology were positive for cancer. The patient underwent an excision of the frontal sinus lesion during the same operative episode. Which is the proper coding (and sequencing if more than one code is assigned) of ICD-9-CM procedure code(s)?
    a. 22.12, 22.42
    b. 22.12
    c. 22.42
    d. 22.42, 22.12

20. The patient fell while climbing a tree, landed on the left side of her body, and sustained a concussion, along with numerous contusions of the left lower leg. (Her face, arms and trunk were protected by clothing.) The patient also sustained a laceration on the left lower leg. Which is the proper coding and sequencing of ICD-9-CM disease codes?
    a. 850.9, 891.0, E884.9
    b. 850.9, 891.0, 923.9, 920, E884.9
    c. 850.9, 891.0, 923.9, 924.5, 920, E884.9
    d. 923.9, 920, 850.9, 891.0, E884.9

ICD-10-CM Coding

1. A patient diagnosed with phlyctenulosis due to tuberculosis received inpatient care. Which is the proper coding (and sequencing if more than one code is assigned) of ICD-10-CM diagnosis code(s)?
    a. A18.52
    b. A18.52, H16.251
    c. H16.251
    d. H16.251, A18.52

2. A symptomatic HIV-positive patient is admitted to the hospital following a motor vehicle accident. The patient is diagnosed as having an open comminuted type I fracture of the left femoral shaft and receives inpatient treatment. The patient also received HIV antiviral medication while in the hospital. Which is the proper coding (and sequencing if more than one code is assigned) of ICD-10-CM diagnosis code(s)?
    a. B20
    b. B20, S72.355B
    c. S72.354B
    d. S72.355B, B20

3. A patient with chronic generalized disseminated choroiditis of the right eye presents with complaints of decreased vision. The patient is diagnosed with cataract due to choroiditis. Which is the proper coding (and sequencing if more than one code is assigned) of ICD-10-CM diagnosis code(s)?
    a. H26.221
    b. H26.221, H30.131
    b. H30.131
    d. H30.131, H26.221

4. A patient was admitted after an accidental industrial explosion occurred where he worked, resulting in an uncontrolled fire occurring in his factory building. As a result of exposure to flames, the patient sustained second-degree burns of the right ear, second- and third-degree burns of the right shoulder, and first- and second-degree burns of the right hand. Thirty-five percent of the body sustained burns,

with 10% third-degree burns, 20% second-degree burns, and 5% first-degree burns. Which is the proper coding and sequencing of ICD-10-CM diagnosis codes?

a. T20.21, T22.351, T23.201, T31.21, X00.0xxA, Y92.63
b. T22.351, T20.21, T23.201, T31.21, X00.0xxA, Y92.63
c. T31.21, T22.351, T20.21, T23.201, X00.0xxA, Y92.63
d. X00.0xxA, T22.351, T20.21, T23.201, T31.21, Y92.63

5. A patient underwent a pre-employment physical examination, which was performed by his family physician. During the office visit, the patient was diagnosed with an external ear infection, right ear. Which is the proper coding (and sequencing if more than one code is assigned) of ICD-10-CM diagnosis code(s)?

a. H60.01
b. H60.01, Z00.10
c. Z00.00
d. Z00.10, H60.01

6. A woman was admitted to the hospital in labor, and she delivered. The final diagnoses included delivery of single full term infant and obstructed labor due to an oversized infant. Which is the proper coding and sequencing of ICD-10-CM diagnosis codes?

a. O33.5xx1, Z37.0
b. O66.2, Z37.0
c. O66.2, O33.5xx1, Z37.0
d. O80, Z37.0

7. A patient previously underwent a mastectomy for treatment of an upper/inner quadrant adenocarcinoma of the left breast. Today the patient was registered as an outpatient and received radiation therapy. Which is the proper coding (and sequencing if more than one code is assigned) of ICD-10-CM diagnosis code(s)?

a. C60.211
b. C60.211, Z51.0
c. Z51.0
d. Z51.0, C60.211

8. A 105-year-old patient is underwent inpatient treatment for traumatic arthritis of the ankle. Which is the proper coding of the ICD-10-CM diagnosis codes?

a. M08.072
b. M11.872
c. M12.572
d. M13.872

9. A patient is admitted with complaints of chest pain and shortness of breath. During the exam, the patient revealed that he had recently come into contact with a white powdery substance in his duties as a postal employee and that a coworker had contracted anthrax. After examination, the physician diagnosed the patient with pneumonia due to pulmonary anthrax. Which is the proper coding (and sequencing if more than one code is assigned) of ICD-10-CM diagnosis code(s)?

a. A22.1
b. A22.1, Y38.6x2A
c. A22.1, Y38.6x2D
d. A22.1, Y38.6x2S

10. Which following is classified by assigning an adverse effect code from the ICD-10-CM Table of Drugs and Chemicals?

a. A patient was admitted in a comatose state. The patient's brother said that an empty bottle of Tylenol with Codeine, which had just been filled that morning, was found on the table beside the patient. The patient had threatened to hurt herself the day before.
b. A patient was prescribed Percocet for back pain due to a muscle injury and was admitted after a motor vehicle accident. The patient claimed that he wasn't getting enough relief from the pain, so he took an "extra dose" that morning and must have fallen asleep at the wheel.
c. A patient who takes prescribed doses of diclofenac for arthritis frequently takes aspirin for headaches. She is admitted to the hospital with gastrointestinal bleeding.
d. A patient with back pain due to a displaced disk was prescribed Darvocet. While taking prescribed doses, the patient experienced extreme fatigue and bradycardia.

11 A patient is diagnosed as having renal and heart disease due to hypertension. Which is the proper coding (and sequencing if more than one code is assigned) of ICD-10-CM diagnosis code(s)?

a. I10
b. I11.9, I12.9
c. I13.10
d. I15.8

12. A pregnant woman underwent outpatient termination of her first trimester pregnancy. The diagnosis was elective abortion due to maternal rubella. Which is the proper coding and sequencing of ICD-10-CM diagnosis codes?
    a. 035.3xx1, Z33.2
    b. 098.511, Z33.2
    c. 035.3xx1, 098.511, Z33.2
    d. Z33.2, 035.3xx1, 098.511
13. A patient was registered as an outpatient and underwent the fitting and adjustment of his partial artificial right arm. The patient had previously experienced a complete traumatic amputation at the level between the right shoulder and right elbow, which was the result of a malfunctioning hay-derrick in the fields at his farm. Which is the proper coding and sequencing of ICD-10-CM diagnosis codes?
    a. S48.111A, Z44.021, W30.2xxA, Y92.73
    b. W30.2xxA, Z44.021, S48.111A, Y92.73
    c. Y92.73, S48.111A, Z44.021, W30.2xxA
    d. Z44.021, S48.111D, W30.2xxD, Y92.73
14. Skilled nursing facility patient received evaluation and management services for senile dementia. Which is the proper coding (and sequencing if more than one code is assigned) of ICD-10-CM diagnosis code(s)?
    a. F02.80, G30.0
    b. F03
    c. F05
    d. R41.81
15. A male newborn was born in the hospital and discharged in excellent condition at 72 hours of age. Which is the proper coding of the ICD-10-CM diagnosis codes?
    a. P00.9
    b. Z00.110
    c. Z37.0
    d. Z38.0
16. Which requires the assignment of an ICD-10-CM screening code?
    a. A seemingly well 52-year-old woman has an encounter for an occult blood test.
    b. A woman has an encounter for a routine postpartum examination.
    c. During an encounter, a patient states that he had poliomyelitis when he was young.
    d. Patient is admitted for observation for suspected tuberculosis.
17. A patient was diagnosed with hiatal hernia by her primary care physician and scheduled for outpatient surgical repair. Which is the proper coding of the ICD-10-CM diagnosis codes?
    a. K44.0
    b. K44.1
    c. K44.9
    d. Q40.1
18. A patient received inpatient breathing treatments due to acute exacerbation of chronic obstructive pulmonary disease (COPD) with moderate persistent asthma. Which is the proper coding (and sequencing if more than one code is assigned) of ICD-10-CM diagnosis code(s)?
    a. J44.0, J45.30
    b. J44.1, J45.30
    c. J44.9, J45.30
    d. J45.901
19. The patient received emergency department services for accelerated angina pectoris. Which is the proper coding of ICD-10-CM diagnosis codes?
    a. I20.0
    b. I21.1
    c. I21.8
    d. I21.9
20. A 60-year-old patient accidentally took too many prescribed skeletal muscle relaxant pills this evening, and she is admitted for treatment of respiratory distress and severe abdominal pain with rigidity. Which is the proper coding and sequencing of ICD-10-CM diagnosis codes?
    a. T48.1x1, J80, R10.0
    b. T48.1x3, J84.8, R10.84
    c. T48.1x4, J84.9, R52
    d. T48.1x2, P22.0, R10.9

Chapter 5
ICD-9-CM and ICD-10-CM/PCS Hospital Inpatient Coding

ICD-9-CM Coding

1. A patient is admitted as a hospital inpatient for open reduction of fractured femur, sustained during a fall at home. The patient was also treated for congestive heart failure during the inpatient stay.

   a. 428.0, 79.25, E888.9, E849.0
   b. 428.0, 821.00, E888.9, E849.0, 79.25
   c. 821.00, 428.0, E888.9, E849.0
   d. 821.00, 428.0, E888.9, E849.0, 79.25

2. A patient underwent total left knee replacement surgery for severe osteoarthritis, left knee, as a hospital inpatient. Her inpatient stay was extended when a postoperative wound infection developed, which cultured as methicillin-resistant *Staphylococcus aureus*. The patient received successful intravenous antibiotic therapy for treatment of the infection and was discharged.

   a. 041.11, 715.96, 998.59, V09.0, 81.54, 99.29
   b. 715.96, 041.11, 998.59, V09.0, 81.54, 99.29
   c. 715.96, 998.59, 041.11, V09.0, 81.54, 99.29
   d. 998.59, 041.11, 715.96, V09.0, 81.54, 99.29

3. A patient underwent below-knee amputation of the left leg as a hospital inpatient due to peripheral vascular disease secondary to type 2 diabetes mellitus.

   a. 250.70, 443.89, 84.15
   b. 443.81, 250.70, 84.15
   c. 250.70, 443.81, 84.15
   d. V49.75, 84.15, 84.3

4. A hospital inpatient underwent sigmoidectomy with creation of temporary colostomy due to obstruction, which was determined to be carcinoma of the sigmoid colon. The patient received his first round of chemotherapy during his inpatient stay.

   a. 560.9, V58.11, 45.76, 46.11
   b. 751.2, V58.11, 45.76, 46.11
   c. 997.4, V58.11, 45.76, 46.11
   d. 153.3, V58.11, 45.76, 46.11

5. A patient is seen in the emergency department for high fever, chills, abdominal pain, and vomiting and is then admitted to the hospital with a diagnosis of severe sepsis due to *Pseudomonas* with septic shock.

   a. 038.43
   b. 038.43, 785.52
   c. 038.43, 995.92, 785.52
   d. 995.92, 038.43, 785.52

6. The patient was admitted to the hospital for acute treatment of decubitus bedsores of both hips.

   a. 707.00, 707.20
   b. 707.04, 707.20
   c. 707.07, 707.20
   d. 707.09, 707.20

7. A patient suffering from weight loss and fatigue is diagnosed with pancreatic cancer and anemia due to impaired absorption. The patient is admitted to the hospital and undergoes radical pancreatectomy.

   a. 157.9, 280.9, 52.7
   b. 157.9, 285.9, 52.7
   c. 157.9, 783.21, 780.79, 285.9, 52.7
   d. 783.21, 780.79, 157.9, 285.9, 52.7

8. A patient with acute cholecystitis was admitted to the hospital and underwent cholecystectomy. Postoperatively, the patient developed adult respiratory distress syndrome (ARDS).

   a. 518.5, 575.0, 51.04
   b. 575.0, 518.5, 51.04
   c. 575.0, 518.5, 51.22
   d. 575.10, 518.5, 51.04

9. A patient was admitted to the hospital for gastric ulcer with hemorrhage and perforation, which resulted in acute anemia.

   a. 285.1, 531.60
   b. 531.60, 285.9
   c. 531.60, 285.1
   d. 531.90, 459.0, 285.9

10. A patient with HIV disease was admitted with a stab wound to the thoracic aorta, which resulted when the patient fell on a pitchfork that was hidden in hay. The patient had been working on his farm property when he sustained the trauma. The wound was repaired with synthetic graft material.
    a. 042, 901.0, E888.0, E920.4, E849.0, 39.57
    b. 042, 901.0, E888.0, E966, E849.0, 39.57
    c. 879.8, 042, E888.0, E920.4, E849.0, 39.57
    d. 901.0, 042, E888.0, E920.4, E849.0, 39.57
11. A female patient is admitted with intrauterine pregnancy at term. Because of cephalopelvic disproportion and obstruction by the mother's bony pelvis during labor and delivery, a cesarean section was performed, and a healthy male infant was delivered.
    a. 653.41, V27.0, 74.99
    b. 653.41, V27.0
    c. 660.11, 653.41, 74.99
    d. 660.11, 653.41, V27.0, 74.99
12. During the same inpatient admission, a full-term infant was born and subsequently developed an upper respiratory infection (URI) and physiologic jaundice.
    a. 465.9, 774.6
    b. 465.9, 774.6, V30.00
    c. V30.00, 465.9
    d. V30.00, 465.9, 774.6
13. A Parkinson patient is admitted to the hospital with a urinary tract infection due to *Escherichia coli* and dehydration. The patient received treatment for all of these conditions.
    a. 332.0, 599.0, 276.51, 041.4
    b. 599.0, 041.4, 276.51, 332.0
    c. 599.0, 041.4, 332.0
    d. 599.0, 276.51, 332.0
14. A patient is admitted to the hospital and undergoes resection of congenital hallux valgus. To stabilize the foot during healing, the patient is fitted for a below-knee cast.
    a. 727.1, 77.59
    b. 735.0, 77.59, 93.53
    c. 755.56, 77.59
    d. 755.66, 77.59, 93.53
15. A 17-hour-old infant weighing 1000 grams and premature at 30 weeks via spontaneous birth was transferred to Alfred State Medical Center's neonatal intensive care unit (NICU). Final diagnoses include female newborn and suspected respiratory disease due to prematurity.
    a. 765.14, 765.25, 769
    b. 765.14, 769
    c. 765.14, 765.25
    d. 765.14, V71.89
16. A patient is admitted with acute coronary insufficiency of the right coronary artery with hypertensive heart disease. Percutaneous transluminal coronary angioplasty (PTCA) with insertion of coronary stent is performed.
    a. 411.89, 402.90, 00.66, 36.06, 00.45, 00.40
    b. 411.89, 402.90, 36.06, 00.45, 00.40
    c. 411.89, 402.90, 36.06, 00.45, 00.40
    d. 411.89, 402.90, 39.50, 36.06
17. A patient was brought to the hospital by ambulance and admitted for cerebrovascular accident (CVA) secondary to cerebral embolism with infarction.
    a. 434.11
    b. 436
    c. 436, 434.11, 437.9
    d. 437.9
18. A patient is admitted to the hospital and undergoes repair of cleft palate. The patient is a child who is severely mentally retarded and receives appropriate treatment for this condition during the hospitalization.
    a. 318.1, 749.00, 27.62
    b. 318.1, 749.00, 27.64
    c. 749.00, 27.64
    d. 749.00, 318.1, 27.62
19. A woman who receives treatment for depression is brought to the emergency department with complaints of acute pelvic pain and nausea, which began one hour prior to admission. She was taken to surgery and underwent left oophorectomy. The postoperative diagnosis was torsion of the ovary. The patient received medication for her depression and for Hashimoto thyroiditis during the hospitalization.
    a. 311, 620.5, 245.2, 65.39
    b. 620.5, 311, 245.2
    c. 620.5, 311, 245.2, 65.39
    d. 620.5, 65.39

20. An unconscious patient is admitted with cerebral anoxia due to previous overdose of sedatives (AHFS 28:24) as a suicide attempt. During this admission, the patient receives treatment for cerebral anoxia.
    a. 348.1, 909.0, E950.2
    b. 348.1, 909.0, E959
    c. 348.1, E950.2
    d. 799.0, 909.0, E959

ICD-10-CM/PCS Coding

21. A patient undergoes open reduction internal fixation of left femoral shaft fracture (closed). The patient fell in the kitchen at her home. The patient was also treated for congestive heart failure during the inpatient stay.
    a. S72.011A, I50.9, 0QS60ZZ
    b. S72.021A, I50.9, 0QSB05Z
    c. S72.091A, I50.9, 0QS9XZZ
    d. S72.301A, I50.9, 0QS804Z
22. A patient underwent outpatient total left knee replacement surgery using a synthetic substitute for severe osteoarthritis of the left knee, as a hospital inpatient. She was admitted as an inpatient when a postoperative wound infection developed, which cultured as methicillin-resistant *Staphylococcus aureus*. The patient received successful intravenous antibiotic therapy for treatment of the infection and was discharged.
    a. B95.6, M17.9, T81.4xxA, Z16, 0SRD0JZ, 3E03329
    b. M17.9, B95.6, T81.4xxA, Z16, 0SRD0JZ, 3E03329
    c. T81.4xxA, B95.6, M17.9, Z16, 0SRD0JZ, 3E03329
    d. Z16, B95.6, M17.9, T81.4xxA , 0SRD0JZ, 3E03329
23. A patient underwent below-knee amputation of the left leg as a hospital inpatient due to peripheral angiopathy secondary to type 2 diabetes mellitus.
    a. E11.51, 0Y6C0Z3
    b. E11.51, 0Y6H0Z3
    c. E11.51, I79.8, 0Y6H0Z1
    d. Z89.52, E11.51, I79.8, 0Y6C0Z3
24. A hospital inpatient underwent open sigmoidectomy with creation of temporary colostomy due to obstruction, which was determined to be carcinoma of the sigmoid colon. The patient received his first round of chemotherapy during his inpatient stay.
    a. C18.7, Z51.11, 0DTN0ZZ, 0D1N0Z4
    b. C18.7, K56.60, Z51.11, 0DTN0ZZ, 0D1N8Z4
    c. C19, Z51.11, 0DTN0ZZ, 0D1N0JN
    d. K56.60, Z51.11, 0DTN0ZZ, 0D1N0ZN
25. A patient is seen in the emergency department for high fever, chills, abdominal pain, and vomiting and is then admitted to the hospital with a diagnosis of severe sepsis due to *Pseudomonas* with septic shock.
    a. A41.52
    b. A41.52, R65.21
    c. A41.9, B96.5, R65.21
    d. R65.21, B96.5
26. The patient was admitted to the hospital for acute treatment of stage III decubitus bedsores of both hips. Patient underwent wound debridement, bilateral hips, using high pressure waterjet with suction.
    a. I96, L89.203, F08G5, 0HD8XZZ
    b. L89.153, 0HDGXZZ, 0HDHXZZ
    c. L89.213, L89.223, I96, 0HD6XZZ
    d. L89.213, L89.223, 0HD9XZZ
27. A patient suffering from weight loss and fatigue is diagnosed with pancreatic cancer and anemia due to impaired absorption. The patient is admitted to the hospital and undergoes radical pancreatectomy.
    a. C25.9, D50.9, F10.99, 0FPG0ZZ
    b. C25.9, D50.9, 0FTG0ZZ
    c. C25.9, F10.99, 0FTG0ZZ
    d. C25.9, 0FPG0ZZ
28. A patient with acute cholecystitis was admitted to the hospital and underwent open cholecystectomy. Postoperatively, the patient developed adult respiratory failure.
    a. J80, K81.0, 0FB40ZZ
    b. K81.0, 0FB40ZZ
    c. K81.0, J95.82, 0FT40ZZ
    d. K81.9, J95.89, 0FT40ZZ
29. A patient was admitted to the hospital with acute gastric ulcer with hemorrhage and perforation. Patient had previously been treated conservatively during a previous hospitalization with nasogastric suction as well as intravenous, pain control, antiulcer medication, and antibiotics. During this admission, patient

underwent open partial gastrectomy. She recuperated postoperatively and was discharged home in stable condition.

a. K25.0, K25.1, 0DB60ZZ
b. K25.2, 0DT60ZZ
c. K25.3, 0DT60ZZ
d. K25.9, 0DB60ZZ

30. A patient with HIV disease was admitted with a puncture wound to the left front wall of the thoracic, penetrating the thoracic cavity and lacerating the thoracic aorta. The patient was working his farm and fell on a pitchfork that was hidden in the hay. Patient underwent open repair of thoracic aorta with insertion of synthetic substitute and open repair of chest skin, subcutaneous tissue, and fascia.

a. B20, S25.01xA, S21.332A, W27.1xxA, Y92.71, 02QW3ZZ, 0JQ60ZZ, 0HR5XZZ
b. S21.332A, S25.01xA, W27.1xxA, Y92.71, Z21, 02RW0JZ, 0JQ60ZZ, 0HQ5XZZ
c. S25.01xA, S21.332A, B20, W27.1xxA, Y92.71, 02UW0JZ, 0JQ60ZZ, 0HQ5XZZ
d. Z21, S21.332A, S25.01xA, W27.1xxA, Y92.71, 02HW0ZZ, 0JQ60ZZ, 0HX5XZZ

31. A female patient is admitted with intrauterine pregnancy at term. A classical cesarean section was performed due to hydrocephalic fetus. A live male infant was delivered.

a. O33.6xx0, Z37.0, 10D00Z0
b. O33.7xx0, Z37.0, 10D00Z1
c. O33.8xx0, Z37.0, 10D00Z2
d. O33.9xx0, Z37.0, 10D00Z8

32. A full-term male was born in the hospital and subsequently developed upper respiratory infection.

a. J06.9, Z38.00
b. J06.9
c. Z38.00
d. Z38.00, J06.9

33. A patient admitted to the hospital for treatment of parkinsonism and urinary tract infection due to *Escherichia coli*. The patient received treatment for all of these conditions.

a. B96.2, G20, N39.0
b. G20, N39.0, B96.2
c. G21.8, N39.0, B96.2
d. N39.0, G20, B96.2

34. A patient diagnosed with bunion, right foot, underwent open bunionectomy, right foot, and was fitted with a below-knee cast.

a. M20.11, 0QBQ0ZZ, 2W3QX2Z
b. M20.1, 0QBL0ZZ, 2W3QX2Z
c. Q66.6, 0QBQ0ZZ, 2W3UX2Z
d. Q66.61, 0QBL0ZZ, 2W3QX2Z

35. A 17-hour-old infant was transferred to Alfred State Medical Center's neonatal intensive care unit (NICU) for treatment of respiratory failure of newborn due to prematurity at 30 weeks' gestation.

a. J96.0, Z38.00, P07.31
b. J96.9, P07.30
c. P28.5, P07.31
d. P28.81, P07.30

36. A patient received inpatient treatment for atherosclerotic heart disease of the native right coronary artery. Patient has been on medication for hypercholesterolemia and atherosclerosis due to lipid-rich plaque. Percutaneous transluminal coronary angioplasty (PTCA), right coronary artery, with insertion of coronary stent was performed.

a. G45.1, E78.0, 02Q00ZZ
b. I24.0, E78.0, 02103D4
c. I24.8, I25.83, 02Q03ZZ
d. I25.10, I25.83, E78.0, 02703DZ

37. A patient received inpatient treatment for cerebral embolism with infarction.

a. G08
b. I24.0
c. I63.30
d. I63.40

38. A patient undergoes open repair of cleft hard palate as a hospital inpatient.

a. Q35.1, 0CQ20ZZ
b. Q35.3, 0CQ30ZZ
c. Q35.5, 0CQ20ZZ, 0CQ30ZZ
d. Q35.9, 0CQ20ZZ

39. A patient undergoes inpatient open oophorectomy, left, for congenital torsion of the left ovary.

a. N83.51, 0UB10ZZ
b. N83.53, 0UC10ZZ
c. Q50.2, 0UT10ZZ
d. Q55.69, 0UDN0ZZ

40. The patient received inpatient treatment for cerebral anoxia, which was the result of a suicide attempt using sedatives approximately three years earlier.

a. R09.01A
b. R09.01S
c. R09.01, T42.72S
d. T42.72S, R09.01

Chapter 6
ICD-9-CM and ICD-10-CM Outpatient and Physician Office Coding

1. Qualified diagnoses are a necessary part of a patient's hospital and office record; however, physician offices are required to report:
   a. qualified diagnoses for inpatients and outpatients.
   b. qualified diagnoses related to outpatient procedures.
   c. signs and symptoms in addition to qualified diagnoses.
   d. signs and symptoms instead of qualified diagnoses.
2. Brenda submitted a Medicare claim on which the first-listed diagnosis code was for encounter for speech therapy and the second-listed code was for aphasia. The Medicare administrative contractor (MAC) denied the claim, stating that its policy was not to pay claims that report health status codes first. Brenda contacted the MAC and explained that she knew this claim was submitted correctly and in accordance with CMS's *Diagnostic Coding and Reporting Guidelines for Outpatient Services: Hospital-Based and Physician Office.* The MAC's representative repeated the policy and would not process the claim to provide reimbursement to the physician. Brenda then contacted her regional CMS office for resolution and relayed the details of the incident. How would you summarize the way Brenda handled this situation?
   a. Brenda's actions were partially warranted, but she should never contact CMS.
   b. Brenda's actions were warranted; but before contacting CMS, she should have provided the MAC with information about the HIPAA provision that requires compliance with the ICD-9-CM official coding guidelines.
   c. Brenda's actions were completely unwarranted because the MAC can decide what claims to reimburse based on internal policies.
   d. Brenda's actions were completely warranted because she knew she had submitted a clean claim and the MAC should stay current regarding HIPAA regulations.
3. If an examination is for administrative purposes (e.g., preemployment physical) and it is not focused on any particular condition, which additional codes may be reported?
   a. chronic conditions
   b. chronic conditions and history of codes
   c. preexisting conditions and history of codes
   d. preexisting conditions, chronic conditions, and history of codes
4. Which is reportable as a first-listed diagnosis code on an outpatient claim?
   a. Infection with drug-resistant microorganisms
   b. Problems with special senses and other special functions
   c. Organ or tissue replaced by transplant
   d. Donors
5. Signs and symptoms should be coded when _______.
   a. a definitive diagnosis has been established by the physician.
   b. a qualified diagnosis has been confirmed by the physician.
   c. they are not routinely associated with the disease process that initiated the encounter.
   d. they are part of the disease process that initiated the encounter.

6. Etiology/manifestation coding may require the assignment of _______.
   a. a history code
   b. a late effect code
   c. an external cause code
   d. more than one code
7. A patient is treated for dysphagia, which is a late effect of the poliomyelitis he had several years ago. How would this be coded in ICD-9-CM?
   a. Assign a code for dysphagia and a code for late effect of poliomyelitis.
   b. Code only the dysphagia.
   c. Report codes for poliomyelitis, dysphagia, and late effect of poliomyelitis, in that order.
   d. Report poliomyelitis as the first-listed code and dysphagia as an additional code.
8. Which describes the condition chiefly responsible for services provided during an outpatient visit?
   a. encounter
   b. first-listed diagnosis
   c. principal diagnosis
   d. qualified diagnosis
9. History codes may be reported as secondary codes if the historical condition or family history has an impact on current care or influences treatment. Reporting history codes _______ reimbursement.
   a. always increases
   b. could increase
   c. decreases
   d. never impacts
10. A patient is seen in the physician's office with the complaint of a sore throat. The physician orders lab tests and documents "pharyngitis, rule out strep infection." The next day the lab results are interpreted by the physician, whose report lists "influenza with pharyngitis" as the diagnosis. Which condition(s) are reported on the outpatient claim?
    a. influenza
    b. influenza with pharyngitis
    c. pharyngitis with strep throat
    d. sore throat
11. Preadmission testing (PAT):
    a. can be performed only for outpatient surgery.
    b. could result in higher reimbursement to a health care facility.
    c. does not facilitate the patient's treatment.
    d. is performed only for inpatient admissions.
12. A patient with pelvic pain underwent outpatient laser laparoscopy for suspected ovarian cysts. During the procedure, no cysts were found; but endometriosis was discovered and documented as the postoperative diagnosis. Which is reported on the outpatient claim?
    a. endometriosis
    b. endometriosis and pelvic pain
    c. ovarian cysts
    d. pelvic pain
13. Which is reported when an outpatient diagnostic test is performed to confirm a suspected condition and the test rules out the condition?
    a. confirmed diagnosis
    b. qualified diagnosis
    c. screening code
    d. signs and symptoms
14. A patient presents with back pain and is referred for magnetic resonance imaging (MRI) to rule out a herniated disk. The interpreted MRI report confirms a herniated disk. However, the encounter was coded as back pain. Which would be an acceptable reason for this code assignment?
    a. The reason for the encounter is all that should be coded.
    b. The coder did not review the entire chart before assigning codes.
    c. The physician's interpretation of the test result is unclear, and the physician was unavailable for clarification.
    d. The report containing the interpretation of the MRI was not available at the time the claim was processed.

15. A patient is referred for an x-ray for suspected rib fracture. After reviewing the x-ray, the interpreting physician confirms the rib fracture and also discovers spots on a lung. How should this be coded?
    a. Only the fractured rib is coded because the spots on the lung are incidental.
    b. Only the spots on the lung are coded because they require immediate intervention.
    c. The fractured rib is coded and reported first, and the spots on the lung are coded and reported second because they are an incidental finding.
    d. The spots on the lung are coded and reported first because they are more serious; the fractured rib is coded and reported second.

16. A patient presents with leg pain and is referred for an x-ray to determine whether there is a fracture. During the performance of the diagnostic test, the interpreting physician noted arthritis in the ankle. The final diagnosis is sprained ankle. Which is the secondary condition?
    a. arthritis
    b. fracture
    c. leg pain
    d. sprained ankle

17. A patient had a colonoscopy performed, and the encounter was reported as a health status code for screening. A code for benign polyp was also reported. Which statement best describes the situation?
    a. The diagnostic test (colonoscopy) was performed in the absence of signs or symptoms, and the polyp was discovered upon screening.
    b. The diagnostic test (colonoscopy) was performed in the absence of signs or symptoms.
    c. There was a qualified diagnosis of benign polyp, which was confirmed by the colonoscopy.
    d. There was a qualified diagnosis of benign polyp, which was not confirmed by the colonoscopy.

18. Which health care service includes both preventative and acute care, is often provided as outpatient care, and is referred to as the point of first contact?
    a. primary health care
    b. principal health care
    c. secondary health care
    d. tertiary health care

19. Ambulatory patients (or outpatients) are treated and released the same day and do not stay overnight in the hospital, which means that their maximum length of stay is:
    a. 23 hours.
    b. 23 hours, 59 minutes, and 59 seconds.
    c. 24 hours.
    d. 24 hours, 59 minutes, and 59 seconds.

20. Which are treated for urgent problems (e.g., trauma) and are either released the same day or admitted to the hospital as inpatients?
    a. ambulatory surgery patients
    b. clinic outpatients
    c. emergency patients
    d. referred outpatients

Chapter 7
HCPCS Level II National Coding System

1. The HCPCS level II national coding system:
   a. describes common medical services and supplies not classified in CPT.
   b. ensures the uniform reporting of diagnoses on submitted claims.
   c. has code descriptors that describe diagnoses, services, and procedures.
   d. is a reimbursement methodology for making coverage and payment determinations.
2. HCPCS level II national codes are:
   a. intended for use by all private and public health insurers.
   b. maintained by the AMA's Editorial Board, which makes decisions about additions, revisions, and deletions.
   c. sometimes replaced by HCPCS level II temporary codes.
   d. updated by CMS when necessary, without participation by the HCPCS National Panel.
3. HCPCS level II temporary codes are:
   a. deleted if not replaced by permanent codes by the HCPCS National Panel within five years.
   b. included as over 50 percent of the HCPCS level II codes.
   c. maintained by the CMS and other members of the HCPCS National Panel, independent of HCPCS level II permanent codes.
   d. updated once a year on January 1.
4. In which section of HCPCS level II would you locate codes for durable medical equipment (DME)-related supplies, accessories, maintenance, and repair?
   a. Administrative, Miscellaneous and Investigational
   b. Durable Medical Equipment
   c. Medical and Surgical Supplies
   d. Outpatient PPS
5. In which section of HCPCS level II would you locate a code for an office visit provided for the sole purpose of monitoring or changing drug prescriptions used in the treatment of mental psychoneurotic and personality disorders?
   a. Diagnostic Radiology Services
   b. Medical Services
   c. Pathology and Laboratory Services
   d. Procedures/Professional Services (Temporary)
6. In which section of HCPCS level II would you locate codes for chemistry, microbiology, and toxicology tests?
   a. Administrative, Miscellaneous and Investigational
   b. Diagnostic Radiology Services
   c. Pathology and Laboratory Services
   d. Procedures/Professional Services (Temporary)
7. In which section of HCPCS level II would you locate codes for exercise equipment, noncovered items and services, nonprescription drugs, and radiopharmaceutical diagnostic imaging agents?
   a. Administrative, Miscellaneous and Investigational
   b. Diagnostic Radiology Services
   c. Drugs Administered Other Than Oral Method
   d. Durable Medical Equipment

8. Which ensures that the provider will receive reimbursement from the patient in the event that medical necessity cannot be established for a procedure, service, or supply?
   a. advance beneficiary notice
   b. HCPCS level II modifiers
   c. *Medicare Carriers Manual* (MCM)
   d. *Medicare National Coverage Determinations Manual*
9. Where can you find clarification about local coverage determinations (LCDs)?
   a. DME MAC medical review policies
   b. *Medicare Benefit Policy Manual*
   c. *Medicare National Coverage Determinations Manual*
   d. *Medicare Program Integrity Manual*
10. Which procedures/services fall under the jurisdiction of the primary MAC only?
   a. dental procedures
   b. enteral and parenteral therapy
   c. hearing and vision services
   d. prosthetic and orthotic procedures
11. A diabetic patient received a J-cell alkaline replacement battery for her home blood glucose monitor.
   a. A4233
   b. A4234
   c. A4235
   d. A4236
12. A pediatric patient received 1 unit (100 calories) of enteral soy-based formula through a feeding tube, nutritionally complete with intact nutrients.
   a. B4102
   b. B4103
   c. B4159
   d. B4160
13. Heavy-duty wheelchair.
   a. K0001
   b. K0003
   c. K0006
   d. K0007
14. Non-removable longitudinal arch support (attached to shoe), left foot.
   a. L3070
   b. L3070-LT
   c. L3090
   d. L3090-LT
15. Halo procedure, cervical halo incorporated into Milwaukee-type orthosis.
   a. L0120
   b. L0810
   c. L0820
   d. L0830
16. Transportation of portable ECG to facility or location, per patient.
   a. G0403
   b. R0070
   c. R0075
   d. R0076
17. Home infusion therapy, peritoneal dialysis, administrative services.
   a. S9330
   b. S9338
   c. S9339
   d. S9353
18. Substance abuse services, skills development.
   a. H0047
   b. H2034
   c. T1010
   d. T1012
19. Assistive listening telecommunication device for the deaf (TDD).
   a. V5267
   b. V5269
   c. V5272
   d. V5273
20. Compression burn garment, chin strap, custom fabricated.
   a. A6501
   b. A6502
   c. A6504
   d. A6512

Chapter 8
Introduction to CPT Coding

1. The regulation that required new, revised, and deleted CPT codes to be implemented each January 1 was a result of the:
   a. American Medical Association CPT Editorial Board's publication of "early release" codes.
   b. Health Insurance, Portability, and Accountability Act (HIPAA).
   c. Medicare Prescription Drug, Improvement, and Modernization Act (MMA).
   d. Omnibus Budget Reconciliation Act (OBRA).
2. The draping and positioning of a patient is coded as:
   a. additions to the standard of practice.
   b. billable services.
   c. integral to the standard of practice.
   d. separately reportable services.
3. The code description for CPT code 70492:
   a. contains the entire description next to the code number.
   b. requires the coder to refer back to code 70490 for the common portion of the code description.
   c. requires the coder to report both codes 70492 and 70490.
   d. results in CPT code 70492 being considered a stand-alone code.
4. Using the CPT index, select the main term, subterm, and qualifier, respectively, that results in the assignment of a code for "transcatheter placement of an intracoronary stent(s), percutaneous, without therapeutic intervention; 2 vessels."
   a. insertion, stent, coronary
   b. percutaneous transluminal angioplasty, artery, coronary
   c. stent, placement, coronary
   d. transcatheter, stent, coronary
5. Using the CPT index, select the main term, subterm, and qualifier, respectively, that results in the assignment of a code for "liver imaging with vascular flow."
   a. hepatic duct, nuclear medicine, imaging
   b. imaging, liver
   c. liver, nuclear medicine, imaging
   d. vascular surgery, unlisted services and procedures
6. Code 45379 defines a colonoscopy with removal of foreign body. Using the CPT index, determine which main term would be used to locate that code.
   a. exploration
   b. foreign body removal
   c. intestine
   d. removal
7. Appendix G contains a summary of CPT codes that include:
   a. add-on codes.
   b. conscious sedation.
   c. genetic testing modifiers.
   d. those exempt from modifier -51.
8. Which symbols identify CPT codes that are listed in its appendices?
   a. bullet, semicolon, bull's-eye
   b. plus, forbidden, bull's-eye
   c. plus, forbidden, bullet
   d. triangle, horizontal triangles, forbidden

9. A triangle symbol located to the left of a CPT code number signifies that the code is:
   a. new.
   b. reported with another code.
   c. revised.
   d. stand-alone.
10. Which symbol indicates that a change has been made to a CPT code, code description, guideline, and/or note when compared with the previous year's coding manual?
    a. bull's-eye
    b. forbidden
    c. semicolon
    d. triangle
11. Headings and subheadings are also called:
    a. categories and subcategories.
    b. main terms and subterms.
    c. sections and subsections.
    d. titles and subtitles.
12. Guidelines, notes, and descriptive qualifiers are found in CPT:
    a. headings only.
    b. sections and headings only.
    c. sections only.
    d. sections, subsections, headings, and subheadings.
13. "Radiology" and "Pathology and Laboratory" are CPT:
    a. descriptive qualifiers.
    b. headings.
    c. sections.
    d. subsections under the "laboratory" section of CPT.
14. If evaluation and management (E/M) services for a patient take longer than normal, which CPT modifier is added to the reported E/M code?
    a. -21
    b. -24
    c. -25
    d. -51
15. Terms found in provider documentation (e.g., difficult, extensive, or unusual) would support adding modifier _______ to a CPT code.
    a. -22
    b. -23
    c. -58
    d. -99
16. An intoxicated patient was brought to the emergency department with a skin laceration, for which he received stitches. The patient became combative and subsequently tore out the stitches, which were repaired by the same physician. Which CPT modifier would be reported for the second stitching procedure?
    a. -55
    b. -58
    c. -76
    d. -77
17. Which CPT modifier(s) are reported when surgery is performed by two surgeons?
    a. -58
    b. -62
    c. -76
    d. -77
18. Which CPT modifier is reported when a procedure is performed on an infant who weighs less than 4 kilograms (kg)?
    a. -54
    b. -59
    c. -63
    d. -66
19. NCCI edits are updated _______ and available to _______.
    a. annually; everyone
    b. annually; Medicare administrative contractors
    c. quarterly; everyone
    d. quarterly; physicians and other providers
20. The National Correct Coding Initiative (NCCI) edits are available as:
    a. paid subscriptions.
    b. paper-based document purchases.
    c. spreadsheets.
    d. telephone inquiry.

Chapter 9
CPT Evaluation and Management

1. Which code reflects a level 5 E/M service?
   a. 99211
   b. 99212
   c. 99214
   d. 99215
2. When an unlisted procedure or service code is reported, a special report must accompany the claim to describe _______ of the procedure or service.
   a. the nature, extent, and need
   b. the place of service and type of service
   c. the type of service and amount of time required
   d. whether the patient is new or established
3. Clinical examples of E/M codes are found in _______ of the CPT coding manual.
   a. Appendix A
   b. Appendix B
   c. Appendix C
   d. Appendix D
4. A patient returns to the physician's office today with neck and back pain. During a previous office visit last month, the patient was diagnosed as having multiple areas of bulging discs. The patient is not considered a surgical candidate at this time. Significant trauma in the past is noted, but C2-12 are intact. Deep tendon reflexes are within normal limits and symmetrical in the upper and lower extremities. Heart, lungs, and abdomen are without significant pathology. There are marked paravertebral spasms throughout the cervical, thoracic, and lumbar regions. HEENT: Patient has bilateral otitis externa noted. Which code is assigned for this level 4 E/M service?
   a. 99203
   b. 99204
   c. 99213
   d. 99214
5. Which terms describe the levels of work involved in medical decision-making?
   a. face-to-face, unit-floor, preencounter, postencounter
   b. minimal, self-limited, low severity, moderate severity, high severity
   c. problem focused, expanded problem focused, detailed, comprehensive
   d. straightforward, low complexity, moderate complexity, high complexity
6. A patient experiencing acute breathing trouble required one hour of direct face-to-face care from the physician. In addition to the appropriate level of E/M service code, which E/M subsection should be referenced to assign an additional code?
   a. Care Plan Oversight Services
   b. Case Management Services
   c. Preventive Medicine Services
   d. Prolonged Services
7. A physician spent approximately two hours on a conference call coordinating activities with members of a transplant team who were preparing to perform an organ transplant on his patient. From which E/M subsection would the code for this service be reported?
   a. Care Plan Oversight Services
   b. Case Management Services
   c. Critical Care Services
   d. Special Evaluation and Management Services

8. A patient was admitted to the hospital on November 4 for reconstructive surgery. After surgery, the physician reviewed the patient's record to determine how the patient was responding to the treatment. The patient was discharged November 6. Under which subsection of Hospital Inpatient Services would the code for the November 6 encounter be located?
   a. Hospital Discharge Services
   b. Initial Hospital Care
   c. Observation or Inpatient Care Services
   d. Subsequent Hospital Care

9. A patient presented with a bruised and swollen finger and was in extreme pain. The patient told the physician that she was loading groceries in her car when her son leaned on the door, causing it to slam shut on her finger. An x-ray was obtained, and the broken finger was put in a splint. After asking about any known allergies, the physician wrote a prescription for the pain and advised the patient to return if symptoms persisted beyond a week. Which type of history was performed?
   a. comprehensive
   b. detailed
   c. expanded problem focused
   d. problem focused

10. Which is considered a consultation and occurs when a surgeon requests that a specialist or another physician examine a patient and indicate whether the patient can withstand the expected risks of a specific surgery?
    a. confirmatory consultation
    b. physician standby services
    c. preoperative clearance
    d. special evaluation and management services

11. A woman is seen in the emergency department for a broken arm she sustained after slipping on ice. A problem-focused history and physical were performed, and medical decision-making was straightforward.
    a. 99201
    b. 99221
    c. 99281
    d. 99282

12. A patient was seen in the office and underwent a baseline physical for the purpose of obtaining medical disability.
    a. 99201
    b. 99211
    c. 99381
    d. 99455

13. A patient is brought to the emergency department with a stab wound in the upper arm. An expanded problem-focused history and examination are performed, and medical decision-making is of moderate complexity.
    a. 99202
    b. 99213
    c. 99232
    d. 99283

14. A patient with a heart condition is scheduled to undergo a cesarean section. Due to the high-risk nature of the delivery, the attending physician requests standby service from a cardiac surgeon; and 45 minutes later the patient delivers a healthy newborn with no complications.
    a. 99026
    b. 99027
    c. 99360
    d. 99360, 99360

15. An inpatient is seen for an initial consultation regarding a cardiac procedure. The consulting physician documented a comprehensive history and exam and spent 80 minutes with the patient. Medical decision-making was of moderate complexity.
    a. 99244
    b. 99254
    c. 99255
    d. 99284

16. An infant is admitted to the neonatal intensive care unit (NICU) shortly after birth on Tuesday morning. The infant remains on life support through Thursday.
    a. 99295, 99296, 99296
    b. 99468, 99469, 99469
    c. 99468
    d. 99468, 99469

17. A nursing facility resident began to experience periods of memory loss and disorientation. The physician performed a detailed interval history and exam. The physician spent 30 minutes talking with the patient and documenting in the medical record.
    a. 99307
    b. 99308
    c. 99309
    d. 99310
18. Dr. Killean called a patient to report the results of his blood test that was performed 10 days ago, and he instructed the patient to lower the dosage of his Coumadin and schedule an appointment to be seen in the office 30 days from now. Medical discussion during this telephone service was 10 minutes in duration.
    a. 99441
    b. 99442
    c. 99443
    d. 99444
19. Physician spent 40 minutes reviewing reports and modifying pain medication and oxygen orders for a 70-year-old hospice patient with terminal lung disease and a do-not-resuscitate order.
    a. 99374
    b. 99377
    c. 99378
    d. 99379
20. The physician documented the history and exam of a normal, healthy newborn admitted and discharged on the same day.
    a. 99221
    b. 99431
    c. 99463
    d. 99499

Chapter 10
CPT Anesthesia

1. Which is loss of pain sensation without loss of consciousness?
   a. analgesia
   b. analgesic
   c. anesthesia
   d. anesthetic
2. Which is the administration of varying amounts of local, regional, and certain mind-altering drugs during a procedure?
   a. conscious sedation
   b. general anesthesia
   c. local anesthesia
   d. monitored anesthesia care
3. The postanesthesia evaluation that is documented by the anesthesiologist or CRNA is _______.
   a. also called postoperative pain management
   b. done prior to the administration of anesthesia
   c. included in the anesthesia services code
   d. reported as a separate anesthesia service
4. When calculating anesthesia fees, which is the dollar amount assigned to a geographic location?
   a. anesthesia conversion factor
   b. anesthesia time unit(s)
   c. base unit value
   d. modifying unit
5. Which indicates the patient's condition at the time anesthesia was administered?
   a. CPT alphabetic modifier
   b. HCPCS level II modifier
   c. physical status modifier
   d. special report
6. Anesthesia services are reported based on time, which:
   a. begins after the patient has received anesthesia and ends when the anesthesiologist or CRNA is no longer in personal attendance.
   b. includes monitoring during administration of regional block anesthesia and during the procedure.
   c. incorporates interval and recovery room times.
   d. is reported in time units for which nonmonitored time is taken into consideration.
7. A diabetic patient who is otherwise healthy has a procedure performed under general anesthesia. The anesthesia services last 45 minutes, and the anesthesia code for this procedure has a base unit value of 5. The conversion factor for the geographic area is $19.20. Which is the correct formula for calculating the anesthesia fee?
   a. (5 + 3 + 1) × $19.20 = $172.80
   b. (5 + 45 + 1) × $19.20 = $979.20
   c. ($19.20 + 3 + 1) × 5 = $116.00
   d. ($19.20 + 5 + 1) × 3 = $75.60
8. Which anesthesia subsection contains the code(s) for surgery on the patella?
   a. knee and popliteal area
   b. pelvis (except hip)
   c. perineum
   d. shoulder and axilla
9. Which anesthesia subsection contains a code for lumbar hernia repair?
   a. intrathoracic
   b. lower abdomen
   c. thorax
   d. upper abdomen

10. Which anesthesia subsection contains the code(s) for myelography?
    a. obstetric procedures
    b. other procedures
    c. radiological procedures
    d. spine and spinal cord
11. An anesthesiologist provides anesthesia services for a right tympanotomy procedure performed on a healthy 6-month-old child.
    a. 00126
    b. 00126, 99100
    c. 00126-P1-AA, 99100
    d. 69420
12. A CRNA provides anesthesia services, with medical direction by a physician, for the reconstructive repair of pectus excavatum on a healthy patient.
    a. 00474
    b. 00474-P1-QX
    c. 00474-P2
    d. 21740
13. A CRNA provides monitored anesthesia care, without medical direction by a physician, during insertion of permanent transvenous pacemaker for a patient with pulmonary valve disorder.
    a. 00530-P3
    b. 00530-P3-QS-QZ
    c. 00530-QS
    d. 33206
14. An anesthesiologist provides anesthesia services for a lumbar sympathectomy on an otherwise healthy patient.
    a. 00630-P1-AA
    b. 00632-P1-AA
    c. 00635-P1-AA
    d. 32664
15. An anesthesiologist provides anesthesia services for a stomach restriction procedure on a patient with morbid obesity.
    a. 00797
    b. 00797-P1-AA
    c. 00797-P2-AA
    d. 00797-P3-AA
16. An anesthesiologist provides anesthesia services for a left femoral artery embolectomy procedure performed on a patient with an embolus in the left femoral artery (mild systemic disease).
    a. 01270
    b. 01272-P2-AA
    c. 01274-P2-AA
    d. 34201-P2-AA
17. A CRNA, with medical direction by a physician, provides anesthesia services to an otherwise healthy patient who undergoes an open elbow-to-shoulder tenotomy, left.
    a. 01710
    b. 01712-P1-QX
    c. 01714
    d. 23405-P1-QX
18. An anesthesiologist provides anesthesia services for a diagnostic arteriography of the left common carotid artery on a patient with possible carotid occlusion.
    a. 01916-P2-AA
    b. 01924-P2-AA
    c. 01926-P2-AA
    d. 01930-P2-AA
19. An anesthesiologist provides anesthesia services to a healthy patient who undergoes neuraxial labor anesthesia for planned vaginal delivery.
    a. 01967
    b. 01967-23
    c. 01967-P1-AA
    d. 01967-P1-23-AA
20. An anesthesiologist provides anesthesia services to a patient with type 1 diabetes mellitus who undergoes transurethral resection of a bladder tumor.
    a. 00910-P2-AA
    b. 00912-P2-AA
    c. 00912-P3-AA
    d. 52500-P3-AA

Chapter 11
CPT Surgery I

1. Which is true about the CPT code descriptions?
   a. CPT code descriptions do not include the numerous activities integral to the procedure, such as the administration of local anesthesia and the initial incision.
   b. CPT code descriptions include all activities integral to the procedure.
   c. If an activity is not listed in the code description, it should be coded separately.
   d. The information in each code description contains all of the information necessary to select the proper code.
2. Which term describes the ablation of benign, premalignant, or malignant tissues by any method?
   a. destruction
   b. excision
   c. removal
   d. repair
3. The CMS national definition for a global surgical package:
   a. categorizes surgeries as major or minor and establishes a postoperative global period for each surgical procedure.
   b. ensures Medicare payments for services that are less comprehensive than intended.
   c. ensures Medicare payments for services that are more comprehensive than intended.
   d. ensures that payments are made consistently for the same services by all third-party payers across the nation.
4. Add-on codes:
   a. allow physicians to bundle procedures and services performed at the same time as the primary procedure.
   b. are usually reported as stand-alone codes because they are performed in addition to another procedure.
   c. can be identified by specific language in the code descriptor, such as "each additional" or "list separately in addition to primary procedure."
   d. sometimes qualify for the multiple procedure concept, which means that modifier -51 must be added to the CPT code.
5. CPT code descriptions that contain the phrase "separate procedure" in parentheses:
   a. are always performed as a separate procedure or service.
   b. are always performed as an integral component of a total service or procedure.
   c. are commonly performed as an integral component of a total service or procedure.
   d. are reported as an additional procedure when performed during the same operative episode as a more comprehensive procedure.
6. During the global period:
   a. complications subsequent to surgery are not reimbursed by the payer.
   b. distinct surgical procedures performed to treat complications during the postoperative period are not reported.
   c. normal, uncomplicated care provided by the surgeon who performed the original procedure is not coded or reported separately.
   d. the surgeon who performed the original procedure reports evaluation and management codes for normal, uncomplicated care.

7. During fine-needle aspiration, imaging guidance is typically used when the cyst or mass is not _______.
   a. malignant
   b. palpable
   c. small
   d. visible
8. Wound repair is coded with the appropriate evaluation and management code when the sole repair material used includes _______.
   a. adhesive strips
   b. staples
   c. sutures
   d. tissue adhesives
9. A biopsy was performed on a woman who did not have an established diagnosis. The results of the biopsy would determine whether to perform a mastectomy. Which is the correct way to report the biopsy?
   a. The biopsy code is not reported.
   b. The biopsy code is separately reported, and modifier -58 may be added to indicate that the biopsy and mastectomy are staged or planned procedures.
   c. The biopsy is coded and separately reported. Modifier -59 may be used appropriately to indicate that the biopsy and the mastectomy are distinct procedural services.
   d. The biopsy is separately reported. Modifier -78 may be used appropriately to indicate a return to the operating room for a related procedure during the postoperative period.
10. Complex repair of 8.5-cm wound, scalp, with extensive debridement of contaminated skin and subcutaneous tissue.
    a. 13121
    b. 13122
    c. 13121, 13122
    d. 13121, 13122, 13122, 11042
11. Excision of 1.5-cm malignant lesion, left ear. Incision and drainage performed to access lesion. Intermediate repair of excision site performed.
    a. 10060-LT, 11642-LT
    b. 11642-LT
    c. 11642-LT, 12031-LT
    d. 11642-LT, 12051-LT
12. Removal of four benign lesions from trunk, each 1.0-cm in size including margins. Simple repair performed.
    a. 11406
    b. 11400, 12002-51
    c. 11401, 11401-59, 11401-59, 11401-59
    d. 11406, 12002-51
13. Adjacent tissue transfer of 3.2-sq cm defect, scalp, after removal of 3.2-cm lesion performed during the same operative session.
    a. 11404, 14000
    b. 14000
    c. 14020
    d. 14020, 11404
14. Bilateral blepharoplasty of upper eyelids.
    a. 15820-50
    b. 15822-50
    c. 15821
    d. 15822
15. Patient presents to the emergency department with multiple lacerations. Simple repair was performed on 7.9-cm laceration of right leg, 6-cm laceration of right arm, 4-cm laceration of right cheek, and 2.5-cm laceration of right ear.
    a. 12002, 12004-51, 12014-51
    b. 12002, 12004, 12013, 12013
    c. 12005, 12013-51
    d. 12005, 12014-51
16. Incision and drainage of three cysts, right buttock.
    a. 10040
    b. 10060
    c. 10061
    d. 10080
17. Escharotomy of chest, three incisions.
    a. 16035
    b. 16036
    c. 16035, 16036
    d. 16035, 16036, 16036

18. Patient underwent 30 minutes of electrolysis.
    a. 17340
    b. 17360
    c. 17380
    d. 17999

19. Bilateral removal of intact mammary implants.
    a. 19316
    b. 19318-50
    c. 19324-50
    d. 19328-50

20. Patient underwent simple repair of the scalp (1.5 cm) and face (1.0 cm).
    a. 12001, 12011
    b. 12002
    c. 12013
    d. 12032

Chapter 12
CPT Surgery II

1. Codes 20900–20938 are reported when _______ tissue (originating in the patient's body) is obtained through separate skin or fascial incisions.
   a. allogenous
   b. autogenous
   c. osteogenesis
   d. rhytides
2. A patient suffered a traumatic amputation in an accident and underwent replantation surgery. A code from the range 20802–20838 was reported. Which procedures are reported with codes in this range?
   a. arthrodesis, cleansing, and debridement
   b. arthrodesis, cleansing, and internal fixation
   c. arthrodesis, cleansing, debridement, internal fixation, and repair of tendons
   d. internal fixation and repair of tendons
3. A surgeon performed an osteotomy and bone graft during the same operative session. Which CPT coding rule applies?
   a. Do not report a separate code for the osteotomy.
   b. Do not report a separate code for the bone graft.
   c. Add modifier -51 (Multiple Procedure) to the bone graft code.
   d. Do not add modifier -51 (Multiple Procedure) to the bone graft code.
4. Which are bundled in the tendon repair codes?
   a. application of immobilization, extension of the excision, and repair and closure of tendon sheath
   b. application of immobilization, repair of nerves or arteries, and repair and closure of tendon sheath
   c. extension of the excision, harvesting and inserting tendon grafts from another site, and repairing nerves or arteries
   d. harvesting and inserting tendon grafts from another site, repairing nerves or arteries, and treating fractures
5. The Pelvis and Hip Joint heading in the Musculoskeletal System subsection includes codes for procedures performed on the:
   a. femur and its tibial plateau.
   b. femur and popliteal bone.
   c. head and neck of the femur.
   d. head, neck, and tibial plateau of the femur.
6. Conversion of previous hip surgery to total hip arthroplasty, left side.
   a. 27130-LT
   b. 27132-LT
   c. 27134-LT
   d. 27137-LT
7. Arthrocentesis was performed for injection of medication, left acromioclavicular joint, for pain relief.
   a. 20600-LT
   b. 20605-LT
   c. 23044-LT
   d. 23130-LT
8. Arthroscopy of the right ankle with fusion of the tibiotalar and fibulotalar joints.
   a. 29894-RT
   b. 29894-RT, 29899-51-RT
   c. 29894-RT, 29899-RT
   d. 29899-RT

9. A 21-year-old male presented to the emergency department with pain in the right hand that began when he pounded his desk this morning after an argument with his boss. He was diagnosed with nondisplaced fractures of the 3rd and 4th right metacarpals. A cast was applied, and the patient was instructed to take Tylenol for pain.
   a. 26600-F7
   b. 26600-F7, 26600-F8
   c. 26600-F7, 26600-51-F8, 29085
   d. 26600-F8, 29085
10. Bilateral reconstruction of medial collateral ligament, elbow, with tendon graft.
   a. 24344-50
   b. 24345-50
   c. 24346-50
   d. 24360-50
11. Three bony plates are located on each side of the entrance to the nasal cavity. These bony plates and the entrance to the nasal cavity are called, respectively, the:
   a. nasal vestibules and septum.
   b. nasal vestibules and turbinates.
   c. septum and nasal vestibule.
   d. turbinates and nasal vestibule.
12. When diagnostic endoscopy is performed, administration of local anesthesia and electrocautery are bundled in the reported code, in addition to access to:
   a. different cavities and extensive shaving/debridement.
   b. different cavities and some shaving/debridement.
   c. one cavity and extensive shaving/debridement.
   d. one cavity and some shaving/debridement.
13. In which situation is a laryngoscopy procedure code separately reported?
   a. diagnostic laryngoscopy only
   b. endotracheal tube for nonemergent reasons
   c. endotracheal tube to provide air passage in an emergency situation
   d. tracheostomy
14. Endoscopy codes 31622–31629 are reported to:
   a. describe multiple procedures performed and reported with codes 31622–31629. (Each code is reported separately, and modifier -51 is added to the subsequent codes.)
   b. describe procedures in codes 31622–31629 that are not distinct surgical procedures and that are considered integral components of one another.
   c. describe procedures that involve use of a bronchoscope, with or without fluoroscopic guidance, to visualize all major lobar and segmental bronchi.
   d. indicate that these procedures do not include obtaining diagnostic specimens as part of the examination.
15. Which is the removal of a portion of lung that is less than a segment?
   a. lobectomy
   b. pneumocentesis
   c. segmentectomy
   d. wedge resection
16. A patient underwent surgical sinus endoscopy on the left frontal sinus. Sinusotomy and diagnostic endoscopy of the left frontal sinus were also performed.
   a. 31070-LT, 31231-LT
   b. 31276-LT
   c. 31276-LT, 31070-LT, 31231-LT
   d. 31276-LT, 31231-LT
17. Bilateral sinusotomy of the frontal, maxillary, and sphenoid sinuses.
   a. 31070, 31020-51, 31050-51
   b. 31070-50, 31020-50, 31050-50
   c. 31090-50
   d. 31090-50-51
18. Partial anterovertical laryngectomy.
   a. 31370
   b. 31375
   c. 31380
   d. 31382
19. Excision of tracheal tumor using cervical approach.
   a. 31750
   b. 31781
   c. 31785
   d. 31786
20. Surgical thoracoscopy with excision of pericardial mass.
   a. 32650
   b. 32658
   c. 32661
   d. 32662

Chapter 13
CPT Surgery III

1. Selective vascular catheterization procedures require separate coding of the:
   a. administration of local anesthesia.
   b. diagnostic procedure and/or therapeutic procedure as well as vascular access.
   c. introduction of the needle or catheter as well as vascular access.
   d. introduction of the needle or catheter or injection of contrast material.
2. Which procedure describes the insertion of a needle to withdraw fluid from the pericardial sac?
   a. pericardiectomy
   b. pericardiocentesis
   c. pericardiotomy
   d. tube pericardiostomy
3. Which is the medical term for the resultant backflow of blood when two valvular flaps do not close properly?
   a. achalasia
   b. atresia
   c. prolapse
   d. stenosis
4. Which is coded as congenital heart defect?
   a. aneurysm
   b. cardiac tumor
   c. coronary arteriovenous fistula
   d. truncus arteriosus
5. When a patient's coronary arteries contain extensive cholesterol plaque, a coronary artery bypass graft (CABG) procedure cannot be performed until the plaque is removed via:
   a. cardiac ablation.
   b. commissurotomy.
   c. coronary endarterectomy.
   d. transmyocardial revascularization.
6. Which is the excision of plaque from inside a blood vessel that involves puncturing the artery with a large needle and inserting a guidewire into the artery?
   a. open transluminal angioplasty
   b. open transluminal atherectomy
   c. percutaneous transluminal angioplasty
   d. percutaneous transluminal atherectomy
7. Bone marrow needle biopsy, right femur.
   a. 38220
   b. 38221
   c. 38230
   d. 38240
8. Transcatheter procedure code 37204 was performed on two vessels from one anatomic structure and another vessel in a different anatomic structure. Which is the correct way to report code 37204 for this procedure?
   a. 37204, 37204
   b. 37204, 37204, 37204
   c. 37204, 37204-59
   d. 37204-51
9. Add-on codes 35685–35686 describe additional procedures or techniques that may be required during a lower extremity bypass graft procedure. They are performed to improve the open and unblocked status of a blood vessel of lower extremity synthetic or autogenous arterial bypass grafts. The terms for the additional procedures and the open and unblocked status are, respectively:
   a. adjacent techniques and patency
   b. adjacent techniques and tunneled
   c. adjuvant techniques and patency
   d. adjuvant techniques and tunneled

10. Which two types of stem cells are located in bone marrow?
    a. hemopoietic and stromal
    b. implanted and tunneled
    c. red and white
    d. red and yellow

11. Transmyocardial laser revascularization, by thoracotomy, performed during pulmonary valve replacement.
    a. 33140, 33475
    b. 33475
    c. 33475, 33140, 33141
    d. 33475, 33141

12. Patient underwent insertion of dual-chamber pacing cardioverter-defibrillator. A left ventricle lead was placed for biventricular pacing.
    a. 33216, 33225-51
    b. 33217
    c. 33217, 33225
    d. 33217, 33225-51

13. Operative incision and reconstruction of atria for treatment of atrial flutter (Maze procedure).
    a. 33250
    b. 33251
    c. 33255
    d. 33261

14. Repair of anomalous coronary artery by graft, with endarterectomy, without cardiopulmonary bypass.
    a. 33503
    b. 33503, 33572
    c. 33504
    d. 33504, 33572

15. Shunt procedure performed from the superior vena cava to the pulmonary artery, with flow to both lungs.
    a. 33750
    b. 33755
    c. 33766
    d. 33767

16. One segment of artery harvested from left arm (for coronary artery bypass graft surgery).
    a. 33508-LT
    b. 35500-LT
    c. 35572-LT
    d. 35600-LT

17. Patient returned to surgery for exploration of postoperative hemorrhage in abdomen.
    a. 35800
    b. 35840
    c. 35840-76
    d. 35840-78

18. Percutaneous carotid catheterization and arteriogram were performed on right side to confirm the need for carotid stenting. The patient then underwent transcatheter placement of an intravascular stent in the right cervical carotid artery, percutaneous, with distal embolic protection.
    a. 36620-RT, 37216-RT
    b. 37215-RT
    c. 37215-RT, 36620-RT
    d. 37216-RT

19. Direct open arteriovenous anastomosis.
    a. 36810
    b. 36821
    c. 36825
    d. 36830

20. A 30-year-old patient underwent repair of acute traumatic diaphragmatic hernia.
    a. 39501
    b. 39503
    c. 39540
    d. 39541

Chapter 14
CPT Surgery IV

1. Which level of lip repair is assigned a code from the Digestive System subsection rather than the Integumentary System subsection?
   a. complex
   b. full-thickness
   c. intermediate
   d. layered
2. Codes for glossectomy procedures are assigned from the _______ heading of the Digestive System subsection.
   a. Dentoalveolar Structures
   b. Palate and Uvula
   c. Tongue and Floor of Mouth
   d. Vestibule of Mouth
3. How is hemorrhage control following a tonsillectomy and adenoidectomy procedure reported?
   a. Do not report a separate code because hemorrhage control is included in the tonsillectomy and adenoidectomy procedure codes.
   b. Report a code for hemorrhage control following tonsillectomy and adenoidectomy procedures and add modifier -59 to that code.
   c. Report a code for the tonsillectomy or adenoidectomy procedure and add modifier -78.
   d. Report a separate code for hemorrhage control following tonsillectomy and adenoidectomy procedures and add modifier -78 to the code.
4. When documentation indicates that enterolysis was extensive and added significantly to the other major procedure performed, report enterolysis code 44005 (freeing of intestinal adhesions) followed by modifier:
   a. -22
   b. -51
   c. -59
   d. -76
5. Bladder irrigation code 51700 is reported:
   a. for irrigation as an independent therapeutic service.
   b. for irrigation with therapeutic agents or for irrigation as an independent therapeutic service.
   c. when performed during a more comprehensive procedure.
   d. when performed to access or visualize the urinary system.
6. Code 44955 is reported for an appendectomy when it is performed _______.
   a. as the primary procedure
   b. during intra-abdominal surgery
   c. for a ruptured appendix with abscess or generalized peritonitis
   d. for an indicated purpose during the same operative session as another major procedure
7. The percutaneous drainage of a liver abscess (47011) includes _______.
   a. final removal of the catheter
   b. initial insertion of the catheter
   c. radiologic guidance
   d. final removal of the catheter, initial insertion of the catheter, and radiologic guidance
8. A patient underwent the surgical treatment of an anal fistula, which required a submuscular fistulectomy. Which description would be documented in the operative report?
   a. excision of multiple fistulas
   b. removal of an anal fistula, including division of the sphincter muscle
   c. removal of an anal fistula, without division of the sphincter muscle
   d. use of a seton to cut through the fistula

9. When multiple endoscopic approaches are performed to accomplish the same procedure, report a code for:
   a. each endoscopic approach performed, adding modifier -51 to each less extensive code.
   b. each endoscopic approach performed.
   c. the least extensive code only.
   d. the successful endoscopic approach only.
10. Urethral catheterization codes (51701–51702) are reported when urethral catheterization is:
    a. necessary for urethral dilation and for accomplishment of a more extensive procedure.
    b. necessary to accomplish a more extensive procedure.
    c. performed independently of another procedure.
    d. performed preceding the scheduled surgery.
11. Diaphragmatic hernia repair performed on neonate.
    a. 39501
    b. 39503
    c. 39540-63
    d. 39541-63
12. Laser-assisted uvulopalatoplasty, second treatment session.
    a. 42145
    b. 42145-51
    c. 42299
    d. 42299, 42299
13. Diagnostic endoscopic retrograde cholangiopancreatography (ERCP) with washing and collection of specimens.
    a. 43260
    b. 43261
    c. 43264
    d. 43269
14. Bilateral posterior vestibuloplasty.
    a. 40840
    b. 40842-50
    c. 40843
    d. 40845
15. Suture of small intestine for perforated ulcer.
    a. 44602
    b. 44603
    c. 44604
    d. 44605
16. Partial proctectomy with anastomosis using transsacral approach.
    a. 45110
    b. 45111
    c. 45113
    d. 45116
17. Donor hepatectomy from cadaver.
    a. 47133
    b. 47140
    c. 47141
    d. 47142
18. Repair of strangulated initial inguinal hernia, 1-year-old child.
    a. 49501
    b. 49507
    c. 49521
    d. 49520
19. Laparoscopic partial nephrectomy.
    a. 50240
    b. 50543
    c. 50545
    d. 50548
20. Aspiration of bladder with insertion of suprapubic catheter with ultrasonic guidance.
    a. 51100, 76942
    b. 51101, 77012
    c. 51102, 77012
    d. 51102, 76942

Chapter 15
CPT Surgery V

1. Which is the abnormal dilation of the spermatic cord veins in the scrotum?
   a. BPH
   b. orchiopexy
   c. TULIP
   d. varicocele
2. Which is included in the delivery service and is therefore not coded and reported separately?
   a. admission to the hospital for observation prior to delivery
   b. delivery of the placenta
   c. treatment of postpartum medical complications
   d. tubal ligation performed after delivery
3. The Endocrine System subsection includes procedures performed on the endocrine glands and the:
   a. carotid body.
   b. pineal glands.
   c. pituitary gland.
   d. carotid body and pineal and pituitary glands.
4. Which causes carpal tunnel syndrome?
   a. compression of the median nerve at the wrist
   b. numbness, pain, and weakness in the hand and wrist
   c. repetitive flexing and extension of the wrist
   d. thickening of the protective sheaths that surround each of the tendons
5. Which is the removal of a portion of the vertebra and adjacent intervertebral disks?
   a. corpectomy
   b. diskectomy
   c. laminectomy
   d. osteophytectomy
6. During a spinal procedure, an incision is made into the area of the affected vertebral segment and the incision is inferiorly curved out to the lateral plane. Paraspinous muscles are mobilized medially (denervating and devascularizing these structures). The muscles are lifted from the spinous process; and they are divided and lifted from the ribs, exposing the vertebral segment. Which surgical approach has been performed?
   a. anterolateral approach
   b. costovertebral approach
   c. lateral extracavitary approach
   d. transpedicular approach
7. Which procedure, classified in the Eye and Ocular Adnexa subsection, includes severing and removing the eyeball from extraorbital muscles and the optic nerve?
   a. enucleation of the eye
   b. evisceration of ocular contents
   c. exenteration of the orbit
   d. extracapsular cataract extraction
8. A common procedure performed to repair facial nerve damage is total nerve decompression, which is used to treat symptoms of:
   a. Bell's palsy.
   b. carpal tunnel syndrome.
   c. orbital implants.
   d. strabismus.
9. An operating microscope is reported in addition to the primary surgical procedure for:
   a. all encounters during which an operating microscope is used.
   b. performance of microsurgery techniques.
   c. procedures where use of an operating microscope is an inclusive component.
   d. visualization with a magnifying loupe or corrected vision.

10. Which involves the removal of skin and deep subcutaneous tissue?
    a. laser ablation of the vulva
    b. radical vulvectomy
    c. simple vulvectomy
    d. volvulus
11. Bilateral epididymovasostomy requiring use of operating microscope.
    a. 54900, 69990
    b. 54900-50
    c. 54901
    d. 54901, 69990
12. Vaginal closure of vesicovaginal fistula; concomitant cystotomy with drainage.
    a. 57310
    b. 57320
    c. 57320, 51040
    d. 57330
13. Patient returns to physician for normal postpartum care after uncomplicated pregnancy, obstetric care, and vaginal delivery using forceps.
    a. 59400
    b. 59409
    c. 59410
    d. 59430
14. Complete thyroidectomy.
    a. 60220
    b. 60240
    c. 60252
    d. 60260
15. Patient with craniosynostosis underwent craniectomy that required a single cranial suture.
    a. 61550
    b. 61552
    c. 61556
    d. 61558
16. Extradural excision of vascular lesion of infratemporal fossa with repair by anastomosis.
    a. 61605
    b. 61605, 61610
    c. 61606
    d. 61607
17. Patient with intracranial lesion underwent creation of burr hole and stereotactic biopsy.
    a. 61140
    b. 61140, 61750
    c. 61750
    d. 61750, 61140
18. Patient with glaucoma underwent sector iridectomy with corneoscleral section.
    a. 66625
    b. 66630
    c. 66635
    d. 66680
19. Removal of superficial foreign body from the conjunctiva of the external eye.
    a. 65205
    b. 65210
    c. 65220
    d. 65222
20. Patient underwent tympanoplasty with mastoidectomy and tympanic membrane repair.
    a. 69641
    b. 69641,69610
    c. 69642
    d. 69643

Chapter 16
CPT Radiology

1. *Coronal, midsagittal, sagittal,* and *transverse* are terms that describe:
   a. components of radiology procedures.
   b. contrast agents.
   c. planes of view.
   d. radiographic projections.
2. Which modifiers are commonly added to radiology codes to indicate the component provided?
   a. -26 and -TC
   b. -50 and -51
   c. -52 and -76
   d. -LT and -RT
3. Component coding:
   a. allows for the reporting of a radiology procedure code and a surgical procedure code to completely describe the service provided.
   b. combines the technical and professional components into a single code.
   c. indicates that a provider owns the equipment and performs both the technical and professional components.
   d. requires that modifier -52 be added to the radiology code reported.
4. Which includes standard radiographs, contrast studies, computed tomography (CT), and magnetic resonance imaging (MRI)?
   a. interventional diagnostic imaging
   b. invasive diagnostic imaging
   c. noninvasive diagnostic imaging
   d. nuclear imaging
5. Which identifies nerve construction or inflammation and the degree of fluid flow in the epidural space?
   a. computed tomography
   b. epidurography
   c. magnetic resonance angiography
   d. mammography
6. A separate code is reported for:
   a. an intrathecal injection.
   b. diagnostic angiography or venography (radiologic supervision and interpretation).
   c. therapeutic nuclear medicine procedures.
   d. therapeutic transcatheter radiologic supervision and interpretation.
7. Which radiologic procedure involves x-rays of different angles to create cross-sectional images of organs, bones, and tissues to visualize blood flow in arterial and venous vessels throughout the body?
   a. computed axial tomography
   b. computed tomography angiography
   c. magnetic resonance angiography
   d. magnetic resonance imaging
8. Amplitude modulation, gray-scale ultrasound, motion mode, and real-time scan are:
   a. planes of view for radiology procedures.
   b. radiographic projections.
   c. tvypes of ophthalmic ultrasound.
   d. ultrasound display modes.
9. Types of radiation oncology treatment devices include:
   a. blocks, breast boards, wedges, and eye shields.
   b. neutron beam and proton beam.
   c. therapeutic port film and megaelectron volts.
   d. treatment volume determination, treatment time/dosage determination, and choice of treatment modality.

10. A patient underwent a procedure that measures thyroid function to determine how much iodine the thyroid absorbs. The type of procedure that the patient had is a(n):
    a. photon absorptiometry.
    b. tomographic single photon emission computed tomography.
    c. uptake test.
    d. vascular flow exam.

11. After being tackled in a football game, a patient with complaints of pain and trouble breathing underwent rib x-rays on both sides. Three views were obtained.
    a. 71100
    b. 71100-51
    c. 71110
    d. 71110-50

12. Myelography of the cervical and thoracic spine, radiological supervision and interpretation.
    a. 72240, 72255
    b. 72270
    c. 72270-51
    d. 72270-52

13. Magnetic resonance imaging of thigh with contrast.
    a. 73718
    b. 73719
    c. 73722
    d. 73725

14. Intravenous (IV) urography with tomography, professional component.
    a. 74400
    b. 74400-26
    c. 74400-26, 74150
    d. 74410-26

15. Angiography of right cervical carotid artery.
    a. 75671-RT
    b. 75676-RT
    c. 75680-RT
    d. 75685-RT

16. A patient in the twentieth week of her pregnancy underwent transabdominal uterine ultrasound, real time with image documentation, for fetal and maternal evaluation, single gestation.
    a. 76801
    b. 76802
    c. 76805
    d. 76810

17. Therapeutic radiology treatment planning with simulation of a single treatment area and no blocking.
    a. 77261
    b. 77262
    c. 77263
    d. 77299

18. Pulmonary perfusion imaging, particulate, with ventilation imaging, aerosol, one or multiple projections.
    a. 78580
    b. 78584
    c. 78585
    d. 78588

19. Radiopharmaceutical therapy, intravenous administration.
    a. 79005
    b. 79101
    c. 79440
    d. 79445

20. Patient underwent magnetic resonance imaging (MRI) of neck without contrast, followed by imaging with contrast.
    a. 70542, 70540
    b. 70543
    c. 70547, 70548
    d. 70549

Chapter 17
CPT Pathology and Laboratory

1. A patient presents with a variety of symptoms for which blood tests are ordered. In the lab, venipuncture is performed. Because the vein collapses prior to completion, a second needle is placed in a different vein. A total of three separate color-coded vials of blood are drawn and labeled for testing. How many codes are reported for specimen collection?
   a. none
   b. one
   c. two
   d. three
2. Which are proteins in the body that are made by the immune system and that fight infection and disease?
   a. adjuvants
   b. analytes
   c. antibodies
   d. antigens
3. A Medicare patient has tests performed at a lab that has a CLIA waiver. Which HCPCS level II modifier is added to pathology and laboratory service codes?
   a. -59
   b. -P1
   c. -QW
   d. -TC
4. The unit of pathology service is a(n):
   a. assay.
   b. block.
   c. section.
   d. specimen.
5. A patient is seen for blood work; and a panel that is performed includes CBC, automated Hgb, Hct, RBC, WBC, and platelet count (85027). Later that day a separate hemoglobin test is run (85018). The coder reports 85027 and 85018-91. Under which condition is it appropriate to report both codes?
   a. Multiple tests are performed as part of a series.
   b. The original panel produces an abnormal hemoglobin result.
   c. The test is repeated due to technician error.
   d. An equipment malfunction occurred during the performance of the test.
6. Organ or disease-oriented panels:
   a. may be reported in addition to individual codes for each lab test performed.
   b. may be reported when most of the component tests have been performed.
   c. were developed for coding purposes only.
   d. were developed for use as clinical parameters.
7. In addition to the Drug Testing and the Therapeutic Drug Assays subsections of pathology and laboratory, CPT codes reported for drug testing are also located in the _______ subsection.
   a. Chemistry
   b. Hematology and Coagulation
   c. Immunology
   d. Urinalysis
8. Test panels from the _______ subsection include the administration of agents that cause production of hormones or other secretions.
   a. Anatomic Pathology
   b. Evocative/Suppression
   c. Immunology
   d. Microbiology
9. Which is the study of microbes?
   a. cytopathology
   b. hematology
   c. immunology
   d. microbiology

10. Which CPT Pathology and Laboratory subsection codes are reported for physician services only?
    a. Anatomic Pathology
    b. Cytogenetic Studies
    c. Organ or Disease-Oriented Panels
    d. Surgical Pathology

11. Glucose tolerance test, six specimens.
    a. 82951
    b. 82951, 82952
    c. 82951, 82951-91
    d. 82951, 82952, 82952, 82952

12. Bilirubin test from feces specimen.
    a. 82247
    b. 82248
    c. 82252
    d. 82270

13. Breath specimen analyzed for urease activity in *Helicobacter pylori,* nonradioactive isotope.
    a. 83009
    b. 83013
    c. 83014
    d. 87338

14. Mutation identification by sequencing, one segment, via molecular diagnostics.
    a. 83903
    b. 83904
    c. 83905
    d. 83906

15. Qualitative analysis of porphyrins in urine.
    a. 84119
    b. 84120
    c. 84126
    d. 84127

16. Manual leukocyte cell count, repeated later in the same day for comparison.
    a. 85032
    b. 85032, 85032-51
    c. 85032, 85032-91
    d. 85048, 85048-91

17. Complete semen analysis, including volume, count, motility, and differential.
    a. 89300
    b. 89310
    c. 89320
    d. 89321

18. Blood culture for bacteria, with isolation and presumptive identification of isolates.
    a. 87040
    b. 87045
    c. 87046
    d. 87075

19. Surgical pathology, gross examination only.
    a. 88300
    b. 88302
    c. 88304
    d. 88305

20. Patient with adrenal insufficiency underwent ACTH stimulation panel including cortisol × 2.
    a. 80400
    b. 80402
    c. 80412
    d. 82024

Chapter 18
CPT Medicine

1. Upon review of ventilator management codes 94002–94005, the note states that these codes are not reported with codes:
   a. 00100–01999
   b. 10021–69990
   c. 99201–99499
   d. 90281–99607
2. Acupuncture is classified in _______-minute increments of face-to-face patient contact.
   a. 10
   b. 15
   c. 20
   d. 30
3. An immune globulin:
   a. contains antigens.
   b. is administered as immunization against infectious agents.
   c. provides long-term protection against infectious agents.
   d. provides temporary protection against infectious agents.
4. Under which heading is the flash symbol found?
   a. Evaluation and Management
   b. Immune Globulins
   c. Immunization Administration for Vaccines/Toxoids
   d. Vaccines/Toxoids
5. Which typically includes a system of desensitization?
   a. behavior-modifying psychotherapy
   b. interactive psychotherapy
   c. psychodynamic psychotherapy
   d. supportive psychotherapy
6. A patient receives ongoing psychotherapy services from a psychologist at a facility and occasionally has an evaluation and management encounter with the resident psychiatrist to evaluate her prescribed medications. When reporting services for this patient, the pharmacologic management service is:
   a. coded and reported separately by the psychiatrist.
   b. coded and reported separately by the psychologist.
   c. included in psychotherapy services reported by the psychologist.
   d. included in the evaluation and management service reported by the psychiatrist.
7. Which service performed during cardiac catheterization is reported separately?
   a. cardiac output measurement
   b. fluoroscopic guidance procedure codes classified by CPT as supervision and interpretation
   c. imaging supervision, interpretation, and documented report for injection procedures
   d. injection procedures during cardiac catheterization
8. Codes for cerebrovascular arterial studies are found in which Medicine subsection?
   a. Cardiovascular
   b. Neurology and Neuromuscular Procedures
   c. Noninvasive Vascular Diagnostic Studies
   d. Pulmonary
9. Which type(s) of allergy sensitivity test(s) identify allergies to insect venom and penicillin?
   a. epicutaneous
   b. intracutaneous
   c. percutaneous and epicutaneous
   d. percutaneous and intracutaneous

10. Which Medicine subsection contains codes for sleep testing?
    a. Biofeedback
    b. Neurology and Neuromuscular Procedures
    c. Other Services and Procedures
    d. Psychiatry
11. End-stage renal disease (ESRD) services for 17-year-old patient with one face-to-face physician visit per month.
    a. 90953
    b. 90957
    c. 90958
    d. 90959
12. Manometric study for gastric motility.
    a. 91010
    b. 91013
    c. 91020
    d. 91022
13. Percutaneous transluminal coronary balloon angioplasty of one vessel.
    a. 92982
    b. 92984
    c. 92986
    d. 92987
14. Under moderate sedation, a patient underwent transesophageal echocardiography in real time with 2D image documentation, including probe placement, image acquisition, interpretation, and report.
    a. 93312
    b. 93312, 99143
    c. 93313
    d. 93318, 99143
15. Patient with acute airway obstruction received two pressurized inhalation treatments.
    a. 94640
    b. 94640, 94640-76
    c. 94640, 94640-51
    d. 94640-76
16. Needle electromyography of both arms and both legs.
    a. 95860
    b. 95861
    c. 95863
    d. 95864
17. Intra-arterial chemotherapy administration, infusion technique, one hour.
    a. 96409
    b. 96413
    c. 96420
    d. 96422
18. Five hours of work hardening/conditioning.
    a. 97545, 97546
    b. 97546, 97546-51
    c. 97545, 97546, 97546, 97546
    d. 97545, 97546, 97546-51
19. A patient received extraspinal manipulation on four regions from a chiropractor.
    a. 98926
    b. 98941
    c. 98943
    d. 98943, 98943, 98943, 98943
20. A therapist administered oxygen therapy to a patient in the patient's home.
    a. 99183
    b. 99503
    c. 99504
    d. 99509

Chapter 19
Insurance and Reimbursement

1. Which of the following eliminated carriers, fiscal intermediaries (FIs), and durable medical equipment regional carriers (DMERCs) and created MACs?
   a. Title I of the Health Insurance Portability and Accountability Act of 1997 (HIPAA)
   b. Title IX of the Medicare Prescription Drug, Improvement, and Modernization Act (MMA)
   c. Title XIX of the Social Security Acts
   d. Title XVIII of the Social Security Acts
2. In 2007, which standard claim form will be submitted by health care institutions to payers for inpatient and outpatient services?
   a. CMS-450
   b. CMS-1500
   c. UB-04
   d. UB-92
3. Which government-sponsored program provides health care services to members of the uniformed services and their families?
   a. CHAMPVA
   b. Military Health System (MHS)
   c. PACE
   d. SCHIP
4. The direct contract model, the individual practice association, and the network model are examples of which type of managed care plan?
   a. closed-panel health maintenance organization
   b. integrated delivery system
   c. open-panel health maintenance organization
   d. triple option plan
5. Which is true of a consumer-directed health plan (CDHP)?
   a. Individuals assume higher cost-sharing expenses after the designated amount has been expended.
   b. Individuals have less freedom in spending health care dollars up to a designated amount.
   c. Individuals receive full coverage for all of their in-network care.
   d. It does not provide individuals with an incentive to control costs of health benefits and health care.
6. Which models are included in the integrated delivery system managed care plan?
   a. flexible spending account, health care reimbursement account, and health reimbursement arrangement
   b. open-panel and closed-panel health maintenance organizations
   c. physician-hospital organization, management service organization, and group practice without walls
   d. point-of-service plan and preferred provider plan
7. Antoinette is preparing to transfer information regarding an inpatient encounter into the hospital's computerized patient accounting system. She uses a document that contains a list of procedures, services, and supplies along with the department code, service code and description, and revenue codes and charges. The document she is referencing is called a(n):
   a. chargemaster.
   b. CMS-1500.
   c. encounter form.
   d. UB-92.

8. The services that Allen received during his inpatient hospitalization resulted in expenses that were much higher than those of other cases in the same diagnosis-related group (DRG). Because these services qualified for additional reimbursement, his case was categorized as a(n):
   a. cost outlier.
   b. day outlier.
   c. exclusion.
   d. indemnification.
9. Which legislation resulted in the implementation of the skilled nursing facility prospective payment system (SNFPPS)?
   a. Balanced Budget Act of 1997
   b. Balanced Budget Refinement Act of 1999
   c. Omnibus Consolidated and Emergency Supplemental Appropriations Act of 1999
   d. Tax Equity and Fiscal Responsibility Act of 1983
10. Leon had some lab work completed as an outpatient on Wednesday in preparation for an inpatient procedure that was to be performed on Thursday. Under the prospective payment system, the lab work will be covered by the diagnosis-related group (DRG) payment. What is the name of the rule that ensures this?
    a. IPPS 3-day payment window
    b. IRF PPS 1-day payment window
    c. LTCH PPS 1-day payment window
    d. OPPS 3-day payment window
11. Which were implemented as a result of the Balanced Budget Act of 1997?
    a. IPPS, HH PPS, and OPPS
    b. IPPS, SNF PPS, and LTCH PPS
    c. OPPS, IRF PPS, and LTCH PPS
    d. SNF PPS, OPPS, and IRF PPS
12. Critical pathways:
    a. are standard procedures developed by hospitals to facilitate management and delivery of care.
    b. focus on the services provided by an individual discipline.
    c. provide opportunities for collaborative practice and team approaches between disciplines.
    d. rarely target clinical services that are high in volume and resource use.
13. The difference between fraud and abuse is the:
    a. concern that fraud involves much greater losses than abuse.
    b. fact that fraud is unintentional while abuse is deliberate.
    c. intent of the individual who committed the act.
    d. resultant damage or loss from fraudulent acts.
14. A provider bills Medicare for services that were never provided to a patient, is found guilty of fraud, and is ordered to pay a fine of $10,000 plus damages. Which of the following supports this decision?
    a. Civil Monetary Penalties Act
    b. Federal Claims Collection Act
    c. Payment Error and Prevention Program (PEPP)
    d. Stark I
15. A claim is submitted that contains codes for reconstruction of a female urethra (53430) and reconstruction of a male urethra (53410). The claim will be denied because 53430 and 53410 are _______ codes.
    a. component
    b. comprehensive
    c. manifestation
    d. mutually exclusive
16. Which is not applicable where there is an indication of fraud?
    a. Civil Monetary Penalties Act
    b. False Claims Act (FCA)
    c. federal antikickback statute
    d. Federal Claims Collection Act of 1966
17. Which resulted from the discovery that some health care organizations were billing Medicare Part B for services that were already paid under Part A?
    a. antikickback statute
    b. Payment Error and Prevention Program (PEPP)
    c. Physicians at Teaching Hospitals (PATH) initiative
    d. safe harbor regulations

18. Which statement describes a characteristic of a flat file?
    a. A flat file consists of a series of variable-length records.
    b. A flat file is not accepted by Medicare administrative contractors for claims submission.
    c. A flat file is used to bill institutional, professional, dental, and drug claims.
    d. Medicare administrative contractors send electronic remittance advices in the flat file format.

19. Which is not considered electronic data interchange (EDI)?
    a. ANSI ASC X12 837
    b. computer-generated paper claim
    c. flat file
    d. National Standard Format (NSF)

20. Locking the record storage areas at all times and limiting access to authorized users is an example of a:
    a. clinical protocol.
    b. confidentiality standard.
    c. privacy measure.
    d. security provision.

ANSWER KEY TO EXAM: CHAPTER 1

1. c
2. a
3. b
4. a
5. a
6. a
7. b
8. a
9. d
10. c
11. c
12. b
13. a
14. a
15. c
16. b
17. a
18. d
19. d
20. d

ANSWER KEY TO EXAM: CHAPTER 2

1. d
2. b
3. a
4. b
5. a
6. a
7. d
8. a
9. a
10. d
11. a
12. b
13. d
14. c
15. d
16. d
17. c
18. d
19. b
20. b

ANSWER KEY TO EXAM: CHAPTER 3

1. a
2. a
3. c
4. d
5. d
6. c
7. d
8. d
9. c
10. b
11. b
12. b
13. a
14. a
15. c
16. a
17. c
18. b
19. c
20. c

ANSWER KEY TO EXAM: CHAPTER 4

ICD-9-CM

1. a
2. d
3. c
4. c
5. d
6. b

Note:

The delivery of an oversized infant requires assignment of fifth digit 1 is assigned to ICD-9-CM code 653.51. The hematoma was a postdelivery complication, which means that fifth digit 2 is assigned to ICD-9-CM code 674.32. (The Pregnancy, Childbirth, and the Puerperium codes in Chapter 15 of ICD-10-CM do not require assignment of a fifth digit to indicate delivery status (e.g., antepartum condition, delivered, postpartum condition, unspecified as to episode of care).

7. d
8. a
9. b
10. d
11. b
12. a
13. b
14. d
15. a
16. a
17. b
18. a
19. d
20. b

Note:

Superficial injuries (e.g., abrasions or contusions) are not coded when associated with more severe injuries to the same site. Because there was a left lower leg laceration (ICD-9-CM code 891.0 or ICD-10-CM code S81.812A), leg contusions (ICD-9-CM code 924.5 or ICD-10-CM code S80.12xA) are not coded.

ICD-10-CM

1. a
2. d
3. b
4. b
5. d
6. b
7. d
8. c
9. b
10. d
11. c
12. d
13. d
14. b
15. c
16. a
17. c
18. b
19. a
20. a

ANSWER KEY TO EXAM: CHAPTER 5

1. d
2. c
3. c
4. d
5. c
6. b
7. a
8. c
9. c
10. d
11. d
12. d
13. b
14. d
15. a
16. a
17. a
18. d
19. c
20. b

ICD-10-CM/PCS Coding

21. a
22. c
23. b
24. b
25. a
26. d
27. b
28. c
29. b
30. c
31. a
32. d
33. b
34. a
35. c
36. d
37. d
38. a
39. c
40. d

ANSWER KEY TO EXAM: CHAPTER 6

1. d
2. b
3. d
4. d
5. c
6. d
7. a
8. b
9. b
10. b
11. b
12. a
13. d
14. d
15. c
16. a
17. a
18. a
19. b
20. c

ANSWER KEY TO EXAM: CHAPTER 7

1. a
2. a
3. c
4. c
5. b
6. c
7. a
8. a
9. a
10. a
11. a
12. c
13. c
14. b
15. d
16. d
17. c
18. d
19. c
20. b

ANSWER KEY TO EXAM: CHAPTER 8

1. c
2. c
3. b
4. a
5. c
6. d
7. b
8. b
9. c
10. d
11. a
12. d
13. c
14. a
15. a
16. c
17. b
18. c
19. c
20. c

ANSWER KEY TO EXAM: CHAPTER 9

1. d
2. a
3. c
4. d
5. d
6. d
7. b
8. d
9. d
10. c
11. c
12. d
13. d
14. c
15. b
16. b
17. c
18. a
19. c
20. c

ANSWER KEY TO EXAM: CHAPTER 10

1. a
2. d
3. c
4. a
5. c
6. b
7. a

Note:

The formula for calculating the anesthesia fee is [code-specific base unit value + anesthesia time unit(s) + modifying unit(s)] × locality-specific anesthesia conversion factor. The code-specific base unit value is 5. Anesthesia services were provided for 45 minutes. Anesthesia time units are counted in 15 minute sections; so (45 ÷ 15) will give you the number of anesthesia time units, which is 3. The patient is healthy; so a physical status modifier of -P1 is assigned, which has a relative value of 1 (the modifying unit). Thus, (5 + 3 + 1) × $19.20 = $172.80.

8. a
9. d
10. c
11. c
12. b
13. b
14. b
15. d

Note:

Morbid obesity is assigned physical status modifier -P3, while obesity would be assigned physical status modifier -P2.

16. c
17. b
18. a
19. c
20. c

ANSWER KEY TO EXAM: CHAPTER 11

1. a
2. a
3. a
4. c
5. c
6. c
7. b
8. a
9. b
10. d
11. d
12. c
13. c
14. b
15. d
16. c
17. d
18. c
19. d
20. a

ANSWER KEY TO EXAM: CHAPTER 12

1. b
2. c
3. d
4. a
5. c
6. b
7. b
8. d
9. b
10. c
11. d
12. b
13. a
14. c
15. d
16. b
17. c
18. c
19. c
20. c

ANSWER KEY TO EXAM: CHAPTER 13

1. b
2. b
3. c
4. d
5. c
6. d
7. b
8. c
9. c
10. a
11. d
12. c
13. c
14. a
15. d
16. d
17. d
18. b
19. b
20. c

ANSWER KEY TO EXAM: CHAPTER 14

1. b
2. c
3. d
4. b
5. b
6. d
7. d
8. b
9. d
10. c
11. b
12. c
13. a
14. c
15. a
16. d
17. a
18. a
19. b
20. d

ANSWER KEY TO EXAM: CHAPTER 15

1. d
2. b
3. a
4. a
5. a
6. c
7. a
8. a
9. b
10. b
11. d
12. c
13. a
14. b
15. a
16. b
17. c
18. b
19. a
20. a

ANSWER KEY TO EXAM: CHAPTER 16

1. c
2. a
3. a
4. c
5. b
6. a
7. b
8. d
9. a
10. c
11. c
12. b
13. b
14. b
15. b
16. c
17. a
18. d
19. b
20. b

ANSWER KEY TO EXAM: CHAPTER 17

1. b
2. c
3. c
4. d
5. b
6. c
7. a
8. b
9. d
10. a
11. d
12. c
13. b
14. b
15. a
16. c
17. c
18. a
19. a
20. a

ANSWER KEY TO EXAM: CHAPTER 18

1. c
2. b
3. d
4. d
5. a
6. d
7. b
8. c
9. d
10. b
11. d
12. c
13. a
14. a
15. b
16. d
17. d
18. c
19. c
20. b

ANSWER KEY TO EXAM: CHAPTER 19

1. b
2. c
3. b
4. c
5. a
6. c
7. a
8. a
9. a
10. a
11. d
12. c
13. c
14. a
15. d
16. d
17. c
18. b
19. b
20. d

SECTION IV

Answer Keys to Workbook Assignments and Reviews

Chapter 1
Overview of Coding

ASSIGNMENT 1.1 – CAREER AS A CODER: INTERVIEW OF A CODING PROFESSIONAL

The student will submit in paragraph format (not Q&A) a two- to three-page word-processed interview of a coding professional. Each paragraph should contain a minimum of three sentences, and the student should write in complete sentences. The paper should contain no typographical or grammatical errors. The last paragraph of the paper should summarize what the student's reaction to the interview was and whether the student would be interested in having this professional's position (along with an explanation of why or why not). Also, the student should "predict the future" by writing about where he or she will be in ten years in terms of employment, family, and so on.

ASSIGNMENT 1.2 – PROFESSIONAL DISCUSSION FORUMS (LISTSERV)

The student will go to http://list.nih.gov and click on "What Is LISTERV?" to learn all about online discussion forums (listservs). The student will also select a professional discussion forum from Table 1-1 in the Workbook and follow its instructions to become a member. If this assignment is completed by the student outside of class, the instructor can require the student to submit a summary of the experience (or if teaching online, post a discussion).

ASSIGNMENT 1.3 – VALIDATING ACCURACY OF ICD CODES

Validating ICD-9-CM Coding Accuracy

(Adapted and reprinted with permission from the American Health Information Management Association. Copyright © 1983 by the American Health Information Association.)

1. Code V55.1 is missing. It should be reported as an other (additional) diagnosis. Correct codes to be reported include V10.04, V55.1, and 44.62.
2. Code 170.9 is incorrect because carcinoma of the bone is considered metastatic spread from an unknown primary; assign codes 198.5 and 199.1 instead of 170.9. Code V67.2 is incorrect because it would be reported for follow-up examination following chemotherapy; delete code V67.2. Code V58.11 (chemotherapy) is missing; add code V58.11.
3. Code 414.0 is missing its fifth digit. The diagnosis arteriosclerotic heart disease (ASHD) does not indicate the type of artery or graft; therefore, assign code 414.00. The coder should query the physician to ask what type of artery or graft is affected by the ASHD. Code 428.0 should be sequenced first as the principal diagnosis because ASHD is a chronic condition and would not result in inpatient hospitalization unless the patient received treatment, such as cardiac catheterization or coronary artery bypass graft surgery. Although congestive heart failure can be considered a chronic condition, it can result in acute inpatient hospitalization with the patient receiving nonsurgical treatment (e.g., respiratory therapy and medications). Correct codes to be reported include 428.0 and 414.00.
4. Code 041.4 should be reported as an other (additional) diagnosis. Correct codes to be reported include 599.0 and 041.4.
5. Never report code 650 with a complicated delivery code (e.g., 653.41). Delivery cases require reporting either code 650 or a complicated delivery code. Although code 653.41 is correctly reported for fetopelvic disproportion, code 660.11 should be assigned and reported first as the principal diagnosis for obstructed labor due to fetopelvic disproportion. Category code 653 contains the instruction to

"Code first any associated obstructed labor (660.1)." Outcome of delivery code V27.0 was not assigned, and it should be reported as an other (additional) diagnosis. Code 74.9 is missing its fourth digit; report 74.99 instead. Correct codes to be reported include 660.11, 653.41, V27.0, and 74.99.

Validating ICD-10-CM and ICD-10-PCS Coding Accuracy

6. Codes Z85.028 and 0DQ67ZZ are correct. However, code Z43.1 is missing, and it should be reported first.
7. Codes Z08 and 3E03305 are correct. However, code C40.80 is incorrect because *secondary carcinoma of the bone* is coded as metastatic spread from an unknown primary; therefore, assign C79.51 (neoplasm, bone, malignant secondary) and C80.1 (neoplasm, unknown or unspecific site, malignant primary) (instead of C40.80).
8. Code I50.9 is correct. However, code I25.1 is missing its fifth digit "0" that classifies the native coronary artery site; assign code I25.10 (instead of I25.1).
9. Code N39.0 is correct; however, code B96.2 should be reported as another (additional) diagnosis to describe the *Escherichia coli* infection.
10. Codes O80 and 10E0XZZ are correct. However, code Z37.0 should also reported to classify the outcome delivery as a single live birth.

ASSIGNMENT 1.4 – COMPUTER-ASSISTED CODING (CAC)

1. a. **Date of procedure:** August 5, 2004

   b. **Preoperative diagnosis:** Right anterior cruciate ligament rupture with possible lateral meniscus tear

   c. **Postoperative diagnosis:** Right knee anterior cruciate ligament rupture with lateral meniscus tear

   d. **Procedures:** Right knee arthroscopy
   Partial lateral meniscectomy and anterior cruciate ligament reconstruction
   Bone-patellar-bone autograft
   Arthroscopy

Note:

The surgeon probably dictated or entered the Arthroscopy *procedure (as the last line of* Procedures *on the bottom half of the CAC demo application's computer screen) in error because* arthroscopy *is previously stated on line one of* Procedures.

2. a. 844.2, 836.1

   b. 836.1

Note:

- Code 836.1 (tear of lateral cartilage or meniscus of knee current) was selected by the coder as the *admitting diagnosis* (abbreviated as A below the *Admitting Diagnosis* heading in Figure 1-1. The *Admitting Diagnosis* box of the screen indicates that the coder originally deleted 836.1 and then set that code as the admission diagnosis.)
- CAC software also assigned 844.2 (sprain of cruciate ligament of knee) as an admitting diagnosis, but the coder did not "set" that code as the admitting diagnosis. Most likely, review of the patient record face sheet and/or responsible physician's admission note resulted in "tear of lateral cartilage or meniscus of knee current" as the reason for surgical admission/encounter.
- CAC software assigned an *admitting diagnosis* and a *reason for admission* because the software option to capture both of these data elements was selected. In future, the health information director might omit the data capture of one of these elements (e.g., electronic health record entry field *reason for admission* is renamed *admitting diagnosis*).

3. a. 844.2, 836.1
   b. 29881-RT, 29888-RT
   c. 29875-RT

Note:

- CAC software most likely displayed code 29875-RT as *Possible*, and upon review of patient record documentation (e.g., operative report) the coder deleted the code.
- Although an arthroscopy was performed, it is already included in the first documented procedure (located in the bottom half of the CAC demo application's computer screen).
- The list of procedures (located in the bottom half of the CAC demo application's computer screen) does not include *synovectomy, limited (e.g., plica or shelf resection) (separate procedure)*, which means that procedure was not performed. (In CPT, *separate procedure* is included in parentheses in code descriptions for procedures that are performed as distinct procedures, not in combination with another procedure.)

ASSIGNMENT 1.5 – FACE VALIDITY OF DATA MANAGEMENT REPORTS

(Permission to reuse granted by the American Health Information Management Association.)

Section A

SERVICE	DISCHARGES	DEATHS	AUTOPSIES[1]		DISCHARGE DAYS	AVERAGE LOS[1]	CONSULTS	MEDICARE PATIENTS		PEDIATRIC PATIENTS	
			#	%				#	DAYS	#	DAYS
Medicine	725	40	8	25%	6,394	9	717	301	3104	0	0
General Surgery	280	10	3	30%	2,374	8	184	80	916	0	0
Cardiac Surgery	64	1	1	100%	1,039	16	35	26	431		0
Hand Surgery	26	0	0	0%	81	3	2	3	10	0	0
Neurosurgery	94	0	0	0%	1,429	15	39	12	266	4	39
Plastic Surgery	46	0	0	0%	319	7	19	7	97	0	0
Dental Surgery	25	0	0	0%	81	3	46	2	11	1	3
Dermatology	20	0	0	0%	289	14	56	6	83	0	0
Neurology	83	0	0	0%	776	9	183	24	284	0	0
Ophthalmology	87	0	0	0%	352	4	98	51	183	0	0
Orthopedics	216	2	0	0%	1,920	9	64	39	563	1	2
Otolaryngology	139	2	0	0%	705	5	87	16	168	4	7
ICU[2]	8	1	1	50%	128	16	1	0		8	127
Psychiatry	126	0	0	0%	3,624	29	97	7	317	1	8
Urology	108	1	1	100%	810	8	74	36	318	0	0
Gynecology	184	2	1	50%	853	5	55	11	93	0	0
Obstetrics	451	2	2	0%	2,099	5	14	0	0	1	2
SUBTOTAL	2682	62	17	27%	23,273	9	1,771	621	6,844	20	189
Newborn	310	0	0	0%	1,191	4	0	0	0	0	0
SCN[3]	38	4	1	25%	742	20	0	0	0	0	0
TOTAL	3030	66	18	27%	25,206	8	1,771	621	6,844	20	189

Section B

DISCHARGE DISPOSITION	# OF PATIENTS
Against medical Advice	15
Home	2,850
Home health care	10
Skilled nursing facility	37
Rehabilitation facility	39
Other hospital	13
Expired	65
TOTAL	3,030

Section C

RESULTS	# OF PATIENTS
Discharged alive	2,964
Not treated	0
Diagnosis only	0
Expired over 48 hours	54
Expired under 48 hours	12
TOTAL	3,029

Section D

TYPE OF DEATH	NUMBER OF DEATHS	AUTOPSIES	
		#	%
Anesthesia	0	0	0%
Postoperative	8	2	25%
Medical examiner	4	3	75%
Stillbirths	4	3	75%
TOTAL	16	8	50%

[1] Round up mathematical calculations to the whole number (e.g., 8.82 is reported as 9).
[2] ICU is the abbreviation for intensive care unit, where patients who need constant monitoring receive care.
[3] SCN is the abbreviation for special care nursery, where premature infants, twins, triplets, and so on receive care.

Section A

Under the Deaths column of the table (Column 3, Row 14), the number of ICU deaths should be 2. Because the Autopsies # data column is accurate and the subtotal of deaths is 62, there is an incorrect data entry in a cell above the Total row. Upon review of the data in each row for Autopsies, # and %, the calculated ICU autopsies % is 50%, which means that there were 2 ICU deaths.

Under the Autopsies column of the table (Column 4, Row 2), the Autopsies % for the Medicine service should be 20%. The Autopsies % in the Medicine service data cell is incorrect because (8 ÷ 40) × 100 = 20% (not 25%).

Under the Autopsies column of the table (Column 4, Row 18), the Autopsies % for the Obstetrics data cell should be 100%. The Autopsies % in the Obstetrics service data cell is incorrect because (2 ÷ 2) × 100 = 100%.

Section B

Under the Discharge Disposition section of the table (Column 2, Row 8, bottom left), the total expired should be 66. The Discharge Disposition, Expired, # of Patients data cell is incorrect because the total expired is correctly reported as 66 in the top portion of the table. (All data located in subtotal and total rows in the upper portion of the spreadsheet are correct.)

Section C

The Results, # of Patients, Total (Column 5, Row 9, bottom middle) should be 3,030. The Results, # of Patients, Total data cell is incorrect because 2,964 + 54 + 12 = 3,030, which also matches the total in the top portion of the table (Column 1) and the bottom portion of the table (Column 1).

REVIEW

Multiple Choice

1. b
2. c
3. b
4. d
5. b
6. a
7. d
8. d
9. d
10. b
11. a
12. a
13. c
14. b
15. b
16. b
17. d
18. a
19. d
20. b

Chapter 2
Introduction to ICD-9-CM and ICD-10-CM/PCS Coding

ASSIGNMENT 2.1 – ICD-9-CM INDEX TO DISEASES AND ICD-10-CM INDEX TO DISEASES AND INJURIES

1. Rheumatoid arthritis — 714.0 (M06.9)
2. Acute myocardial infarction (Infarct, infarction) — 410.90 (I21.3)
3. *Pseudomonas pneumonia* — 482.1 (J15.1)
4. Type 2 diabetes mellitus — 250.00 (E11.9)
5. Congestive heart failure — 428.0 (I50.9)
6. Crush injury of right index finger — 927.3 (S67.19-)
7. Sickle cell disease with crisis — 282.62 (D57.00)
8. Comminuted fracture, traumatic, of lower end of tibia (Fracture, traumatic in ICD-10-CM) — 824.8 (S82.30)
9. Congenital cleft lip, incomplete, unilateral — 749.12 (Q36.9)
10. Hypertensive heart disease (Hypertension, hypertension disease in ICD-9-CM or disease – *see* Hypertension in ICD-10-CM) — 402.90 (III.9)

ASSIGNMENT 2.2 – ICD-9-CM INDEX TO PROCEDURES AND ICD-10-CM INDEX

1. Incision and drainage of skin abscess (Incision (and drainage) in ICD-9-CM, Incision, Abscess—*see* Drainage in ICD-10-CM) — 86.04 (0H97)
2. Low cesarean section — 74.1 (10D0)
3. Laparoscopic cholecystectomy (Cholecystectomy—*see* Resection, Gallbladder in ICD-10-PCS) — 51.23 (0FT4)
4. Transurethral laser-induced prostatectomy (Prostatectomy—*see* Resection, Prostate in ICD-10-PCS) — 60.21 (0VT0)
5. Extracorporeal shock wave lithotripsy of kidney, left (Lithotripsy—*see* Fragmentation in ICD-10-PCS) — 98.51 (0TF4)
6. Loop electrosurgical excision procedure of cervix — 67.32
7. Colostomy closure (Closure—*see* Repair in ICD-10-PCS) — 46.52 (0DQM)
8. Knee arthroscopy (Arthroscopy—*see* Inspection, Lower Joints in ICD-10-PCS) — 80.26 (0SJ)
9. Extracapsular cataract (lens) extraction, right — 13.59 (08DJ3ZZ)
10. Abdominal hysterectomy (Hysterectomy—*see* Resection, Uterus in ICD-10-PCS) — 68.49 (0UT9)

ASSIGNMENT 2.3 – GENERAL EQUIVALENCY MAPPING (GEMs)

	Column 1	Column 2	Column 3	Column 4	Column 5
	ICD-9-CM Code	GEM ICD-9-CM Diagnosis Code	GEM ICD-10-CM Diagnosis Code	ICD-10-CM Diagnosis Code	GEM ICD-10-PCS Procedure Code(s)
1.	003.24	00324	A0229	A02.29	n/a
2.	001.0	0010	A001	A00.1	n/a
3.	002.1	00021	A012	A01.2	n/a
4.	00.01	0001	n/a	n/a	
5.	00.03	0003	n/a	n/a	

Note:

- ICD-10-CM codes contain three characters, a decimal, and up to four additional characters.
- ICD-10-PCS codes are seven characters in length, and they do *not* contain decimals.

ASSIGNMENT 2.4 – ICD-10-PCS INDEX AND TABLES

1. Nuclear medicine
2. Section qualifier
3. Qualifier
4. Radiation oncology
5. Root type
6. 01U0
7. second qualifiers "cranial" and "pelvic" located below the subterm contain ICD-10-CM characters
8. 00160J2
9. 001U077
10. False. The index entry for "bypass, cavity, cranial" includes just six characters (0W110J). The coder would refer to ICD-10-PCS Table 0W1 to determine the seventh character. An ICD-10-PCS code is always seven characters in length.

REVIEW

Multiple Choice

1. c
2. b
3. d
4. c
5. b
6. d
7. d
8. d
9. d
10. d
11. b
12. c
13. c
14. d
15. b
16. c
17. c
18. d
19. c
20. c
21. c
22. b
23. b
24. c
25. b
26. c
27. b
28. d
29. b
30. c

Chapter 3
ICD-9-CM and ICD-10-CM/PCS Coding Conventions

ASSIGNMENT 3.1 – APPLYING ICD-9-CM CODING CONVENTIONS

Format

1. 176.4 (C46.51)
2. 285.1 (D62)
3. 365.21 (H40.232)
4. 772.2 (P52.5)
5. 584.6 (N17.1)
6. 732.8 (M42.12)
7. 391.8 (I01.8)
8. 300.11 (F45.8)
9. 388.31 (H93.11)
10. 088.81, 320.7 (A69.21)
11. 49.31 (0DBQ8ZZ)
12. 58.31 (0T5D8ZZ)
13. 45.02 (0D9840Z)
14. 09.41 (087Y7ZZ, 3E1CX8Z)
15. 15.7 (08QM0ZZ)

Eponyms

16. 272.7 (E75.249)
17. 767.6 (P14.0)
18. 346.20 (G44.099)
19. 422.91 (I40.1)
20. 114.0 (B39.0)
21. 690.8 (L30.3)
22. 100.89 (A77.3)
23. 270.0 (E72.04)
24. 015.00, 720.81 (A18.01)
25. 426.9 (45.9)

Note:

There are no ICD-10-PCS codes for #26–30 because eponyms *do not appear in the ICD-10-PCS index or tables.*

26. 83.88
27. 05.29
28. 44.66
29. 77.99
30. 52.7

NEC and NOS Abbreviations

31. 482.30 (J15.4)
32. 724.4 (M51.16)
33. 999.5 (T80.6xxA)
34. 098.2 (A54.9)
35. 008.47 (A04.8)
36. 374.82 (H02.841)
37. 253.2 (E23.0)
38. 296.90 (E39)
39. 455.6 (I84.20)
40. 514 (J81.1)

Note:

There are no ICD-10-PCS codes for #41–45 because NEC and NOS abbreviations *do not appear in the ICD-10-PCS index or tables.*

41. 43.99
42. 09.59
43. 67.12
44. 83.09
45. 77.58

Punctuation

46. 458.9 (I95.9)
47. 730.20 (M86.9)
48. 242.00, 376.22 (E05.00)
49. 284.01 (D61.01)
50. 250.50, 362.01 (E11.319)
51. 250.40, 581.81 (E11.21)
52. 027.0 (A32.0)
53. 284.1 (D61.81)
54. 486 (J18.9)
55. 472.0 (J31.0)

Note:

There are no ICD-10-PCS codes for #56–60 because of the limited use of punctuation *in the ICD-10-PCS index.*

56. 08.42
57. 27.69, 29.4
58. 22.60
59. 39.29
60. 74.3

Boxed Notes

Note:

ICD-9-CM codes only *are assigned to to #61–75 because* boxes notes *do not appear in the ICD-10-CM or ICD-10-PCS indexes.*

61. 824.8
62. 813.32
63. 250.02
64. 807.05
65. 550.92
66. 915.3
67. 923.10
68. 715.95
69. 851.83
70. 303.00
71. 90.33
72. 81.06, 81.62
73. 55.69, 00.91
74. 90.49
75. 33.6, 39.61, 00.93

Tables

Note:

Codes in # 76 to 80 are from the ICD-9-CM Hypertension Table, codes in # 81 to 85 are from the ICD-9-CM and ICD-10-CM Neoplasm Table, and codes in # 86 to 90 are from the ICD-9-CM and ICD-10-CM Table of Drugs and Chemicals.

Note:

There are no ICD-10-CM codes for #76–80 because the Hypertension Table *does not appear in the ICD-10-CM index.*

76. 405.99, 592.0
77. 405.09, 255.0
78. 572.3
79. 402.10
80. 404.90
81. 162.5 (C34.31)
82. 234.8 (D09.3)
83. 197.8 (C78.89)
84. 212.1 (D14.1)
85. 237.9 (D43.3)
86. 983.9, E980.6 (T54.1x1A)
87. 995.29, E935.4 (T39.1x5A)
88. 969.4, E950.3 (T42.4x2A)
89. 962.7, E858.0 (T38.1x1A)
90. 693.0, E930.0 (T36.0x5A, L27.0)

Includes and Excludes Notes and Inclusion Terms

91. 277.39 (E85.1)
92. 451.81 (I80.211)
93. 013.30 (A17.81)
94. 726.19 (M75.82)
95. 098.40 (A54.31)
96. 518.89 (J09.4)
97. 736.79 (M21.071)
98. 572.2 (K72.91)
99. 362.70 (H35.50)
100. 334.9 (G11.9)

Note:

There are no ICD-10-PCS codes for #101–105 because includes and excludes notes and inclusion terms *do not appear in the Tables.*

101. 60.5
102. 57.71
103. 46.10
104. 43.19
105. 27.63

Other, Other Specified, and Unspecified Codes

106. 729.90 (M70.90)
107. 576.8 (K83.8)
108. 529.8 (K14.8)
109. 459.89 (I87.8)
110. 274.9 (M10.9)
111. 006.9 (A06.9)
112. 319 (F79)
113. 241.9 (E04.9)
114. 110.9 (B35.9)
115. 259.9 (IE34.9)

Note:

There are no ICD-10-PCS codes for #116–120 because other, other specified, and unspecified codes *do not appear in the Tables.*

116. 47.99
117. 36.99
118. 48.76
119. 85.89
120. 93.39

Etiology and Manifestation Rules

121. 282.62, 517.3 (D57.01)
122. 536.41, 041.11 (K94.22, B95.6)
123. 710.0, 582.81 (M32.14, N08)
124. 590.10, 041.2 (N10, B95.3)
125. 421.0, 041.00 (I33.0, B95.3)
126. 334.0, 425.8 (G11.1, I43)
127. 006.8, 595.4 (A06.81)
128. 117.5, 321.0 (B45.1)
129. 608.0, 041.02 (N49.0, B95.1)
130. 202.30 (C86.0)
131. 015.00, 737.43 (A18.01)
132. 099.3, 711.11 (M02.312)
133. 693.0, E930.0 (L27.0, T36.0x5A)
134. 510.9, 041.81 (J86.9, B96.0)
135. 290.40, 437.0 (F01.50, I67.2)

And

136. 474.11 (J35.1)
137. 513.1 (J85.3)
138. 523.33 (K05.20)
139. 565.1 (K60.5)
140. 592.1 (N20.1)
141. 616.10 (N76.0)
142. 627.1 (N95.0)
143. 749.23 (Q37.4)
144. 776.4 (P61.1)
145. 680.2 (L02.229)
146. 682.4 (L02.511)
147. 472.2 (J31.1)
148. 427.42 (I49.02)
149. 372.75 (H11.441)
150. 344.02 (G82.52)

Due to

151. 371.24 (H18.211)
152. 525.11 (K08.119)
153. 708.2 (L50.2)
154. 767.8 (P15.2)
155. 032.89 (A36.89)
156. 482.81 (J15.8)
157. 103.2 (A67.2)
158. 537.3 (K56.2, K31.5)
159. 598.1 (N35.010)
160. 117.9 (J32.2, B49)
161. 039.1 (A42.0)
162. 773.1 (P55.9)
163. 364.04 (H40.021)
164. 275.03 (K74.69, E83.11)
165. 130.2 (B58.01)

With

166. 381.4 (H65.92)
167. 583.7 (N17.2)
168. 571.2 (K70.2)
169. 780.60 (R50.9)
170. 276.4 (R06.89, E87.4)
171. 398.0 (I09.0)
172. 379.05 (H15.041)
173. 287.33 (Q87.2)
174. 707.10, 785.4 (L97.913, I96)
175. 282.2 (D55.1)
176. 810.02 (S42.022A)
177. 466.19 (J21.9)
178. 115.95 (B39.2, J17)
179. 094.0 (A52.19)
180. 487.1 (J10.1)

Cross References: *See, See Also, See* Category, *See Condition*

181. 363.20 (H30.92)
182. 424.90 (I38)
183. 520.1 (K00.1)
184. 526.4 (M27.2)
185. 927.3 (S67.01xA)
186. 386.48 (H83.11)
187. 441.02 (I71.02)
188. 944.00 (T23.001A)
189. 537.89 (K29.40)
190. 566 062.3 (A83.3)
191. 83.89 (0JQ03ZZ)
192. 93.08 (4A0FX3Z)
193. 88.75 (BT40ZZZ)
194. 99.43 (3E0234Z)
195. 80.47 (0M8Q0ZZ)

REVIEW

Multiple Choice

1. d
2. d
3. a
4. b
5. c
6. a
7. b
8. c
9. b
10. d
11. d
12. a
13. a
14. b
15. b
16. c
17. c
18. b
19. c
20. b
21. c
22. d
23. c
24. a
25. c

Chapter 4
ICD-9-CM and ICD-10-CM Coding Guidelines

ASSIGNMENT 4.1 – ICD-9-CM OFFICIAL GUIDELINES FOR CODING AND REPORTING

1. 380.10, 785.6 (H60.392, R59.0)

Note:

- Do not assign codes to hearing loss (symptom) or fever (sign), which are the result of otitis externa. (A symptom is a condition the patient complains about, such as sore throat, chest pain, or difficulty urinating. A sign is a condition that the provider can observe, such as throat erythema (redness), tight chest, or blood in the urine.
- Be sure to assign a code to the "swollen axillary lymph nodes" because "axillary" is the medical term for "of armpit," and it is likely that the patient has another problem that has to be worked up due to this sign.

2. 345.50 (G40.009)
3. 250.00 (E11.9)
4. V10.87 (Z85.850)
5. 786.05 (R06.02)
6. 728.71 (M72.2)
7. 250.60, 357.2 (E11.40)

Note:

In ICD-9-CM, refer to main term "diabetes, diabetic" in the index, and locate subterm "neuropathy." The index entry includes two codes: 250.6 [357.2]. *Verify code 250.6 in the tabular list to assign fifth digit 2 (type 2, not stated as uncontrolled), and sequence code 250.60 first. Code 357.2 is located in slanted brackets in the index; therefore, it is sequenced second because it is a manifestation of the diabetes. (A manifestation is a condition the patient develops as the result of already having another condition, such as diabetic cataracts. The index provides the clue to proper sequencing of codes because the manifestation code in slanted brackets is always sequenced second.)*

8. 601.9 (N41.9)
9. 614.0, 614.1 (N70.03, N70.13)
10. 483.1 (J16.0)
11. 591, 600.90 (N13.39, N40.0)

Note:

In ICD-10-CM, code N40.0 is assigned (instead of N40.1) because hydronephrosis *is not associated with the lower urinary tract system (LUTS).*

12. 438.12 (I69.321)
13. 715.94, 906.4 (M19.142, S67.22S)

Note:

In ICD-9-CM, the residual condition is sequenced first, followed by the code for late effect. In ICD-10-CM, the residual condition is also sequenced first, followed by the late effect code. In ICD-10-CM, the late effect code is classifed as the original injury code with 7th character S *for* sequela.

14. 411.1 (I20.0)
15. 086.9, 321.3 (B56.9, G02)
16. 789.03 (R10.31)
17. 908.3 (S09.0xxS)
18. 034.0 (J03.00)
19. 277.02, 041.7 (E84.0, B96.5)
20. 710.0, 583.81 (M32.14, N00.9)

ASSIGNMENT 4.2 – ICD-9-CM DISEASE CODING

Infectious and Parasitic Diseases

1. 091.0 (A51.0)
2. 045.92 (A80.9)
3. 008.67 (A08.4, B97.12)
4. 005.1 (A05.1)
5. 030.9 (A30.9)
6. 034.1 (A38.9)
7. 053.9 (B02.9)
8. 070.53 (B17.2)
9. 072.2 (B26.2)
10. 077.2 (B30.2)

Neoplasms

11. 224.4 (D31.11)
12. 211.3 (D12.6)
13. 212.1 (D14.1)
14. 227.0 (D35.02)
15. 228.04 (D18.3)
16. 140.4 (C00.4)
17. 208.00 (C95.00)
18. 202.50 (C96.0)
19. 191.3 (C71.3)
20. 183.0 (C56.1)

Endocrine, Nutritional, Metabolic, Immunity

21. 246.8 (E03.4)
22. 253.3 (E23.0)
23. 267 (E54)
24. 279.11 (D82.1)
25. 270.1 (E70.0)
26. 256.31 (E28.319)
27. 257.1 (E89.5)
28. 251.3 (E89.1)
29. 254.1 (E32.1)
30. 255.12 (E26.01, D35.0)

Diseases of the Blood and Blood-Forming Organs

31. 285.0 (D64.3)
32. 288.3 (D72.1)
33. 283.10 (D59.4)
34. 282.49 (D56.9)
35. 281.1 (D51.1)
36. 282.62, 517.3 (D57.01)
37. 284.09 (D61.09)
38. 286.2 (D68.1)
39. 286.6 (D65)
40 289.4 (D73.1)

Mental Disorders

41. 291.3 (F10.951)
42. 290.20 (F03)
43. 295.50 (F21)
44. 300.21 (F40.01)
45. 304.00 (F11.29)
46. 301.7 (F60.2)
47. 307.46 (F51.4)
48. 307.23 (F95.2)
49. 306.4 (F45.8)
50. 307.81 (G44.209)

Diseases of the Nervous System and Sense Organs

51. 320.82 (G00.8, B96.5)
52. 331.11 (G31.01)
53. 336.1 (G95.19)
54. 362.18 (H35.061)
55. 339.00 (G44.009)
56. 361.12 (H33.191)
57. 356.3 (G60.1)
58. 355.5 (G57.52)
59. 372.13 (H10.44)
60. 354.3 (G56.32)

Diseases of the Circulatory System

61. 397.0 (I36.1)
62. 455.4 (I64.02)
63. 443.0, 785.4 (I73.01)
64. 446.5 (G31.6)
65. 427.31, 427.32 (I48.0, I48.1)
66. 429.6 (I51.2)
67. 429.2 (I25.10)
68. 428.0 (I50.9)
69. 412 (I25.2)
70. 401.1 (I10)

Diseases of the Respiratory System

71. 474.10 (J35.3)
72. 482.84 (A48.1)
73. 478.6 (J38.4)
74. 494.1 (J47.1)
75. 513.1 (J85.3)
76. 518.84 (J96.2)
77. 518.3 (J82)
78. 491.0 (J41.0)
79. 478.26 (J39.2)
80. 477.2 (J30.81)

Diseases of the Digestive System

81. 523.40 (K05.30)
82. 524.62 (M26.62)
83. 530.5 (K22.4)
84. 529.5 (K14.5)
85. 536.41, 041.4 (K94.22, B96.2)
86. 551.01 (K41.41)
87. 572.1 (K75.1)
88. 579.1 (K90.1)
89. 560.31 (K56.3)
90. 526.81 (M27.8)

Diseases of the Genitourinary System

91. 593.6 (R80.2)
92. 600.00 (N40.0)
93. 611.5 (N64.89)
94. 599.5 (N36.8)
95. 593.0 (N28.83)
96. 599.82 (N36.42)
97. 588.0 (N25.0)
98. 581.1 (N04.1)
99. 590.2 (N15.1)
100. 595.1 (N30.10)

Complications of Pregnancy, Childbirth, and the Puerperium

101. 666.04 (072.0)
102. 669.32 (090.4)
103. 630 (001.9)
104. 633.80 (000.8)
105. 635.52 (004.81)
106. 634.91 (003.4)
107. 672.04 (086.4)
108. 674.14 (090.0)
109. 651.01, V27.2 (030.003, Z37.2)
110. 644.21, V27.0 (060.120, Z37.0)

Diseases of the Skin and Subcutaneous Tissue

111. 690.11 (L21.0)
112. 707.07, 707.23 (L89.623)
113. 706.8 (L85.3)
114. 709.1 (L81.7)
115. 701.4 (L91.0)
116. 703.8 (L60.3)
117. 705.1 (L74.0)
118. 694.0 (L13.0)
119. 692.77 (L55.2)
120. 695.3 (L71.9)

Diseases of the Musculoskeletal System and Connective Tissue

121. 729.30 (M79.3)
122. 736.05 (M21.331)
123. 737.20 (M40.46)
124. 710.2 (M35.00)
125. 712.95 (M11.851)
126. 714.81 (M05.10)
127. 727.42 (M67.411)
128. 726.32 (M77.02)
129. 726.90 (M77.9)
130. 730.06 (M86.162)

Congenital Anomalies

131. 743.33 (Q12.0)
132. 746.86 (Q24.6)
133. 744.23 (Q17.2)
134. 748.0 (Q30.0)
135. 749.14 (Q36.0)
136. 754.61 (Q66.5)
137. 755.31 (Q72.31)
138. 755.02 (Q69.2)
139. 758.2 (Q91.3)
140. 757.32 (Q82.5)

Certain Conditions Originating in the Perinatal Period

141. 760.71 (P04.3)
142. 770.3 (P26.8)
143. 767.2 (P13.4)
144. 777.3 (P78.2)
145. 779.82 (P29.11)
146. 765.02, 765.23 (P07.02, P07.22)
147. 277.4, 774.31 (E80.4, P59.8)
148. 775.3 (P72.1)
149. 779.33
150. 779.5 (P92.09)

Symptoms, Signs, and Ill-Defined Conditions

151. 793.1 (R91)
152. 790.4 (R74.0)
153. 789.59 (R18.8)
154. 796.2 (R03.0)
155. 794.4 (R94.4)
156. 798.0 (R99)
157. 797 (R41.81)
158. 789.05 (R10.33)
159. 790.93 (R97.2)
160. 790.1 (R70.0)

Injury and Poisoning

161. 951.5 (S04.62A)
162. 807.4 (S22.53xA)
163. 806.03 (S12.101A, S14.122A)
164. 811.02 (S42.134A)
165. 833.00 (S63.005A)
166. 967.0, E980.1 (T42.3x4A)
167. 824.4 (S82.844A)
168. 826.1 (S93.53B, S92.52B, S91.104A)
169. 836.0 (S83.211A)
170. 803.03 (S02.91A, S06.0x3A)

Factors Influencing Health Status and Contact with Health Services

171. V10.60 (Z85.6)
172. V17.2 (Z82.0)
173. V43.3 (Z95.2)
174. V53.32 (Z45.02)
175. V58.64 (Z79.1)
176. V57.3 (Z51.89)
177. V65.3, 250.00 (Z71.3, E11.9)
178. V69.4 (Z72.820)
179. V70.4 (Z02.83)
180. V77.6 (Z13.228)

External Causes of Injury and Poisoning

181. E837.3 (V91.01xA)
182. E870.6 (Y65.8)
183. E904.0 (T74.02A)
184. E968.7 (Y04.1xxA)
185. E960.0 (Y04.1xxA)
186. E905.3 (T63.441A)
187. E908.4 (X37.3xxA)
188. E876.0 (Y65.0)
189. E853.2 (T42.4x1A)
190. E884.2 (W07.xxxA)

REVIEW

Multiple Choice

1. b
2. a
3. b
4. a
5. b

Note:

According to the AHA Coding Clinic for ICD-9-CM, "Secondary arthritis is confined to joints of one area, and is due to some external or internal injury or disease process." To locate code 715.24, index main term "arthritis" directs you to see "osteoarthrosis." Then, locate subterms "localized" and "secondary," and locate code 715.2 in the tabular list (and assign fifth digit 4 for "hand)."

6. c
7. a
8. a
9. c
10. b
11. a
12. b
13. a
14. a
15. c
16. c
17. d
18. b
19. a
20. d

Chapter 5
ICD-9-CM and ICD-10-CM/PCS Hospital Inpatient Coding

ASSIGNMENT 5.1 – PHYSICIAN QUERY PROCESS

1. c

Note:

- Alcohol use and gallstones are the most common causes of acute pancreatitis.
- Do not assign codes to symptoms (e.g., midabdominal pain) when a definitive diagnosis is established. In this case, the patient was definitively diagnosed with acute pancreatitis and cholecystitis.
- Do not assign a code to cholelithiasis because this condition was not evaluated during the admission; it will be evaluated on an outpatient basis.

2. c

Note:

- Do not assign codes to symptoms such as fatigue, shortness of breath, and chest pain when a definitive diagnosis has been established. In this case, the patient was diagnosed with congestive heart failure.
- According to the AHA's *Coding Clinic for ICD-9-CM,* "Pleural effusion is commonly seen with congestive heart failure . . . pleural effusion documented only as an x-ray finding without the physician having made such a diagnosis should not be reported." In this case, generate a physician query to ask if the "pleural effusion" should be documented as the principal diagnosis (instead of congestive heart failure).

3. d

Note:

Documentation indicates that the patient was administered insulin during the hospitalization, and the patient is discharged with a prescription for insulin. Although the patient receives insulin during the hospitalization and continues to receive insulin upon return to the nursing facility, a physician query should be generated to ask if the patient's diabetes is type I or II.

4. c

Note:

Elevated blood urea nitrogen (BUN) and creatinine levels are indicative of possible renal disease, and the physician should be asked if a diagnosis should be added for coding purposes.

5. c

Note:

- The diagnosis of "ectopic pregnancy" does not include the type (e.g., interstitial). The physician should be asked to document the type so a specific code can be assigned.
- Pelvic tenderness is a symptom of an ectopic pregnancy, and it is not assigned a code.

6. Upon review of this case, the coder should query the physician to ask whether knee joint effusion should be assigned a code because that condition was addressed by a consultant but it is not listed as a final diagnosis.
7. Upon review of this case, the coder should assign codes to HIV and lymphadenopathy because the physical examination, diagnostic workup, and final diagnosis justify assigning those codes.
8. Upon review of this case, the coder should query the physician to ask that he or she document the patient's final diagnosis on the record because it is inappropriate to assign codes for conditions based on review of the record when the physician has not documented established diagnoses.
9. Upon review of this case, the coder should query the physician to ask that a diagnosis related to the prescribed antibiotics be documented (e.g., cystitis) because benign prostatic hypertrophy is not typically associated with an infection.

Note:

Cystitis can be caused by urinary retention associated with benign prostatic hypertrophy (BPH). Antibiotic treatment would be indicated for cystitis, and the patient's symptom of painful urination also supports this diagnosis.

10. Upon review of this case, the coder should query the physician to confirm that "microscopic fractures at T1 and L5" should be coded. The physician should also be asked whether the patient has "possible osteoporosis" because fractures noted on x-ray were not confirmed as a diagnosis by the attending physician. (The diagnosis of compression fractures plus the performance of bone density testing indicates "possible osteoporosis.")

Note:

The age of the patient and the microscopic fractures provide clues that a physician query should be generated to ask if "possible osteoporosis" should be documented on the record. However, even if "possible osteoporosis" is documented, do not assign a code to this condition because it is a qualified diagnosis. (For an outpatient case, code signs and/or symptoms instead of qualified diagnoses.)

ASSIGNMENT 5.2 – ICD-9-CM PROCEDURE CODING

Procedures and Interventions, Not Elsewhere Classified

1. 00.22
2. 00.51
3. 00.62, 99.10
4. 00.33
5. 00.03
6. 00.12
7. 00.22
8. 00.50
9. 00.53
10. 00.11

Operations on the Nervous System

11. 03.51
12. 04.81
13. 07.72
14. 04.01
15. 03.53
16. 03.31
17. 01.59
18. 02.12
19. 03.95
20. 01.11

Operations on the Endocrine System

21. 06.4
22. 07.11
23. 07.62
24. 07.44
25. 06.95
26. 06.39
27. 07.52
28. 06.7
29. 07.16
30. 07.54

Operations on the Eye

31. 08.42
32. 09.81
33. 11.22
34. 16.21
35. 16.72
36. 14.54
37. 11.60
38. 13.19
39. 08.21
40. 09.21

Operations on the Ear

41. 19.9
42. 20.61
43. 20.23
44. 18.71
45. 19.53
46. 20.42
47. 18.12
48. 18.79
49. 18.11
50. 20.31

Operations on the Nose, Mouth, and Pharynx

51. 21.21
52. 23.19
53. 27.0
54. 27.62
55. 28.3
56. 29.4
57. 21.03
58. 21.61
59. 22.11
60. 23.09

Operations on the Respiratory System

61. 31.92
62. 34.02
63. 34.83
64. 32.22
65. 33.22
66. 33.27
67. 34.24
68. 34.74
69. 33.99
70. 31.1

Operations on the Cardiovascular System

71. 35.91, 39.61
72. 35.81
73. 37.28
74. 39.51
75. 37.0
76. 35.23
77. 39.30
78. 38.94
79. 38.22
80. 35.34, 39.61

Operations on the Hemic and Lymphatic System

81. 41.43
82. 41.91
83. 40.23
84. 41.31
85. 41.5
86. 40.63
87. 40.54
88. 41.06
89. 41.33
90. 40.11

Operations on the Digestive System

91. 45.16
92. 45.73
93. 48.0
94. 49.73
95. 49.22
96. 51.11
97. 51.23
98. 52.7
99. 53.71
100. 54.59

Operations on the Urinary System

101. 55.21
102. 55.7
103. 57.32
104. 56.85
105. 58.93
106. 58.0
107. 58.23
108. 55.69, 00.92
109. 55.23
110. 57.6

Operations on the Male Genital Organs

111. 60.21
112. 60.97
113. 62.5
114. 60.96
115. 60.11
116. 60.62
117. 62.3
118. 61.91
119. 63.73
120. 64.11

Operations on the Female Genital Organs

121. 65.24
122. 66.11
123. 68.79
124. 67.33
125. 66.8
126. 70.22
127. 71.3
128. 69.09
129. 68.16
130. 68.31

Obstetrical Procedures

131. 74.1
132. 75.38
133. 75.93
134. 72.4
135. 73.6
136. 73.01
137. 72.71
138. 75.4
139. 75.61
140. 75.1

Operations on the Musculoskeletal System

141. 77.47
142. 79.73
143. 81.11
144. 83.86
145. 77.23
146. 80.51
147. 81.54
148. 81.43
149. 83.01
150. 83.14

Operations on the Integumentary System

151. 86.27
152. 86.07
153. 85.21
154. 85.94
155. 86.24
156. 86.09
157. 86.28
158. 86.25
159. 86.11
160. 86.64

Miscellaneous Diagnostic and Therapeutic Procedures

161. 89.19
162. 93.05
163. 94.32
164. 95.03
165. 96.33
166. 99.07
167. 97.82
168. 97.23
169. 95.41
170. 96.14

ASSIGNMENT 5.3 – ICD-10-PCS PROCEDURE CODING

(Adapted from the *ICD-10-PCS Reference Manual*. Permission to reuse in accordance with http://www.cms.hhs.gov Content Reuse and Linking policy.)

Root Operation: Destruction

1. 0H5GXZZ
2. 0C5T3ZZ
3. 02583ZZ
4. 095KXZZ
5. 0V508ZZ
6. 065Y3ZZ
7. 0U524ZZ
8. 085G3ZZ
9. 0B5P3ZZ, 3E0L3TZ
10. 01533ZZ, 3E0T3TZ

Root Operation: Detachment

11. 0X6B0ZZ
12. 0Y6H0Z1
13. 0X6K0Z8
14. 0Y620ZZ
15. 0X6L0Z3
16. 0X6J0Z0
17. 0Y6N0Z9
18. 0X680Z2

19. 0Y6W0Z1
20. 0Y6C0Z3

Excision

21. 0HB2XZZ
22. 0UB14ZZ
23. 0TB03ZX
24. 0DB68ZX
25. 03BJ0ZZ
26. 0CB1XZZ
27. 0FBG0ZZ
28. 0KBS3ZX
29. 0DBN8ZZ
30. 0LBN0ZZ

Root Operation: Extraction

31. 0CDWXZ2, 0CDXXZ2
32. 0HDQXZZ
33. 08DJ3ZZ
34. 0UDN4ZZ
35. 0HDMXZZ

Root Operation: Resection

36. 0DTH0ZZ
37. 0GT00ZZ
38. 0TT10ZZ
39. 07T60ZZ
40. 0UT9FZZ
41. 0HTT0ZZ
42. 02TD0ZZ
43. 0VT00ZZ
44. 0FT44ZZ
45. 09TQ4ZZ, 09TR4ZZ

Root Operation: Drainage

46. 0T9B70Z
47. 0D9QXZZ
48. 0W9G3ZZ
49. 0U914ZZ
50. 0F9100Z
51. 0S9C00Z
52. 0W9B3ZZ
53. 059F3ZZ

54. 0W9930Z
55. 099V4ZZ

Root Operation: Extirpation

56. 08C8XZZ
57. 03C83ZZ
58. 0DC68ZZ
59. 0HCGXZZ
60. 0TCB8ZZ
61. 09CKXZZ
62. 0DCV4ZZ
63. 08CX0ZZ
64. 0UCG7ZZ
65. 0JCR0ZZ

Root Operation: Fragmentation

66. 0TF6XZZ, 0TF7XZZ
67. 0FF98ZZ
68. 02FN0ZZ
69. 0TFB8ZZ
70. 0UF68ZZ

Root Operation: Division

71. 0L8V3ZZ
72. 02883ZZ
73. 0P8N0ZZ
74. 0D848ZZ
75. 018R3ZZ

Root Operation: Release

76. 0TN60ZZ
77. 0HNDXZZ
78. 0CN7XZZ
79. 0MN14ZZ
80. 02NG0ZZ
81. 0LNP3ZZ
82. 0DNW4ZZ
83. 0RNJXZZ
84. 01NG0ZZ
85. 0UN14ZZ, 0UN64ZZ

Root Operation: Reattachment

86. 0HM0XZZ
87. 09M0XZZ

88. 0KMT0ZZ
89. 0CMXXZ1
90. 0XMK0ZZ

Root Operation: Reposition

91. 0QSG0ZZ
92. 0DS64ZZ
93. 0MSP4ZZ
94. 01S40ZZ
95. 0QS634Z

Root Operation: Transfer

96. 0LX70ZZ
97. 01X64Z5
98. 0JXM0ZC
99. 0XXP0ZM
100. 0JX43ZZ
101. 00XK4ZM
102. 0LXP4ZZ
103. 0HX0XZZ
104. 0KXK0Z6, 0KXL0Z6
105. 0HX6XZZ

Root Operation: Transplantation

106. 0FY00Z0
107. 02YA0Z2
108. 0BYK0Z0
109. 0DYE0Z0
110. 0FYG0Z0, 0TY10Z0

Root Operation: Bypass

111. 0D160ZA
112. 031S0JG
113. 0B113F4
114. 02103D4
115. 041L0KL
116. 00160J6
117. 0D1L0Z4
118. 0T170ZC
119. 02100Z9
120. 0W190JG

Root Operation: Dilation

121. 0F798ZZ
122. 02703DZ, 02703ZZ

123. 0T7C8ZZ
124. 047L0ZZ
125. 0D717ZZ
126. 03773ZZ
127. 087X7DZ
128. 0U778ZZ
129. 0B718ZZ
130. 0T778DZ

Root Operation: Occlusion

131. 06L33ZZ
132. 03LL3DZ
133. 0UL74CZ
134. 03L80ZZ
135. 03LG3DZ

Root Operation: Restriction

136. 0UVC7ZZ
137. 02VR0CZ
138. 07VK3DZ
139. 03VG0CZ
140. 08VX7DZ

Root Operation: Change

141. 0S2YX0Z
142. 0B21XFZ
143. 0W2BX0Z
144. 0020X0Z
145. 0T2BX0Z

Root Operation: Insertion

146. 0JH80M7, 0JP0MZ
147. 02H73MA, 02PA3MZ
148. 0JH60P2
149. 05HM33Z
150. 09HE0S3
151. 02HV32Z
152. 0BH081Z
153. 0JH73VZ
154. 0QHY0MZ
155. 0VH081Z

Root Operation: Removal

156. 01PY0MZ
157. 02PYX2Z
158. 0FPG00Z
159. 0BP1XEZ
160. 0DP6XUZ
161. 0UPH71Z
162. 0QPN04Z
163. 0TP98DZ
164. 0DP6X0Z
165. 0PPJX5Z

Root Operation: Replacement

166. 0HRDX73
167. 0QR70K
168. 08R83KZ
169. 0HRV0JZ
170. 04R00JZ
171. 0SRC0JZ
172. 0HRV076
173. 0LRS0KZ
174. 02RG08Z
175. 08RJ3JZ

Root Operation: Revision

176. 02WYX2Z
177. 0SW90JZ
178. 02WA3MZ
179. 0QWH04Z
180. 0JWT0WZ

Root Operation: Supplement

181. 02UF0JZ
182. 0YU64JZ
183. 01U547Z
184. 0SUS09Z, 0SPB09Z
185. 0UUG0JZ
186. 02UA0JZ
187. 0WUF0JZ
188. 0LU207Z, 0LBL0ZZ
189. 08U9XJZ
190. 0SUR0BZ

Root Operation: Inspection

191. 0WJ90ZZ
192. 0CJS8ZZ
193. 0SJD0ZZ
194. 0UJD8ZZ
195. 0DJD7ZZ
196. 0RJJ4ZZ
197. 09JY4ZZ
198. 0FJ00ZZ
199. 0TJB8ZZ
200. 0DJD8ZZ

Root Operation: Map

201. 00K83ZZ
202. 02K83ZZ
203. 00K00ZZ
204. 00K74ZZ
205. 02K80ZZ

Root Operation: Control

206. 0W3R8ZZ
207. 0X3F0ZZ
208. 0W3H0ZZ
209. 0W3C0ZZ
210. 0Y3F4ZZ

Root Operation: Repair

211. 01Q60ZZ
212. 0DQ90ZZ
213. 0WQN0ZZ
214. 0LQ30ZZ
215. 0WQF0ZZ

Root Operation: Alteration

216. 0W020ZZ
217. 0H0V0JZ
218. 090K07Z
219. 0W0F0ZZ
220. 0J0L3ZZ, 0J0M3ZZ

Root Operation: Creation

221. 0W4N0K1
222. 0W4M0J0
223. 0W4N071

224. 0W4M070
225. 0W4N0J1

Root Operation: Fusion

226. 0RGP04Z
227. 0SG1031
228. 0RGQ0KZ
229. 0SG507Z
230. 0SGQ34Z

Section: Obstetrics

231. 10A07ZW
232. 10E0XZZ
233. 10A07ZX
234. 10J07ZZ
235. 10D00Z2
236. 10903ZA
237. 10Y04ZS
238. 10Q00ZK
239. 10T24ZZ
240. 10P073Z

Section: Placement

241. 2Y42X5Z
242. 2W6MX0Z
243. 2W5AX1Z
244. 2W32X3Z
245. 2Y04X5Z
246. 2W44X5Z
247. 2W27X4Z
248. 2Y50X5Z
249. 2W18X7Z
250. 2W0PX6Z

Section: Administration

251. 3E1M39Z
252. 3E0P7LZ
253. 3E0436Z
254. 3E0G8GC, 0DJ68ZZ
255. 3E1U38Z
256. 3E0S33Z
257. 3E0L3TZ
258. 30263V1

259. 3E0P3Q1
260. 30243G0

Section: Measurement and Monitoring

261. 4A02XM4
262. 4A0C85Z
263. 4A1Z7KZ
264. 4A04XJ1
265. 4A12X45
266. 4A09XCZ
267. 4A1H7CZ
268. 4A07X7Z
269. 4A133B3
270. 4A08X0Z

Section: Extracorporeal Assistance and Performance

271. 5A1935Z
272. 5A1C00Z
273. 5A2204Z
274. 5A09358
275. 5A1D60Z

Section: Extracorporeal Therapies

276. 6A550Z2
277. 6A801ZZ
278. 6A4Z0ZZ
279. 6A650ZZ
280. 6A930ZZ
281. 6A0Z1ZZ
282. 6A221ZZ
283. 6A750ZZ
284. 6A551Z3
285. 6A210ZZ

Section: Osteopathic

286. 7W06X8Z
287. 7W00X5Z
288. 7W07X6Z
289. 7W04X4Z
290. 7W01X0Z

Section: Other Procedures

291. 8E023DZ
292. 8E09XBG, 09BU0ZZ
293. 8E0WXY8

294. 8E0ZXY6
295. 8E0W0CZ, 0VT00ZZ

Section: Chiropractic

296. 9WB3XGZ
297. 9WB9XCZ
298. 9WB6XDZ
299. 9WB4XJZ
300. 9WB0XKZ

Section: Imaging

301. BW21ZZZ
302. B342ZZ3
303. BW03ZZZ
304. BF43ZZZ
305. BG34YZZ
306. BD11YZZ
307. BP0JZZZ
308. BY4DZZZ
309. BB240ZZ
310. B41G1ZZ

Section: Nuclear Medicine

311. C226YZZ
312. CT631ZZ
313. CP151ZZ
314. CH22SZZ
315. C23GQZZ
316. CW1BLZZ
317. C050VZZ
318. CD15YZZ
319. C030BZZ
320. C763HZZ

Section: Radiation Oncology

321. D8Y0FZZ
322. D0011ZZ
323. DDY5CZZ
324. DV109BZ
325. DM013ZZ
326. DWY68ZZ
327. D9Y57ZZ
328. DF034ZZ

329. D016B9Z
330. DWY5GFZ

Section: Physical Rehabilitation and Diagnostic Audiology

331. F13Z31Z
332. F0DZ8UZ
333. F07L0ZZ
334. F00ZHYZ
335. F0FZ8ZZ

Section: Mental Health

336. GZ58ZZZ
337. GZGZZZZ
338. GZJZZZZ
339. GZB1ZZZ
340. GZ2ZZZZ
341. GZ13ZZZ
342. GZFZZZZ
343. GZ10ZZZ
344. GZ61ZZZ
345. GZ72ZZZ

Section: Substance Abuse Treatment

346. HZ94ZZZ
347. HZ63ZZZ
348. HZ81ZZZ
349. HZ54ZZZ
350. HZ2ZZZZ
351. HZ47ZZZ
352. HZ53ZZZ
353. HZ3CZZZ
354. HZ5CZZZ
355. HZ42ZZZ

ASSIGNMENT 5.4 – SELECTING AND CODING PRINCIPAL DIAGNOSIS AND OTHER (ADDITIONAL) DIAGNOSES

1.

	ICD-9-CM & ICD-10-CM/PCSCode(s)
Principal Diagnosis:	162.3 (C34.11)
Other (Additional) Diagnosis(es): (e.g., comorbidities, complications, and secondary diagnoses)	V15.82 (Z87.891)
Principal Procedure:	33.27 (0BBC8ZX)
Other Significant Procedure(s):	(0BJK8ZZ)

Note:

The patient's symptoms of shortness of breath and chest discomfort are not assigned codes because a reason for these symptoms was documented (non-small cell lung carcinoma). The patient's history of tobacco use is assigned a code to reflect an increased risk factor for the non-small cell lung carcinoma disease. The patient's family history was not assigned codes because his complaints and the final diagnosis were related to body systems other than those associated with diabetes and hypertension.

2.

ICD-9-CM & ICD-10-CM/PCS Code(s)	
Principal Diagnosis:	V30.00 (Z38.00)
Other (Additional) Diagnosis(es): (e.g., comorbidities, complications, and secondary diagnoses)	755.01 (Q69.0) 755.02 (Q69.2)
Principal Procedure:	86.26 (0H5FXZZ)
Other Significant Procedure(s):	(0H5GXZZ) (0H5MXZZ) (0H5NXZZ)

Note:

- For newborn records, the principal diagnosis code always indicates newborn or new birth status.
- The condition of extra digits is called polydactyly. Because there is no combination code for polydactyly of fingers and toes, classify each separately. Do not assign ICD-10-CM code Q69.1, accessory thumb(s). Because there is no mention of that condition in the case.
- To build an ICD-10-PCS code for *ligation of extra digits, both hands and feet*, go to index main term *Destruction*, which means the *physical eradication of all or a portion of a body part by the direct use of energy, force, or a destructive agent*. The extra digits on both hands and feet are skin (because X-ray results reveal no bony involvement in the extra digits), which were *tied off* (ligation); thus, the ICD-10-PCS root operation is destruction because tying off the extra skin uses force.
- If bony involvement in the extra digits had been seen upon X-ray, surgical removal would be required, and ICD-10-PCS index main term *Excision* (cutting out or off, without replacement, a *portion* of a body part) would be referenced to assign the codes.

3.

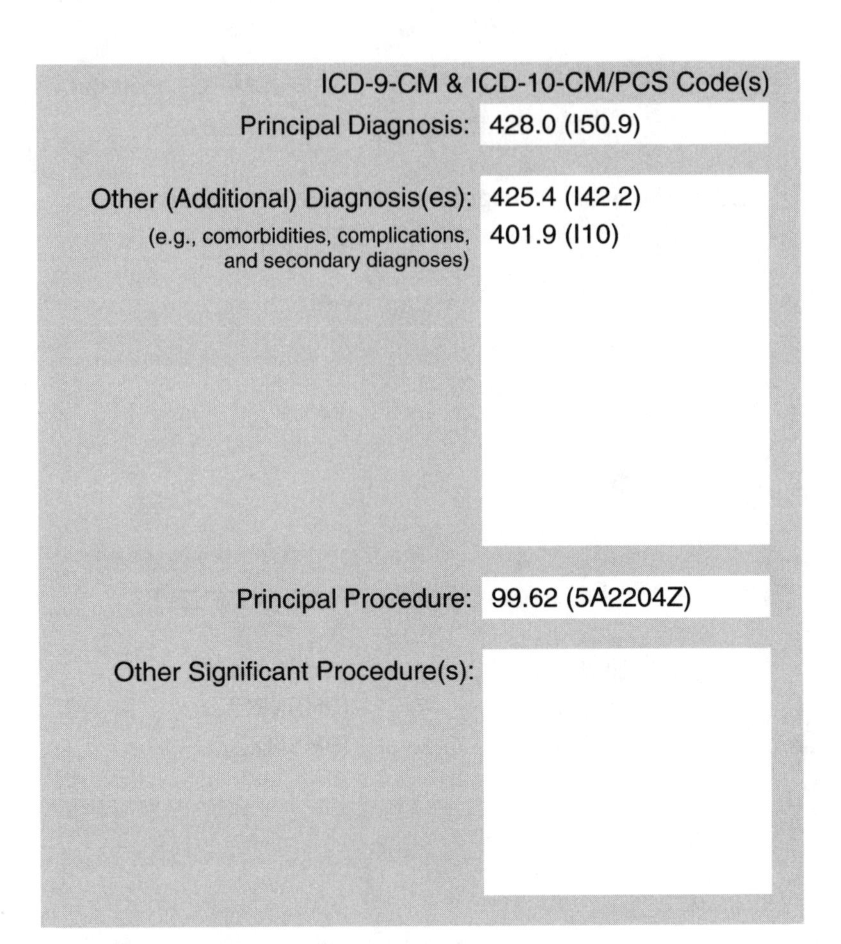

ICD-9-CM & ICD-10-CM/PCS Code(s)

Principal Diagnosis:	428.0 (I50.9)
Other (Additional) Diagnosis(es): (e.g., comorbidities, complications, and secondary diagnoses)	425.4 (I42.2) 401.9 (I10)
Principal Procedure:	99.62 (5A2204Z)
Other Significant Procedure(s):	

Note:

The signs and symptoms of respiratory distress, which include distended neck veins, systolic murmur, ventricular hypertrophy, and leg edema, are not assigned codes. All of these conditions are signs and symptoms of the patient's diagnoses: congestive heart failure and nonobstructive hypertrophic cardiomyopathy.

4.

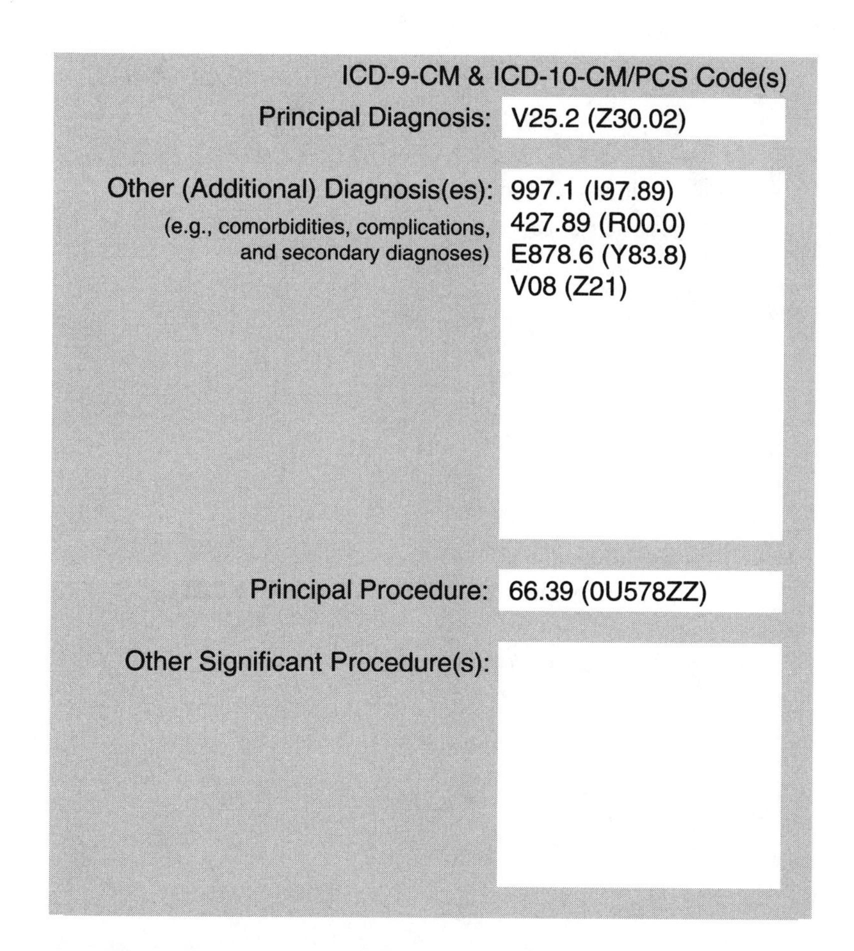

ICD-9-CM & ICD-10-CM/PCS Code(s)

Principal Diagnosis: V25.2 (Z30.02)

Other (Additional) Diagnosis(es): (e.g., comorbidities, complications, and secondary diagnoses)
997.1 (I97.89)
427.89 (R00.0)
E878.6 (Y83.8)
V08 (Z21)

Principal Procedure: 66.39 (0U578ZZ)

Other Significant Procedure(s):

Note:

- Assign ICD-9-CM codes 997.1, 427.89, and E878.6 (or ICD-10-CM codes I97.89, R00.0, and Y83.8) for postoperative complication of bradycardia.
- ICD-9-CM code V08 (or ICD-10-CM code Z21) is assigned to indicate the patient's HIV-positive status.
- The ICD-9-CM ligation procedure code can be located by referring to main term *Sterilization* in the Index to Procedures. An alternative to locating the procedure code is to refer to main term *Ligation*. In ICD-10-PCS, go to index main term *Destruction* to locate the appropriate female reproductive system Table.

5.

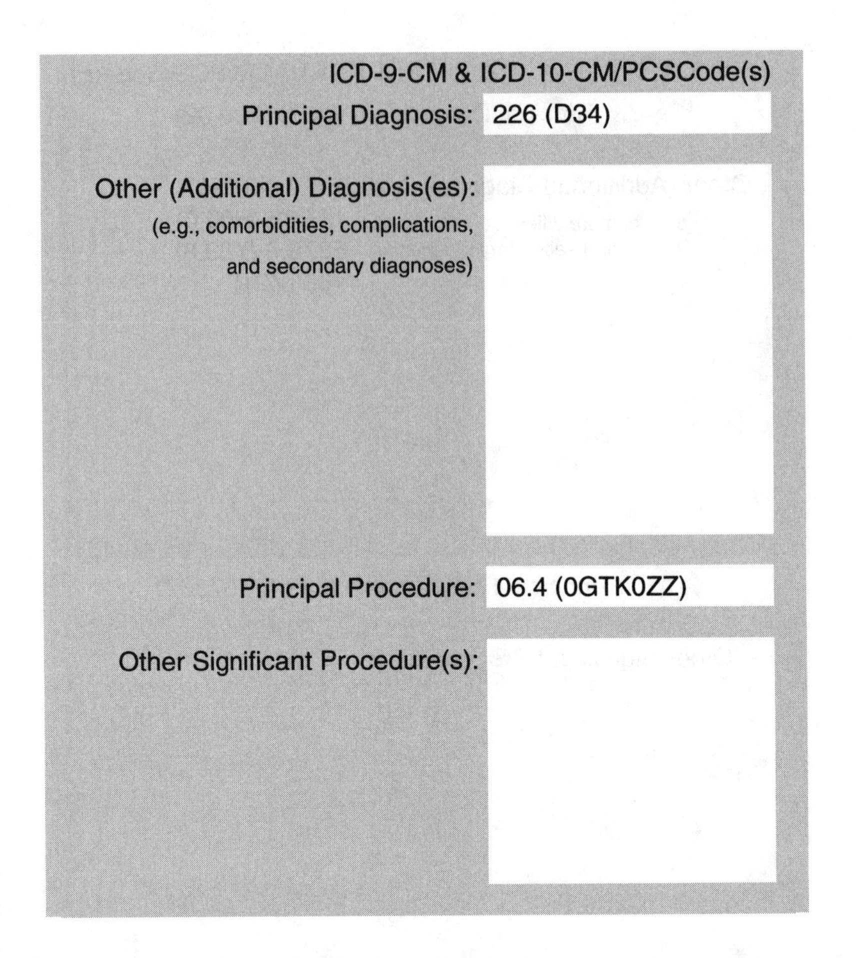

ICD-9-CM & ICD-10-CM/PCSCode(s)	
Principal Diagnosis:	226 (D34)
Other (Additional) Diagnosis(es): (e.g., comorbidities, complications, and secondary diagnoses)	
Principal Procedure:	06.4 (0GTK0ZZ)
Other Significant Procedure(s):	

Note:

The coder should locate the diagnosis code in the ICD-9-CM or ICD-10-CM index under main term Papilloma. *From there, the coder is directed to the Neoplasm Table,* benign, *and the specific site.*

6.

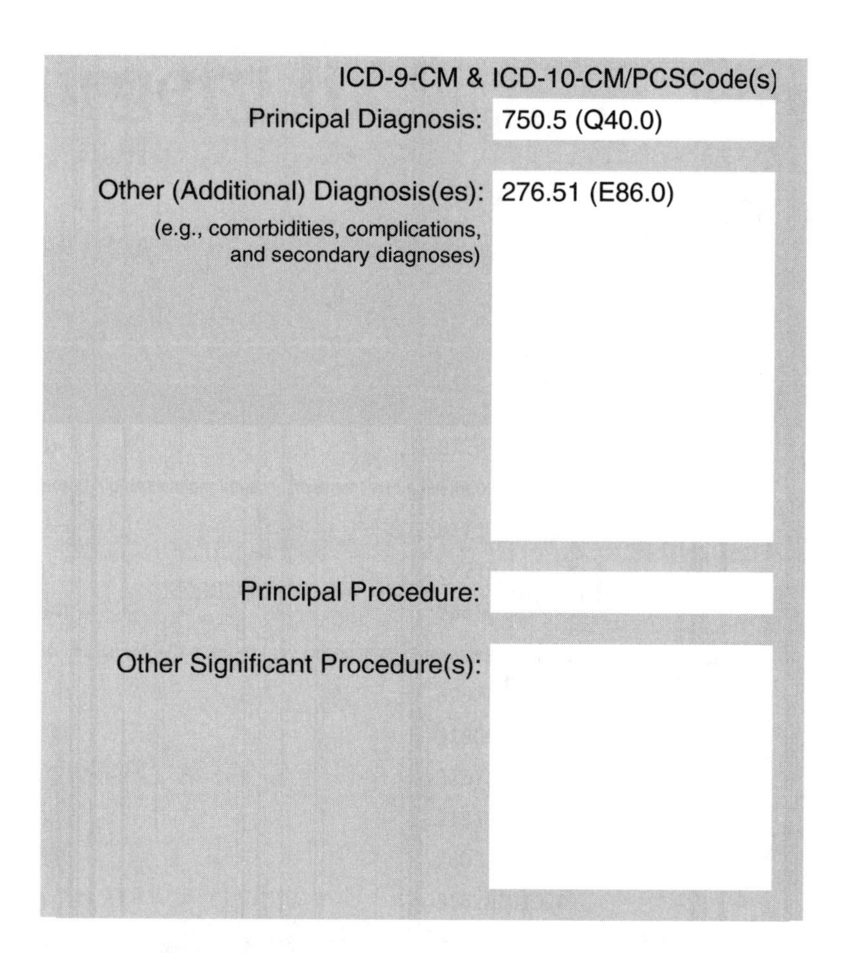

ICD-9-CM & ICD-10-CM/PCSCode(s)

Principal Diagnosis:	750.5 (Q40.0)
Other (Additional) Diagnosis(es): (e.g., comorbidities, complications, and secondary diagnoses)	276.51 (E86.0)
Principal Procedure:	
Other Significant Procedure(s):	

Note:

In the ICD-9-CM or ICD-10-CM index, refer to main term Stenosis, *subterm* pylorus (hypertrophic), *and 2nd qualifier* Infantile *to locate code 750.5 (or Q40.0). The patient in this case is 12 weeks old.*

7.

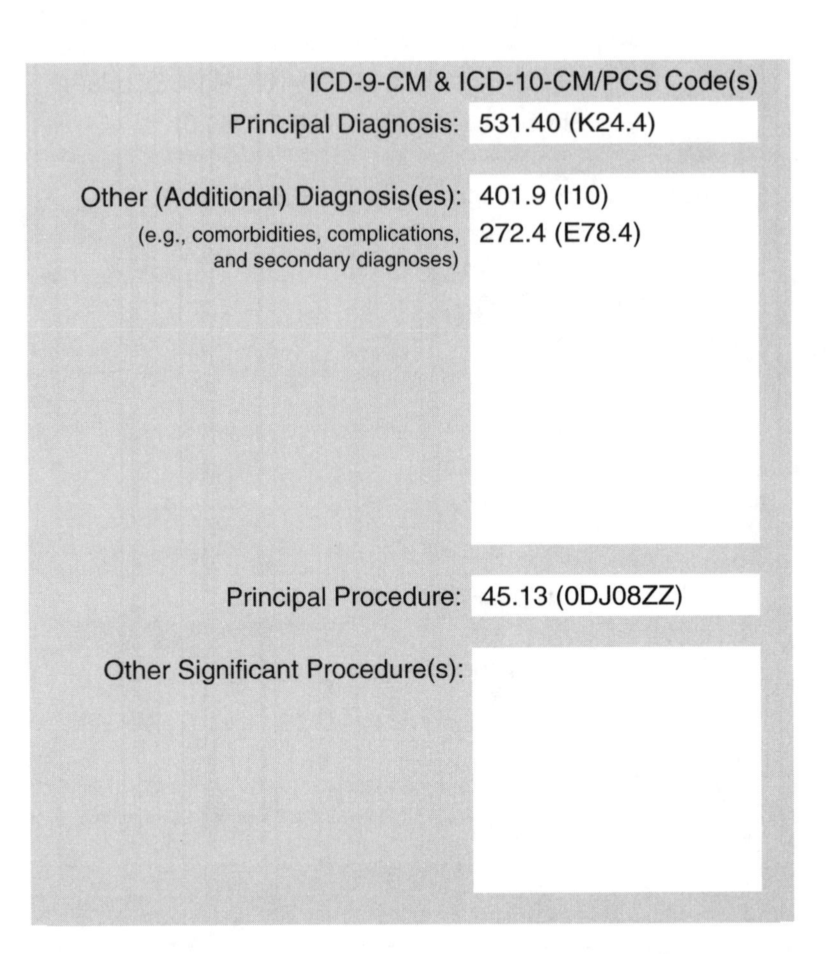

ICD-9-CM & ICD-10-CM/PCS Code(s)

Principal Diagnosis:	531.40 (K24.4)
Other (Additional) Diagnosis(es): (e.g., comorbidities, complications, and secondary diagnoses)	401.9 (I10) 272.4 (E78.4)
Principal Procedure:	45.13 (0DJ08ZZ)
Other Significant Procedure(s):	

Note:

- The prepyloric peptic ulcer is described as "with acute hemorrhage," which means that ICD-9-CM combination code 531.40 (or ICD-10-CM code K25.4) is assigned. To assign the correct ICD-9-CM or ICD-10-CM code, locate main term "ulcer," subterm "prepyloric," which directs you to "ulcer, stomach." Do not assign the code for "ulcer, peptic" because it states "site unspecified." In this case, the site is "prepyloric."
- The comorbidities of hypertension and hyperlipidemia are assigned codes because the patient's medication for these conditions was continued on this inpatient admission.

8.

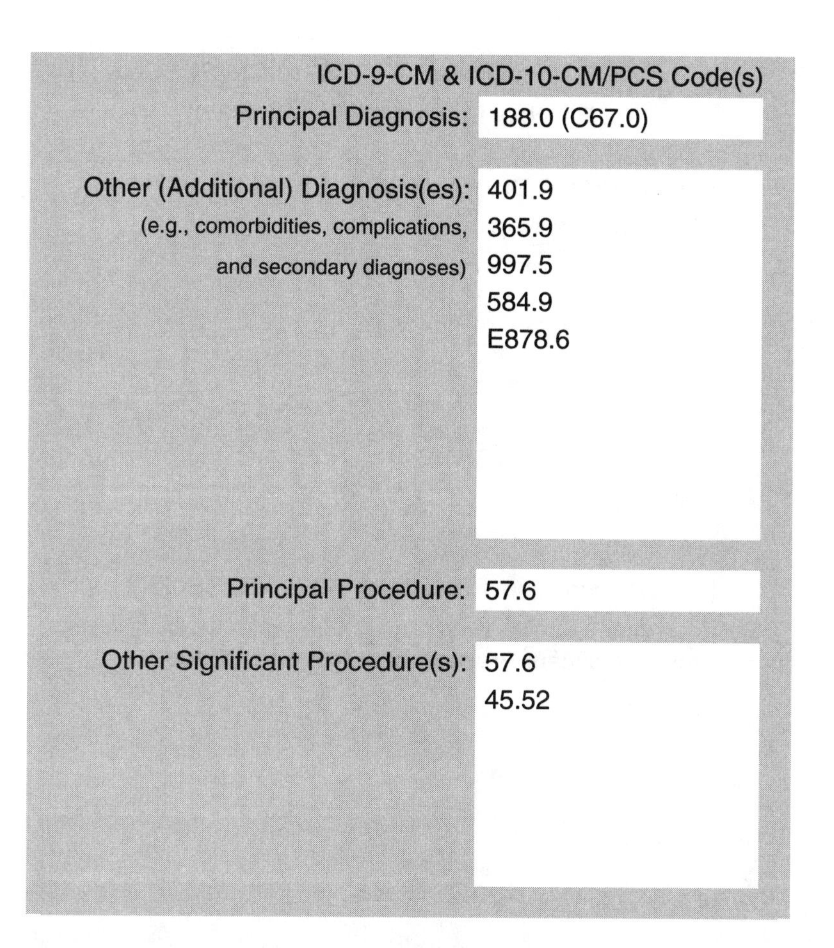

ICD-9-CM & ICD-10-CM/PCS Code(s)

Principal Diagnosis: 188.0 (C67.0)

Other (Additional) Diagnosis(es): (e.g., comorbidities, complications, and secondary diagnoses)
401.9
365.9
997.5
584.9
E878.6

Principal Procedure: 57.6

Other Significant Procedure(s):
57.6
45.52

Note:

- Assign ICD-9-CM code 584.9 (or ICD-10-CM N17.9) for acute renal failure to indicate the specific type of postoperative complication; an external cause code is also assigned (ICD-9-CM code E878.8 or ICD-10-CM code Y83.6).
- To assign ICD-9-CM code 57.87 for "partial cystectomy with enterocystoplasty, using part of the sigmoid colon," go to "reconstruction, bladder" in the procedure index. The patient underwent a reconstruction procedure because a bit of the colon was used to repair the bladder after the diseased portion of the bladder was removed.
- ICD-9-CM code 57.87 contains a "code also" instruction to assign code 45.52 for resection of the colon (intestine). In this case, a portion of the sigmoid colon was used to repair the bladder after the partial cystectomy was performed.
- To build ICD-10-PCS code 0TBB0ZZ, go to main term *Excision* and subterm *Bladder* in the index.
- To build ICD-10-PCS code 0TQB0ZZ, go to main term *Repair* and subterm *Bladder* in the index.
- To build ICD-10-PCS code 0DB0NZZ, go to main term *Excision* and subterm *Intestine* (because a *portion* of the small intestine was removed). (Do not go to ICD-10-PCS index subterm *Resection* to code the removal of a portion of the intestine because a resection is performed to remove an entire organ.)

9.

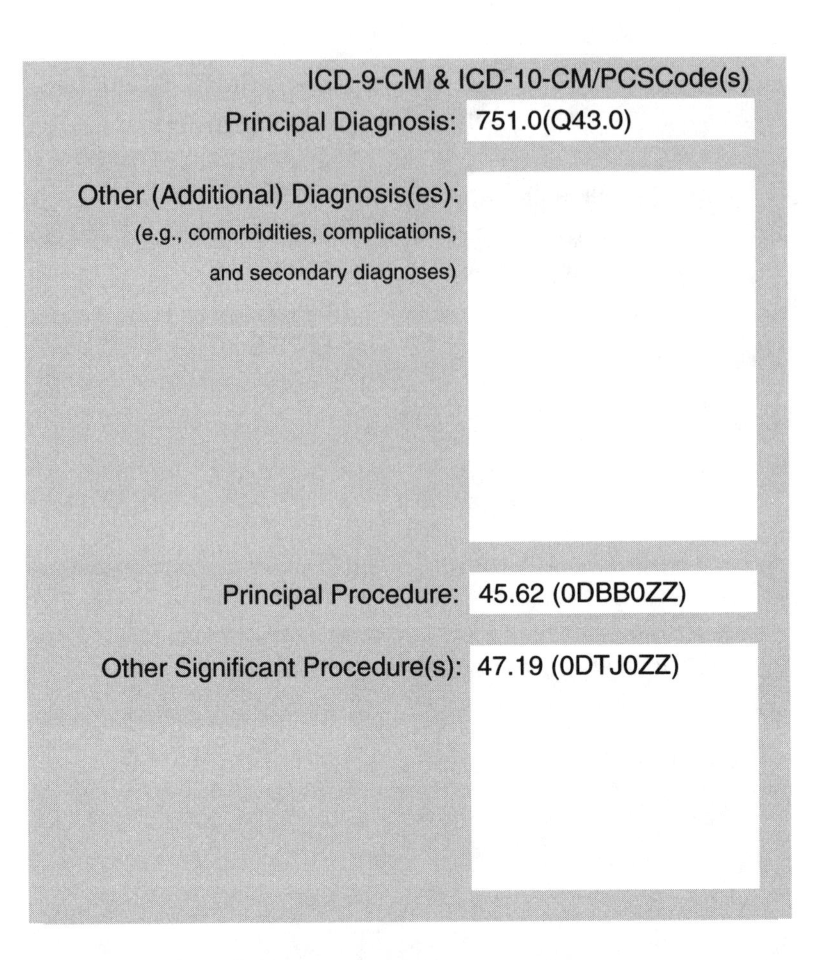

ICD-9-CM & ICD-10-CM/PCSCode(s)	
Principal Diagnosis:	751.0(Q43.0)
Other (Additional) Diagnosis(es): (e.g., comorbidities, complications, and secondary diagnoses)	
Principal Procedure:	45.62 (0DBB0ZZ)
Other Significant Procedure(s):	47.19 (0DTJ0ZZ)

Note:

Do not assign a code to the exploratory laparotomy *because that procedure resulted in the open resection of the appendix and excision of a portion of the ileum. (In ICD-9-CM, the* open resection of the appendix *is called an* incidental appendectomy.*)*

In ICD-10-PCS, go to main term Excision *and subterm* ileum *to build code 0DBB0ZZ (because a* portion *of the ileum was removed). To build ICD-10-PCS code 0DTJ0ZZ, go to index main term* Resection *and subterm* Appendix *(because the* entire *appendix was removed).*

10.

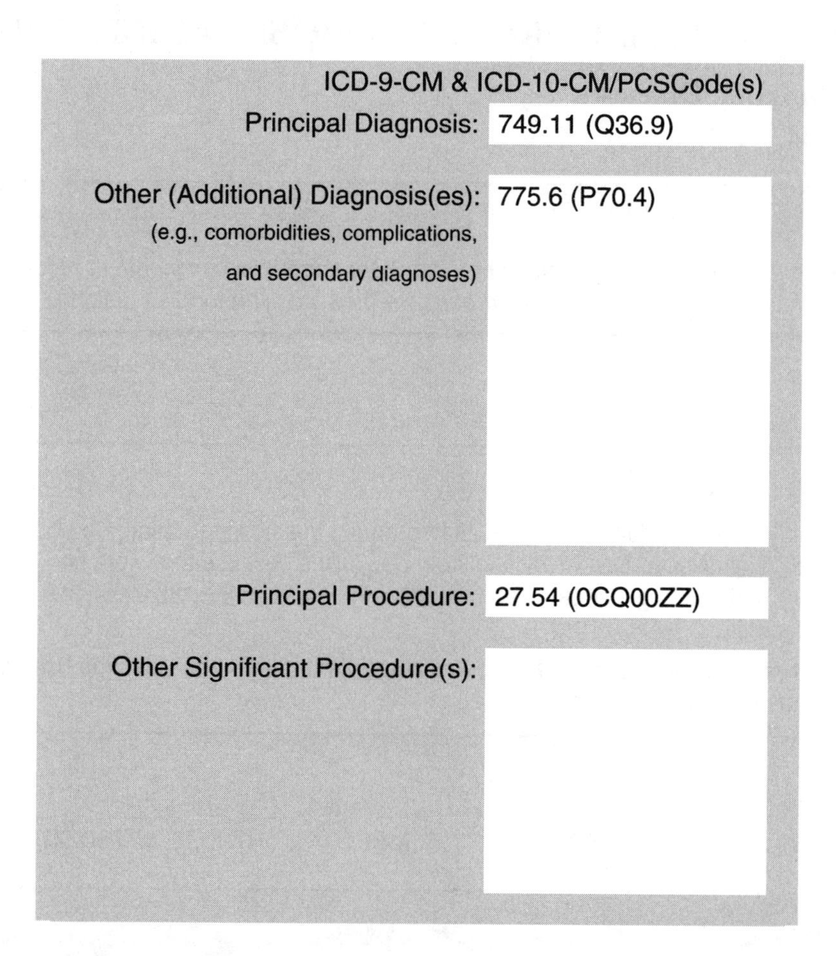

ICD-9-CM & ICD-10-CM/PCSCode(s)	
Principal Diagnosis:	749.11 (Q36.9)
Other (Additional) Diagnosis(es): (e.g., comorbidities, complications, and secondary diagnoses)	775.6 (P70.4)
Principal Procedure:	27.54 (0CQ00ZZ)
Other Significant Procedure(s):	

Note:

- A code from ICD-9-CM category V30 (or ICD-10-CM category Z38) is not assigned for this patient's discharge from Children's Hospital because the infant was not born during this admission.
- The condition of insulinoma was ruled out and is not coded. The code for hypoglycemia can be found by locating main term *Hypoglycemia* and the subterm *neonatal* in the ICD-9-CM (or ICD-10-CM) index. There is no documentation that the infant's mother is a diabetic; therefore, do not assign ICD-9-CM code 775.0 (or ICD-10-CM codes P70.0 or P70.1) to this case. Also, because the patient is an infant, do not assign ICD-9-CM code 251.2 (or ICD-10-CM code E16.2) for this case.

ASSIGNMENT 5.5 – CODING PRACTICE – HOSPITAL INPATIENT CASES

Infectious and Parasitic Diseases

1. 084.6, 034.0 (B54, J02.0)

Note:

Qualified diagnoses (e.g., probable exacerbation of malaria) are coded only on inpatient records. This means that back pain, low-grade fever, and chills are not coded because they are symptoms of malaria.

2. 021.9 (A21.9)

Note:

- Tularemia was the only diagnosis documented as treated during this hospitalization. Do not assign codes for the other (additional) diagnoses to past medical history diagnoses because they were not documented as treated. Do not assign codes to night sweats, fever, headache, poor appetite, dizziness, and weakness; they are symptoms of the tularemia.
- Although the chest x-ray documented arteriosclerotic changes in the aorta, because the condition was not treated during this hospitalization, it is not coded.

Neoplasms

3. 174.4, 196.3, M8010/3, 85.43 (C50.412, C77.3, M8010/3, 0HTU0ZZ, 07T60ZZ)

Note:

- Don't forget to assign morphology codes (e.g., M8010/3) to inpatient cancer cases.
- Although the chest x-ray indicated some calcification of the mitral valve and dilation of the aorta, because there is no documentation that it was treated, it is not coded.
- Although lab results indicated a cholesterol level of 304, because there is no documentation that it was treated, it is not coded.
- Do not assign a procedure code for removal of breast tumor because that diagnostic procedure was followed by modified radical mastectomy, left during the same operative episode. Assign a code for the modified radical mastectomy, left.

4. 154.1, M8140/3, 48.50, 45.95 (C20, M8140/3, 0DTP0ZZ, 0D1N0Z4, 0D1B0Z4)

Note:

- Because there is no documentation that coronary artery disease and gastroesophageal reflux disease were treated, do not code them.
- To locate ICD-9-CM code 48.50, locate main term *Resection* and subterm *abdominoendorectal* in the ICD-9-CM Index to Procedures.
    - The Tabular List of Procedures contains an instructional note to to "code also any synchronous anastomosis other than end-to-end," which means that code 45.95 is also assigned.
    - However, the "includes" note below code 48.5 states "with synchronous colostomy." An ileostomy is a type of colostomy; it is a surgical opening created through the abdominal wall into the ileum so waste can be discharged from the body without going through the colon. Because the ileostomy was performed during the same operative episode as the lower abdominal resection, it is not separately coded.
- In ICD-10-PCS, each surgical procedure performed during the operation is coded separately: resection of rectum (0DTP0ZZ), sigmoid coloanal anastomosis (0D1N0Z4), and ileostomy (0D1B0Z4). Notice that cutaneous is selected as the 7th-character value (4) for ICD-10-PCS code 0D1N0Z4; a separate value for anus is not listed at the 7th-character level because the anus contains specialized tissue called anoderm (a type of cutaneous tissue).

Endocrine, Nutritional, and Metabolic Diseases and Immunity Disorders

5. 250.02, 446.20, 447.6, V58.67, 38.21 (E11.69, M35.9, I77.6, Z79.4, 03BT3ZX)

Note:

- Pain in the hands is not coded because it is a symptom of collagen vascular disease and the qualified diagnosis (probable vasculitis of both hands).
- ICD-9-CM code V58.67 (or ICD-10-CM code Z79.4) classifies the long-term (current) use of insulin.
- Do not code demineralization of bones as found on hand X-rays because there was no treatment of this condition.

6. 276.8, E944.4, 462, 401.9, V58.69 (T50.2x5A, E87.6, J02.9, I10, Z79.899)

Note:

- This patient sustained an adverse effect due to her diuretic medication. For ICD-9-CM, sequence the adverse effect (hypopotassemia) first, followed by a code for the drug causing the adverse effect (diuretic). For ICD-10-CM, sequence the code selected from the Table of Drugs and Chemicals first, followed by the the adverse effect (hypopotassemia).
- Fever and chills are not assigned codes because they are symptoms of acute pharyngitis.

Diseases of the Blood and Blood-Forming Organs

7. 998.11, 287.31, E878.8, 27.52 (K91.840, D69.3, Y83.8, 0CQ4XZZ)

Note:

- The case states that the hemorrhage is likely due to the idiopathic thrombocytopenic purpura. However, the bleeding occurred postoperatively; therefore, it is classified as a postoperative complication. (The oral cavity is part of the digestive system.)
- Do not mistakenly assign ICD-9-CM code 86.59 for the mouth suture; ICD-9-CM code 27.52 is correct.

Mental Disorders

8. 969.5, E853.9, 300.00 (T43.501A, F41.9)

Note:

- An overdose is considered a poisoning. In ICD-9-CM, refer to the Table of Drugs and Chemicals in the Index to Diseases to assign two separate codes: one code for the poisoning (overdose) and another code for the external cause (tranquilizer tablets). The patient states that she was not trying to hurt herself; therefore, the E code is selected from the Accident column. A third ICD-9-CM code is assigned for anxiety.
- In ICD-10-CM, a code from the poisoning (accidental) column in the Table of Drugs and Chemicals is sequenced first, followed by the anxiety code. Notice that in ICD-10-CM, a combination code classifies the poisoning and external cause.

Diseases of the Nervous System and Sense Organs

9. 780.39, 437.0 (R56.9, I67.2)

Note:

Do not code the possible lung tumor, as reported by the radiologist, because it was not treated.

Diseases of the Circulatory System

10. 437.7, 401.9 (G45.4, I10)

Note:

- The patient was evaluated and treated for transient global amnesia. She was also given medication for hypertension while hospitalized. Both conditions are coded.
- The physician could be queried about the patient's elevated blood glucose level to determine if it is clinically significant and if it was treated.

11. 438.22, 438.11, 429.2, 440.9, 412, 250.00, 332.0 (I69.353, I69.320, I25.10, I25.2, E11.9, G20)

Note:

- The patient sustained cerebrovascular accident (CVA) in the past and is treated during this admission for residuals of CVA (hemiplegia and aphasia), which are late effects of the CVA. (In ICD-9-CM, refer to main term *Late* in the Index to Diseases.) (In ICD-10-CM, refer to main term *Hemiplegia* in the Index to Diseases and Injuries.)
- Previous subendocardial myocardial infarction is coded as 412 (ICD-9-CM) or I25.2 (ICD-10-CM).
- The patient's conditions of atherosclerotic cardiovascular disease, Parkinson's, and adult-onset diabetes mellitus were treated during this admission, and they are coded.

12. 410.11, 496, 429.2, 440.9, 412 (I21.09, J44.9, I25.10, I25.2)

Note:

Code the status post myocardial infarction (in addition to the current STEMI) due to its clinical presentation during this admission and because this condition is significant to the patient's medical history.

Diseases of the Respiratory System

13. 482.31, 428.0, 707.03, 707.20 (J15.4, I50.9, L89.150)

Note:

- IV Ancef, chest physical therapy, and IPBB were done to treat pneumonia.
- Lasix treated congestive heart failure.
- Betadine and sugar compound treated the sacral decubitus. A physician query would be generated to obtain documentation of the pressure ulcer's stage.
- Pleural effusion is a common symptom of congestive heart failure and is not coded unless specifically treated (e.g., chest tube insertion to drain the pleural effusion).

14. 493.22 (J44.1)

Note:

- Cough, shortness of breath, and difficulty breathing are symptoms of asthma; therefore, they are not coded.
- Chronic obstructive pulmonary disease is a chronic condition that was treated with Lasix and oxygen. However, ICD-9-CM code 496 contains a note that states *this code is not to be used with any code from categories 491–493*.

15. 518.81, 276.51, 414.00 (J96.0, E86.0, I25.10)

Note:

- Shortness of breath is not coded because it is a symptom of acute respiratory failure.
- In this case, peripheral cyanosis and hypotension are not coded because they are signs of acute respiratory failure and dehydration.
- Atelectasis, noted on chest x-ray, is an abnormal finding that was not specifically treated during this admission; therefore, do not code it.

Diseases of the Digestive System

16. 276.51, 261, 486, 331.0, 599.0, 041.00 (E86.0, E46, J18.9, G30.9, N39.0, B95.5)

Note:

- The patient's condition of Alzheimer's is coded due to its impact on her care during this admission and the fact that it resulted in dehydration and severe malnutrition.

17. 562.01, V15.29, 45.25 (K57.12, Z98.84, 0DJD8ZZ, 0DBN8ZX)

Note:

- Diagnostic evaluation revealed jejunal diverticulitis.
- An ICD code for personal history of gastric bypass surgery can be assigned.
- An ICD-9-CM combination code is assigned for colonoscopy with biopsy. Separate ICD-10-PCS codes are assigned for the colonoscopy and the biopsy procedures.

Diseases of the Genitourinary System

18. 591, V13.01, 55.51 (N13.30, Z87.43, 0TT10ZZ)

Note:

- The conditions of TIA, hyperlipidemia, and hypertension are not coded because there is no documentation that they were treated on this admission.
- The patient's nonfunctioning kidney is due to hydronephrosis. Nonfunctioning kidney is coded as V13.01.

Complications of Pregnancy, Childbirth, and the Puerperium

19. 642.51, V27.0, V25.2, 74.1, 66.32 (O14.13, Z37.0, Z30.2, 10D00Z1, 0UL70ZZ)

Note:

- Although the patient delivered at 34 weeks, she did not experience "spontaneous early onset of delivery" or "premature labor;" therefore, ICD-9-CM code 644.21 is *not* reported.
- Severe pre-eclampsia is documented as treated with magnesium sulfate as seizure prophylaxis.
- All delivery records must have a code assigned to identify the outcome of delivery; in this case, a single liveborn infant.
- The patient's wish for elective sterilization following delivery is coded, along with assignment of a procedure code.

20. 658.21, 664.01, V27.0, 75.69 (O42.02, O70.0, Z37.0, 0HQ9XZZ)

Note:

- This patient underwent induction of labor after her membranes ruptured over 24 hours prior to delivery, which is classified as delayed delivery.
- The patient also had a tear of her anterior perineum fourchette area during delivery. When an obstetrical patient undergoes episiotomy and sustains a perineal tear, code only the tear. (If the tear was repaired, a procedure code would also be reported.)
- All delivery charts must have a code to identify the outcome of the delivery; in this case, a single liveborn infant.

Diseases of the Skin and Subcutaneous Tissue

21. 682.6, 278.01, 86.28 (L03.116, E66.01, 0HDLXZZ)

Note:

- Obesity is assigned a code because it contributed to the development of her cellulitis.
- The debridement of this patient's cellulitis was done via whirlpool, which is coded as a nonexcisional debridement. In the ICD-10-PCS index, main term *Debridement* and subterm *Nonexcisional* include the instructional note to *see* Extraction, which results in code 0HDLXZZ.
- In ICD-10-PCS, whirlpool therapy provided as an activity of daily living is hydrotherapy. It is classified in the Physical Rehabilitation and Diagnostic Audiology, table F08, which contains an axis for *wound management*. The patient in this case underwent whirlpool debridement on the day of discharge, and it is not considered an activity of daily living. If the patient had undergone *wound management* as part of a physical rehabilitation program to learn how to care for her wound at home, an ICD-10-PCS code from table F08 would be assigned.

22. 873.51, E819.1, 86.59, 98.22 (S01.421A, V49.9xxA, 0HQ1XZZ, 0HC1XZZ)

Note:

- Because glass (foreign body) was embedded in the laceration, in the ICD-9-CM Index to Diseases, locate *Wound, open, cheek, complicated.*
- The fifth digit in ICD-9-CM code E819.x reflects that this patient was a passenger in the motor vehicle.

Diseases of the Musculoskeletal System and Connective Tissue

23. 733.19, 591, V13.01 (M84.48, N13.30, Z87.43)

Note:

Right upper quadrant abdominal pain is a symptom of the pathological rib fractures; therefore, do not code it.

24. 722.10, 846.0, 93.39 (M51.26, S39.012A, F07L6ZZ)

Note:

There is no documentation of any injury in this case; therefore, do not assign an external cause code.

Congenital Anomalies

25. 753.14, 599.0, 041.4 (Q61.19, N39.0, B96.2)

Note:

- The patient was admitted for reevaluation of his polycystic kidney disease, which is reported as the principal diagnosis.
- The urinary tract infection due to *Escherichia coli* found during admission is coded as an other diagnosis; two codes are required to report this condition.

Certain Conditions Originating in the Perinatal Period

26. 558.9, 779.81 (K52.9, P29.12)

Note:

- Although the infant is just two weeks old, assign ICD-9-CM code 558.9 (or ICD-10-CM code K52.9) for gastroenteritis (because there is no code for this condition in the Certain Conditions Originating in the Perinatal Period chapter). Lytren, Questran, and Nutramigen are antidiarrheal medications. Impending dehydration is not documented as having occurred and is not coded. Diarrhea is a symptom of gastroenteritis and is not coded. Urinary tract infection is not coded because the first culture proved to be contaminant.
- The perinatal period begins at birth and lasts through the 28th day following birth, which means that ICD-9-CM code 779.81 (or ICD-10-CM code P29.12) is assigned for neonatal bradycardia.

Symptoms, Signs, and Ill-Defined Conditions

27. 780.60, 278.01, 780.39 , 93.22 (R50.9, E66.01, R56.9, F07Z9ZZ)

Note:

- The obesity resulted in difficult ambulation, and treatment was physical therapy.
- The seizure disorder was treated with continuation of oral medications.

Injury and Poisoning

28. 973.3, E858.4, E849.0 (T47.4x1A, Y92.00)

Note:

- Fleet enema is a sodium phosphate intended to promote bowel elimination. ICD-9-CM code 973.3 is found by locating main term *Sodium,* subterm *phosphate,* and assigning a code from the Poisoning column in the Table of Drugs and Chemicals, then referring to the Accidental column to locate the E code. (In ICD-10-CM, combination code T47.4x1 is located in the Table of Drugs and Chemicals by locating main term *Sodium* and subterm *basic phosphate*, and 7th character A is added to the code to indicate *initial encounter.*)
- An external cause code is also assigned to indicate the place of occurrence (home).
- This patient did not exhibit any signs or symptoms during this admission; therefore, no additional diagnosis codes are provided.

29. 964.0, 787.03, 787.91, E858.2, E849.0, 96.33, 96.39 (T45.4x1A, R11.10, R19.7, Y92.00, 3E1G78Z, 3E1H78C)

Note:

- This case documents an accidental poisoning. Locate main term *Iron* in the ICD-9-CM Table of Drugs and Chemicals and assign the code from the Poisoning column; then assign the E code from the Accidental column. In ICD-10-CM, combination code T45.4x1A is assigned for the accidental poisoning due to ingesting iron tablets.
- An external cause code is also assigned to indicate the place of occurrence (home).
- Additional codes are assigned to describe manifestations, symptoms, or signs of the poisoning; in this case, codes for vomiting and diarrhea are assigned.
- Signs/symptoms are coded because they are documented and provide a "clinical picture" of the patient's condition from a coding perspective.

30. 807.01, 831.04, 486, 511.9, E819.1 (S22.32xA, S43.102A, J18.9, J90, V49.9xxA)

Note:

Velosef is an antibiotic used to treat the pneumonia. The shoulder dislocation and rib fracture were treated with analgesics. Qualified diagnoses (e.g., possible dislocation) are coded as if they were confirmed on inpatient records.

REVIEW

Multiple Choice

1. d

> **Note:**
>
> *The Uniform Hospital Discharge Data Set (UHDDS) includes definitions of specific inpatient coding terms such as* principal diagnosis, other (additional) diagnoses, principal procedure, *and* significant procedure.

2. d

> **Note:**
>
> *The insertion of a central line in this case is a significant procedure. The coronary artery bypass graft surgery is the principal procedure.*

3. c

> **Note:**
>
> *This case is an example of coding and reporting a symptom as principal diagnosis, followed by codes for comparing and contrasting diagnoses.*

4. c

> **Note:**
>
> *The principal diagnosis is the condition established after study to be the cause for admission. In this case, the principal diagnosis is the herniated lumbar disk.*

5. a

> **Note:**
>
> *Comorbidities are coexisting conditions, which means that the patient was diagnosed with them prior to hospital admission and those conditions were treated and/or medically managed during the hospitalization. They are, therefore, reported on the hospital claim as other (additional) diagnosis codes.*

6. c

> **Note:**
>
> *The principal diagnosis is the condition established after study to be the cause for admission. In this case, the nosebleeds and headaches are symptoms of hypertension.*

7. d

> **Note:**
>
> *In an inpatient setting, qualified diagnoses (e.g., possible) are coded as confirmed conditions.*

8. b

Note:

This question is an example of an abnormal finding documented on an ancillary report. In this case, the atelectasis is not coded because the patient did not receive treatment or medical management of the condition. To code the atelectasis, the attending physician would need to have documented its clinical significance and/or treated the condition.

9. d

Note:

Both conditions (myocardial infarction and dilated cardiomyopathy) were present at admission, and both were treated equally. Per coding guidelines, either condition can be reported as the principal diagnosis.

10. c

Note:

Correct codes to be reported include V30.00 and 754.60.

11. b

Note:

Per coding guidelines, the code for AIDS (042) is sequenced first, followed by the code for disseminated toxoplasmosis (130.8). The conditions of fever, headache, fatigue, and sore throat are not coded or reported because they are symptoms of the toxoplasmosis.

12. c

Note:

The final diagnosis of "likely fibromyalgia" is coded as if confirmed and reported as principal diagnosis. The symptoms of musculoskeletal pain of the neck, back, and shoulders are not coded or reported because these are common symptoms of fibromyalgia.

13. b

Note:

Adrenal hypofunction is also called Addison's disease. The admission diagnoses are symptoms of this disease, and they are not coded.

14. a

Note:

Acute pancreatitis is coded as 577.0.

15. c

Note:

The combination code for asthma with status asthmaticus is 493.91.

16. d
17. a

Note:

Students may ask why the procedure statement did not include "partial" or "total" cholecystectomy so that a more specific code could be assigned. Explain that the intent of this review question was to determine whether students would carefully read the statement and code only to the extent documented. They should not infer anything more in the procedure statement. This is an application of the rule If it wasn't documented, it wasn't done, *which means do not code something that was not documented as having been performed. If a more specific code is assigned, that is considered* overcoding.

18. d
19. c
20. c
21. c
22. a

Note:

Do not assign code 99.10 because it is reported for hypodermic (below skin), intramuscular (within muscle), or intravenous (into vein) injections only.

23. d
24. c
25. c
26. c

Note:

Assign code P71. to newborn *dehydration.*

27. d

Note:

Aortic value stenosis is not *documented as rheumatic in origin.*

28. c

Note:

Although the fracture is closed, *the* treatment is open.

29. b

Note:

Postoperative bradycardia is classified as a complication of surgery.

30. c

Note:

Maxillary sinusitis is documented as chronic *(not acute).*

Chapter 6
ICD-9-CM and ICD-10-CM Outpatient and Physician Office Coding

ASSIGNMENT 6.1 – PHYSICIAN QUERY PROCESS

1. d

Note:

Even though the radiologist documented "frontal sinusitis" on the radiology report, the attending physician should be asked if she concurs that "frontal sinusitis" is the diagnosis that should be coded. Official coding guidelines state that abnormal findings (e.g., x-ray results) are not coded and reported unless the physician indicates their clinical significance. If the findings are outside the normal range and the physician has ordered other tests to evaluate the condition or prescribed treatment, it is appropriate to ask the physician whether the abnormal finding should be added. Also do not assign codes to the headache and facial pain because they are symptoms of the frontal sinusitis.

2. a

Note:

The patient's record clearly documents past history of type 2 diabetes mellitus and hypertension (HTN), which was also documented as medically managed during the visit. Type 2 diabetes mellitus justifies medical necessity for the blood glucose level, and HTN justifies medical necessity for the physician's writing a refilled prescription for Verelan.

3. a

Note:

This case is properly documented. A Colles' fracture involves the lower end of the radius with displacement of the distal fragment dorsally.

4. b

Note:

Assign a code for the toxic effect first (spider bite) and then the nature of the toxic effect (rash). The physician also has to be queried about whether the spider was venomous or not so the proper ICD-9-CM E code (or ICD-10-CM external cause code).

5. b

Note:

The surgeon documented "obstructive cholecystitis" and "chronic cholecystitis with cholelithiasis" as the postoperative diagnosis on the operative report. Even though the surgeon did not document these diagnoses in the final diagnosis on the face sheet, the coder can assign codes to these diagnoses because the surgeon is the attending physician on this case. (If the diagnosis documented on the face sheet and the postoperative diagnosis on the operative report were different from that documented on the pathology report, the coder would query the surgeon because official coding guidelines state that abnormal findings (e.g., pathology results) are not coded and reported unless the physician (in this case, the surgeon) indicates their clinical significance.)

6. Upon review of this case, the coder should query the physician as to whether a code for actinic keratosis should be assigned because official coding guidelines state that abnormal findings (e.g.,pathology results) are not coded and reported unless the attending physician indicates their clinical significance.
7. Upon review of this case, the coder should assign a code for the skin tag, which was removed, because the skin tag was clearly documented in the case.
8. Upon review of this case, the coder should query the physician to ask whether symptoms of fatigue, blurred vision, and weight gain should be assigned codes because the diagnoses of hypertension and osteoarthritis do not account for the symptoms documented for this case. (NOTE: Do not assign a code to the osteoarthritis because it was not medically managed during this encounter.)
9. Upon review of this case, the coder should query the physician to verify that codes should be assigned to symptoms of flank pain, abdominal pain, and dysuria because although no diagnosis is documented, the ED physician may have established a definitive diagnosis based on examination and the results of ancillary tests.
10. Upon review of this case, the coder should query the physician because the type of burn (first-, second- or third-degree) is not documented. Due to documented blistering, the physician should be asked whether it would be appropriate to document for second-degree burns so a more specific code can be assigned.

ASSIGNMENT 6.2 – DIAGNOSTIC CODING AND REPORTING GUIDELINES FOR OUTPATIENT SERVICES – HOSPITAL-BASED AND PHYSICIAN OFFICE

Note:

If multiple codes are listed in the answer, they are presented in the correct order based on coding principles.

1. 463 (J03.90)
2. 786.50 (R07.9)
3. 466.0, 401.9, V16.1 (J20.9, I10, Z80.1)

Note:

When acute and chronic conditions are treated during the same encounter, report the acute condition code first. In this case, report acute bronchitis code first.

4. 214.1 (D17.24)
5. 493.92 (J45.901)
6. V72.31, V76.47 (Z01.419, Z12.4)
7. 881.00, 924.8 (S51.811A)

Note:

"Rule out" conditions are qualified diagnosis and are not assigned codes for outpatient care.

8. V22.0 (Z34.02)
9. 592.0 (N20.0)

Note:

Do not report a code for hematuria, which is a sign of renal calculi.

10. V57.21, V12.59 (Z59.89, I69.20)
11. 382.9, 784.1, 228.01 (H66.90, D18.01)

Note:

Do not code fever or throat pain because they are signs and symptoms of acute otitis media.

12. 075 (B27.00)
13. 003.0 (A02.0)
14. 428.0 (I50.9)
15. 790.21 (R73.01)
16. 530.81 (R73.01)
17. 477.9 (J30.9)
18. 577.0, 681.00, 785.0 (K85.9, L03.011, R00.0)
19. 711.06, 041.5 (M00.861, B96.3)
20. 017.90, 420.0 (A18.84, I32)

ASSIGNMENT 6.3 – ICD-9-CM CODING GUIDELINES FOR OUTPATIENT DIAGNOSTIC TESTS

1. 715.97 (M19.071)
2. 369.8 (H54.7)
3. V74.2, V01.89 (Z11.2, Z20.09)

Note:

"No bacterium found" in the diagnostic statement indicates that the patient underwent testing for Hansen's disease.

4. 620.2, 796.2 (N83.20, R03.0)

Note:

Assign a code from the signs and symptoms chapter for "BP reading 175/90." Another option is to generate a physician query to ask if a diagnosis should be documented for "BP reading 175/90."

5. 042, 136.3 (B20, B59)
6. 599.70 (R31.9)
7. 218.9 (D25.9)
8. 253.5 (E23.2)

Note:

All of the symptoms and signs in this case are included in the diagnosis, diabetes insipidus. Therefore, do not code them separately.

9. 255.0 (E24.0)

Note:

- The signs and lab values in this case are included in the diagnosis, Cushing's syndrome. Therefore, do not code them separately.
- Lab tests often include determining cortisol levels in blood. Cortisol is a corticosteroid hormone produced by the adrenal cortex (of the adrenal gland).

10. 442.81, 351.0 (I72.9, G51.0)
11. V76.11, V16.3 (Z12.31, Z80.3)
12. 836.0 (S83.211A)
13. V72.83, 401.9 (Z01.812, I10)
14. 173.3 (C44.31)
15. 959.01 (S09.90A)
16. 860.0, 807.01 (S27.0xxA, S22.31xA)
17. 286.0, 356.9 (D66, G62.9)
18. 728.2, 728.87 (M62.81, M62.50)
19. 422.90 (I40.9)
20. 845.00 (S93.401A)

ASSIGNMENT 6.4 – SELECTING THE FIRST-LISTED DIAGNOSIS AND LINKING DIAGNOSES WITH PROCEDURES/SERVICES FOR MEDICAL NECESSITY

Selecting the First-Listed Diagnosis

1. Pain, left knee
2. Gastroesophageal reflux disease
3. Hypertension
4. Sore throat
5. Lipoma

Linking Diagnoses with Procedures/Services for Medical Necessity

6. e
7. b
8. a
9. c
10. g
11. i
12. j
13. f
14. h
15. d

ASSIGNMENT 6.5 – CODING PRACTICE

Ambulatory Surgery Center (ASC)

1. 246.1 (E07.1)
2. 550.90, 752.51 (K40.90, Q53.10)

Note:

ICD-9-CM code 550.90 (or ICD-10-CM code K40.90) is assigned for right inguinal hernia because there is no documentation that the hernia is recurrent.

3. 550.90, 214.4 (K40.90, D17.6)
4. 574.31 (K80.41)
5. 608.1 (N43.42)

Chiropractic Office

6. 353.0 (G54.0)

Note:

The patient's complaints of neck and shoulder pain are not assigned ICD codes because they are symptoms of thoracic outlet syndrome.

7. 724.3 (M54.31)

Note:

The patient's complaint of gluteal pain with radiation is not assigned a code because it is a symptom of sciatica.

8. 724.4 (M54.16)

Note:

The patient's complaint of low back pain is not assigned a code because it is a symptom of lumbar radiculitis.

9. 729.1 (M79.1)

Note:

The patient's complaints of neck and back pain are not assigned codes because they are symptoms of myalgia.

10. 847.0 (S16.1)

Note:

- When main term *Strain* is located in the ICD-9-CM index, the coder is referred to *sprain*. (In ICD-10-CM, main term *Strain* contains a list of subterms with codes.)
- The patient's complaints of neck pain and muscle spasms are not assigned codes because they are symptoms of cervical sprain and cervical subluxation.

Hospital Emergency Department

11. 530.3 (K22.2)
12. 709.00 (L81.9)

Note:

- Locate code 709.00 by referring to the ICD-9-CM or ICD-10-CM index main term *Lesion* and subterm *pigmented (skin).*

13. 883.1 (S61.242D)

Note:

The patient sustained an open wound to his finger when some PVC pipe entered the finger. The patient removed the piece of PVC pipe on his own. The open wound then became infected. In ICD-9-CM, infected open wounds are coded by going to main term Wound, *subterm* finger, *and 2nd qualifier* complicated *to assign the code to this case. Do not assign ICD-9-CM code 958.3 (wound infection) to this case because the excludes note directs you to main term Wound. In ICD-10-CM, the condition is classified as a subsequent encounter by adding letter D to the S61.242 puncture wound code. (The original ED visit was assigned ICD-10-CM code S61.242A because it was an initial encounter.)*

14. 729.5 (M79.671)

Note:

In the ambulatory setting, the statement, sprain of right great toe versus early gout *is a qualified diagnosis, and the conditions are not coded as confirmed conditions. The patient's symptom of right foot pain coded instead.*

15. 780.2 (R55)

Hospital Outpatient Department

16. V56.0, 585.6, 250.41, 583.81, 303.90, V64.1 (N18.6, Z99.2, E10.21, F10.20, Z53.09)

Note:

- The reason for care is dialysis treatment, coded as V56.0 in ICD-9.CM, followed by code 585.6 (ESRD). In ICD-10-CM, codes N18.6 (ESRD) and Z99.2 (Dependence on renal dialysis) are assigned.
- *Diabetic nephropathy due to type 1 diabetes mellitus* is assigned codes 250.41 and 583.81 in ICD-9-CM and combination code E10.21 in ICD-10-CM. (The case does not specify that ESRD is due to type 1 diabetes mellitus.)
- The patient has documented chronic alcoholism; the patient is documented as being drunk during treatment, but the type of drunkenness is not stated. Do not assign a code for "acute alcoholic intoxication and unspecified drunkenness." The condition "acute alcoholic intoxication" does not mean that the patient has alcoholism. (For example, many people who were occasionally acutely intoxicated on alcohol during their youth were not later diagnosed with alcoholism.)
- The patient is drunk, and the treatment is cancelled, which means ICD-9-CM code V64.1 (or ICD-10-CM code Z53.09) is reported.

17. 784.0 (R51)

18. 575.8, 789.01, 790.29, 790.6, V18.59 (K82.8, R10.11, R73.9, R79.89, Z83.79)

Note:

Qualified diagnoses (e.g., probable) are not coded for ambulatory or outpatient care. Instead, the patient's signs and symptoms are coded. Family history of digestive disorders (such as gallbladder disease) is also assigned a code.

19. 378.9 (H50.9)

20. 780.60, 462 (R50.9, J02.9)

Note:

Qualified diagnoses (e.g., probable) are not coded for ambulatory or outpatient care. Instead, the patient's signs and symptoms are coded.

Hospital Same Day Surgery

21. 226, 401.9 (D34, I10)

Note:

Hypertension is not documented by the physician as a postoperative complication. The documentation does not specify a type of hypertension. Thus, the coder cannot presume that the hypertension is malignant even though a blood pressure reading of 200/110 was documented. The hypertension is coded as unspecified.

22. 585.9, 596.3, 600.00 (N18.9, N32.3, N40.0)
23. 474.10, V12.09 (J35.3, Z86.19)
24. 836.0 (S83.211S)
25. 185 (C61)

Note:

ICD-9-CM Index to Diseases (or ICD-10-CM Index to Diseases and Injuries) main term Adenocarcinoma *refers the coder to "Neoplasm, by site, malignant." This entry is located under the Malignant column in the Neoplasm Table.*

Physician Office

26. 883.0 (S61.235A)
27. 381.4 (H65.92)
28. 871.4, 368.8 (S05.32D, H53.8)
29. 490 (J40)

Note:

Laryngitis and cough are not assigned codes because they are symptoms of bronchitis.

30. 843.9, 847.2 (S73.101A, S33.5xxA)

Stand-Alone Radiology Center

31. 722.0 (M50.22)
32. 723.1 (M54.2)
33. 721.0 (M47.22)
34. 719.47 (M25.572)
35. 496 (J44.9)

Note:

Qualified diagnoses (e.g., possible, probable) are not coded for ambulatory or outpatient care. Instead, the patient's signs and symptoms are coded.

Stand-Alone Urgent Care Center

36. 346.90 (G43.909)
37. 836.2 (M23.92)

Note:

This case is coded as a current injury, "internal derangement of the left knee," based on documentation provided in the case.

38. 413.1 (I20.1)
39. 873.0 (S01.01A)
40. 284.1, 789.2 (D61.81, R16.1)

REVIEW

Multiple Choice

1. c
2. c
3. a
4. a
5. a
6. b
7. b
8. b
9. c
10. d
11. b
12. a
13. c
14. b
15. d
16. c
17. a
18. a
19. b
20. d

Chapter 7
HCPCS Level II National Coding System

ASSIGNMENT 7.1 – HCPCS LEVEL II INDEX

1. Breast pump
2. Chemotherapy administration (OPPS)
3. Dialysate solution
4. External defibrillator electrode
5. Fracture orthosis
6. Liquid gas system
7. Oral antiemetic
8. Pneumatic nebulizer administration set
9. Pneumococcal vaccination administration
10. Wheelchair shock absorber

ASSIGNMENT 7.2 – HCPCS LEVEL II MODIFIERS

1. a
2. e
3. d
4. f
5. i
6. 8
7. c
8. j
9. h
10. b

ASSIGNMENT 7.3 – ASSIGNING HCPCS LEVEL II CODES

Transport Services Including Ambulance (A0000–A0999)

1. A0100
2. A0428
3. A0225
4. A0160
5. A0433

Medical and Surgical Supplies (A4000–A8999)

6. A4349
7. A4338
8. A4367
9. A4458
10. A4556

Administrative, Miscellaneous, and Investigational (A9000–A9999)

11. A9503
12. A9517
13. A9150
14. A9300
15. A9700

Enteral and Parenteral Therapy (B4000–B9999)

16. B9004
17. B4082
18. B4103
19. B4176
20. B4102

C Codes for Hospital OPPS (C1000–C9999)

21. C1722
22. C1880
23. C1785
24. C1750
25. C9363

Dental Codes (D0000–D9999)

26. D0274
27. D0475
28. D0330-EP
29. D1110
30. D3910

Durable Medical Equipment (E0100–E9999)

31. E0730
32. E0850
33. E0303
34. E1520
35. E0325

Procedures/Professional Services (Temporary) (G0000–G9999)

36. G0105
37. G0117
38. G0268
39. G0403
40. G0156 × 8

Note:

Code G0156 is reported for each 15 minutes of assistance.

Alcohol and/or Drug Abuse Treatment Services (H0001–H2037)

41. H2001
42. H0014

Note:

To locate the correct code, go to main term Alcohol *in the HCPCS level II index and locate subterm* abuse service. *Then when verifying that code, review all codes in that section of the HCPCS level II tabular list to locate correct code H0014. (The HCPCS level II index is not as extensive as ICD's index, and coders must review tabular listings to locate correct codes.)*

43. H0030
44. H2014 × 2

Note:

Code H2014 is reported for each 15 minutes of training and development.

45. H0009

Drug Codes (J0000–J9999)

46. J0690
47. J0587
48. J0735
49. J2271
50. J3301, J3301

Temporary Durable Medical Equipment (K0000–K9999)

51. K0108
52. K0006
53. K0606
54. K0105
55. K0462

Orthotic Procedures (L0000–L4999)

56. L3001-LT
57. L1830
58. L3510
59. L2260
60. L1500

Prosthetic Procedures (L5000–L9999)

61. L8001
62. L8614
63. L6310
64. L6708
65. L8670

Medical Services (M0000-M0301)

66. M0301
67. M0076
68. M0300
69. M0075
70. M0064

Pathology and Laboratory Services (P0000–P9999)

71. P9057
72. P9010
73. P9022
74. P9043
75. P3000

Q Codes: Temporary Codes (Q0000–Q9999)

76. Q0113
77. Q4033
78. Q4049
79. Q0085
80. Q2004

Diagnostic Radiology Services (R0000–R5999)

81. R0076
82. R0070
83. R0075
84. R0070-UR
85. R0075-UN

Temporary National Codes (Non-Medicare) (S0000–S9999)

86. S9439
87. S2053
88. S0612
89. S3850
90. S9075

National T Codes Established for State Medicaid Agencies (T1000–T9999)

91. T1013

Note:

Code T1013 is reported for each 15 minutes of service.

92. T1027 × 2

Note:

Code T1027 is reported for each 15 minutes of training.

93. T2030
94. T1502-TE
95. T1000-TD × 2

Vision Services (V0000–V2999)

96. V2756
97. V2600
98. V2020
99. V2785
100. V2750 × 2

Note:

Code V2750 is reported for each lens that receives antireflective coating.

Hearing Services (V5000–V5999)

101. V5362
102. V5270
103. V5008
104. V5244
105. V5254

ASSIGNMENT 7.4 – HCPCS LEVEL II CODING CASE STUDIES

1. G0204-GH

Note:

Patient was seen for scheduled screening mammography. A suspicious lesion was found, and the patient underwent additional radiographic views. The patient's screening mammogram was converted to a diagnostic mammogram; therefore, add modifier -GH to the HCPCS code for diagnostic mammogram.

2. S0612, Q0091

Note:

Established patient presented for an annual gynecological examination, which included a screening annual Pap smear. In the HCPCS level II index, go to "Screening, gynecological, established patient" to locate the "annual gynecological examination" code. The CBC, thyroid panel, and complete metabolic panel are reported with codes from the Pathology and Laboratory section of CPT.

3. L8049-RT

Note:

Patient presents for modification of right ocular prosthesis device. Add modifier -RT to the HCPCS level II code to identify on which side of the body the prosthesis device is located.

4. S3841

Note:

This case documents two patients who are presenting for genetic testing for retinoblastoma. Report code S3841 on each patient's health insurance claim.

5. D2740

Note:

This case documents the placement of a porcelain crown. There is no documentation that it was fused onto a metal; therefore, code D2740 is reported.

REVIEW

Multiple Choice

1. c

> **Note:**
>
> *Ambulance origin and destination modifiers are located at the beginning of the Transportation Services Including Ambulance section of HCPCS level II.*
>
> - Modifier -S refers to "scene of accident or acute event."
> - Modifier -H refers to "hospital."

2. d
3. b
4. b
5. a deleted
6. b
7. c
8. b
9. c
10. d D Code
11. b
12. a
13. b
14. d
15. c
16. d
17. b
18. d
19. c
20. c

Chapter 8
Introduction to CPT Coding

ASSIGNMENT 8.1 – CPT INDEX

Identification of Main Term in CPT Index

1. Laparoscopic jejunostomy
2. Removal of a foreign body embedded in the conjunctival of the eye

Note:

The main term can also be Removal.

3. Suture of a wound of the kidney

Note:

The main term can also be Suture.

4. Kasai procedure
5. Repair of an inguinal hernia

Note:

"Repair of an inguinal hernia" is indexed under main term Repair *or main term* Hernia.

Identification of Procedure or Service as Main Term in CPT Index

6. Postpartum dilation and curettage
7. Ileum endoscopy via stoma
8. Clamp circumcision of newborn
9. Arthrotomy of toe, interphalangeal joint
10. Gastrostomy with vagotomy

Identification of Organ or Other Anatomic Site as Main Term in CPT Index

11. Repair of diaphragm laceration
12. Excision of heel spur
13. Excision of cyst of pericardium
14. Pulmonary valve replacement
15. Excision of epiphyseal bar of radius

Identification of Condition as Main Term in CPT Index

16. Toe polydactyly reconstruction
17. Repair of sliding inguinal hernia; patient is a 35-year-old male
18. Drainage of cyst of liver
19. Drainage of hip hematoma
20. Destruction of kidney calculus

Note:

The main term can be "calculus," which is the condition of the kidney as specified in the area of the exercise (16 to 20). An alternative main term is "kidney," which is the anatomical location.

Identification of Synonym as Main Term in CPT Index

21. Albarran test
22. Binding globulin, testosterone-estradiol
23. Digital slit-beam radiograph
24. Energies, electromagnetic
25. Urine test for epinephrine

Identification of Eponym as Main Term in CPT Index

26. Blom-singer prosthesis
27. Waldius procedure
28. Dupuytren's contracture
29. Lee and White test
30. Ober-Yount procedure

Identification of Abbreviation as Main Term in CPT Index

31. Manual sedimentation rate of RBCs

Note:

RBCs is the abbreviation for red blood cells.

32. MRA of the leg

Note:

MRA is the abbreviation for magnetic resonance angiography.

33. Urine pH

Note:

The abbreviation for potential of hydrogen is pH, which is a measure of acidity and alkalinity.

34. Standard EEG

Note:

EEG is the abbreviation for electroencephalography.

35. Complete MRI of the heart

Note:

MRI is the abbreviation for magnetic resonance imaging.

CPT Index Code Ranges

75840–75842 36. Adrenal venography

61697–61708 37. Intracranial artery aneurysm repair

Note:

To locate this CPT code range, first index the word "repair," then "aneurysm," and finally "intracranial"; this will then identify the code range.

84702–84703 38. Chorionic gonadotropin

15300–15336 39. Allograft burns

33420–33422 40. Mitral valve valvotomy

Use of the Directional Term *See* in the CPT Index

41. *See* Clotting Factor
42. *See* Fundoplasty, Esophagogastric
43. *See* Esophagomyotomy
44. *See* Chlamydia
45. *See* Antibody, Tetanus

ASSIGNMENT 8.2 – CPT APPENDICES

Appendix A

1. b
2. b
3. d
4. c
5. a

Appendix B

6. b
7. b
8. c
9. d
10. c

Appendix C

11. b
12. d
13. c
14. c
15. d

Note:

CPT Appendix C code 99205 contains examples of cases that involve initial office or other outpatient consultation with patients who present with established diagnoses (made by another physician) or with an onset of symptoms that require a high level of service. In this case, the patient presents with recent onset of severe symptoms and the endocrinologist ordered a series of tests to evaluate the patient.

Appendix D

16. c
17. a
18. b
19. a
20. c

Appendix E

21. a
22. d
23. b
24. c
25. a

Appendix F

26. c
27. c
28. a
29. d
30. d

Appendix G

31. b
32. c

Note:

EPS is the abbreviation for electrophysiological studies.

33. c
34. c
35. d

Appendix H

36. b
37. a
38. c
39. b
40. b

Appendix I

41. b
42. c
43. b
44. b
45. a

Appendix J

46. d
47. c
48. b
49. c
50. c
51. d
52. b
53. b
54. c
55. d

Appendix K

56. c
57. c
58. a
59. b
60. c

Appendix L

61. c
62. d
63. b
64. d
65. a

Appendix M

66. b
67. c
68. a
69. a
70. b

ASSIGNMENT 8.3 – CPT SYMBOLS

1. c
2. a
3. d
4. d
5. a
6. c
7. b
8. d
9. a
10. b

ASSIGNMENT 8.4 – CPT SECTIONS, SUBSECTIONS, CATEGORIES, AND SUBCATEGORIES

1. d
2. c
3. b
4. a
5. b
6. b
7. b
8. b
9. d
10. c

ASSIGNMENT 8.5 – CPT MODIFIERS

1. c
2. a
3. d
4. b
5. b
6. c
7. c
8. c
9. b
10. a
11. c
12. d
13. c
14. a
15. d
16. d
17. b
18. b
19. c
20. b

REVIEW

Multiple Choice

1. d
2. a
3. d
4. b
5. d
6. b
7. c
8. d
9. a
10. b
11. b
12. c
13. a
14. b
15. b
16. c
17. c
18. c
19. b
20. a

Chapter 9
CPT Evaluation and Management

ASSIGNMENT 9.1 – LEVELS OF EVALUATION AND MANAGEMENT SERVICES

1. Subsequent
   Hospital Inpatient Services, Subsequent Hospital Care
2. New
   Office or Other Outpatient Services, New Patient
3. Not applicable (For emergency department services, no distinction is made between new and established patients.)
   Emergency Department Services
4. Established
   Preventive Medicine Services, Established Patient
5. New
   Nursing Facility Services
6. Detailed history
7. Expanded problem focused examination
8. Expanded problem focused history
   Problem focused examination
9. Expanded problem focused history
   Expanded problem focused examination
   Low complexity of medical decision making
10. Expanded problem focused history
    Expanded problem focused examination
    Straightforward complexity of medical decision making

ASSIGNMENT 9.2 – ASSIGNING EVALUATION AND MANAGEMENT CODES

	ICD Codes	CPT Codes
1.	782.1 (R21)	99254

NOTE:

- The "rash due to allergy" is
- When a patient is seen at the request of another physician, consultation services are provided. Because this consultation took place during an inpatient admission, refer to codes 99251 to 99255. (NOTE: For Medicare patients, consultation codes are not reported. Instead, report either an inpatient hospital visit or an office or other outpatient E/M code.)

	ICD Codes	CPT Codes
2.	948.32, 946.3, 250.00, 427.1, E890.3, E849.0 (T31.32, T30.0, E11.9, I47.2, X00.0xxA, Y92.00)	99284, 99291, 99292

NOTE:

- Although the patient was primarily treated for his burns, there is also documentation of treatment of ventricular tachycardia and diabetes. Therefore, ICD codes are assigned to each condition; and each justifies medical necessity for the evaluation and management and critical care services provided.
- The case does not include the burn site; therefore, ICD-9-CM code 948.32 (or ICD-10-CM code T31.32) is reported for the burn. In a health care facility, the coder should review the record to determine the burn site and/or initiate a physician query.
- The emergency department (ED) physician provided ED services to the patient, which is reported with code 99284. The physician documented 80 minutes of time administering critical care services to the patient; therefore, report codes 99291 and 99292.

	ICD Codes	CPT Codes
3.	780.79 (R53.83)	99213
4.	493.90, 462, 783.0 (J45.909, J02.9, R63.0)	99203

NOTE:

- Because sore throat and loss of appetite are unrelated to the asthma condition, all three conditions are assigned ICD codes. Each ICD code also justifies medical necessity for the evaluation and management services provided.
- Before assigning the CPT code, determine the level of history and examination and complexity of medical decision making. For a new patient office visit, three of three key components must be met or exceeded. The level of history for this case is detailed because the following were documented:
  - History of present illness that contained five elements (location, duration, severity, associated signs and symptoms, and modifying factors)
  - Complete review of systems
  - One element of the past/family/social history

Per the case, the level of examination is detailed and medical decision making was of moderate complexity.

	ICD Codes	CPT Codes
5.	842.00, E884.9, E849.0 (S63.502A, W17.81xA, Y92.017)	99283

NOTE:

- Code the wrist sprain but not the wrist pain because it is a symptom of the sprain.
- Patients treated in the emergency department are not classified as new or established, and three of three key components must be met or exceeded to assign the appropriate code.
- Do not assign a CPT code for wrapping the sprained wrist with an Ace bandage because that service is included in the evaluation and management code.

	ICD Codes	CPT Codes
6.	780.50, 331.0 (G47.9, G30.9)	99308

NOTE:

- "Difficulty sleeping" is located in the ICD index under main term *Disturbance* and subterm *sleep*.
- A code for Alzheimer disease is assigned to this case because the physician reviewed the patient's prescription medications to ensure that an adverse reaction would not occur when the patient was administered the newly prescribed sleep medication. Each ICD code justifies medical necessity for the evaluation and management services provided.
- Follow-up nursing facility care is called "subsequent nursing facility care" in CPT, and just two of three key components must be met or exceeded to assign the appropriate code.

	ICD Codes	CPT Codes
7.	560.9 (K56.60)	99221

NOTE:

- Assign an ICD code to the intestinal obstruction, but do not assign an ICD code to bone cancer because there is no documentation that it was treated or that the intestinal obstruction is related to the cancer.
- For initial hospital (inpatient) care, three of three key components must be met or exceeded to assign the appropriate code.

	ICD Codes	CPT Codes
8.	728.87, 368.2 (M62.81, H53.2)	99243

NOTE:

- Assign ICD codes to muscle weakness and diplopia, both of which justify medical necessity for evaluation and management services.
- For office or other outpatient consultations, three of three key components must be met or exceeded to assign the appropriate

	ICD Codes	CPT Codes
9.	729.1 (M79.7)	99214

NOTE:

- Assign an ICD code to fibromyalgia, but not aching muscles because that is a symptom of fibromyalgia.
- An established patient office or other outpatient service requires that just two of three key components be met or exceeded to assign the appropriate code.

	ICD Codes	CPT Codes
10.	466.0 (J20.9)	99239

NOTE: Hospital discharge services include a final examination of the patient, discussion of the hospital stay with the patient and/or family, instructions for continuing care, preparation of discharge records (e.g., dictating the discharge summary), prescriptions, and referral forms. A key factor in selecting the appropriate code is the length of time the physician spent performing hospital discharge services.

ASSIGNMENT 9.3 – CODING PRACTICE

	ICD Codes	CPT Codes
1.	401.9 (I10)	99211
2.	959.01, 780.97, E880.9, E849.0 (S09.90xA, R41.0, W10.8xxA, Y92.010)	99219

NOTE:

- Refer to *injury,* head to assign the ICD code.
- CPT initial observation care codes require all three key components be met or exceeded to assign the appropriate code.

	ICD Codes	CPT Codes
3.	453.40 (I82.40)	99222, 93965

NOTE:

- Edema of the ankle and calf is a symptom of the suspected deep venous thrombosis and is not coded. Because this is an inpatient case, the suspected condition is coded as if confirmed.
- CPT initial hospital care codes require all three key components be met or exceeded to assign the appropriate code.
- The plethysmography procedure performed on this patient is classified in the CPT Medicine section.

	ICD Codes	CPT Codes
4.	427.9 (I49.9)	99244
5.	821.01 E884.9, E849.4 (S72.302a, W09.2, Y92.830)	99283
6.	518.81 (J96.0)	99291, 99292

NOTE:

- An ICD code is assigned to the acute respiratory arrest because that condition was treated by the respiratory care physician hospitalist. Do not assign ICD codes to chronic obstructive pulmonary disease with acute exacerbation, which is being treated by her attending physician during the inpatient stay. (A hospitalist is a staff physician employed by the hospital.)
- Code 99291 is reported for up to the first 74 minutes of critical care, and code 99292 is reported for each additional 30 minutes. (Code 99291 is reported just once on each date of service.) The patient in this case received a total of 105 minutes of critical care services. Therefore, report code 99291 for up to the first 74 minutes and code 99292 for the next 31 minutes.

	ICD Codes	CPT Codes
7.	779.5, 765.07, 765.26 (P96.1, P07.17, P07.31)	99468
8.	715.96 (M17.9)	99325
9.	278.01 (E66.01)	99349
10.	V70.0, 401.9 (Z00.01, I10)	99397, 99354

NOTE:

- ICD-9-CM code V70.0 (or ICD-10-CM code Z00.01) (annual examination) justifies medical necessity for the annual physical (CPT code 99397).
- ICD-9-CM code 401.9 (or ICD-10-CM code I10) (hypertension) justifies medical necessity for prolonged services (CPT code 99354).
- Code 99354 is reported for up to the first 60 minutes of prolonged services provided by the physician. (A third-party payer might require an office or another outpatient service evaluation and management code to be reported instead of the prolonged services code.)

	ICD Codes	CPT Codes
11.	079.4 (B97.7)	99441
12.	414.00 (I25.10)	99375
13.	V20.0 (Z76.1)	99392
14.	V30.01 (Z38.01)	99464
15.	V70.3 (Z02.6)	99450

REVIEW

Multiple Choice

1. a
2. d
3. d
4. c
5. d

Note:

This patient is at a high level of severity for presenting problem due to the intra-abdominal bleeding. If this medical condition is not addressed, the possibility for mortality is high due to blood loss.

6. d
7. d
8. c
9. c
10. a
11. a
12. b
13. a
14. b
15. d
16. b

Note:

The code range for this encounter is 99211 to 99215 since this is an established patient being seen in the physician's office. For established patient's, two out of three levels must be met or exceeded for a level to be assigned. An expanded problem focused exam and a MDM of moderate complexity met or exceeded the requirements for code 99213. (Code 99214 cannot be assigned because the physician did not document a detailed examination.)

17. c

Note:

All patients receiving ED E/M services are viewed as new patients; therefore, three out of three levels must be met or exceeded to assign a specific E/M code. Based on documentation, the ED physician exceeded the requirements for both examination and history; but code 99284 met the requirement of MDM for that level.

18. a

Note:

Initial inpatient consultations require that three out of three levels be met or exceeded. Based on the documentation, the consulting physician exceeded the requirement for the history and medical decision making component code 99253. The examination provided by the physician met the requirement of a detailed level, which is why code 99253 is assigned (and not a higher E/M, such as 99254).

19. d

Note:

For an established patient home visit, just two out of the three key components must be met or exceeded for a code to be assigned.

20. b

Note:

For an initial hospital care visit, all three key components must be met or exceeded.

Chapter 10
CPT Anesthesia

ASSIGNMENT 10.1 – DETERMINING ANESTHESIA SERVICE PAYMENTS

1. 01967-P2-AA (Code and modifiers)
   5 (Base unit value)
   3 (Anesthesia time units; 45 ÷ f15 = 3)
   0 (Relative value)
   $16.52 (Conversation factor, Arkansas)
   $132.16 (Anesthesia service payment)

Note:

The formula is (5 + 3 + 0) × $16.52 = $132.16.

2. 01967-P2-AA, 01968-P2-AA, 99140 (Codes and modifiers)
   11 (Base unit value)

Note:

Reimbursement for multiple anesthesia services is based on the sum of base unit values because code 01968 is an add-on code. Anesthesia code 01967 has a base unit value of 5, and code 01968 has a base unit value of 6. Thus, the total base unit value is 11.

   5 (Anesthesia time units; 75 ÷ 15 = 5)

Note:

Modifier -P2 has a relative value of 0, and code 99140 has a relative value of 2. Total relative value is 2.

   2 (Relative value)
   $17.83 (Conversion factor, Arizona)
   $320.94 (Anesthesia service payment)

Note:

The formula is (11 + 5 + 2) × $17.83 = $320.94.

3. 00210-P5-AA, 99140 (Codes and modifiers)
   10 (Base unit value)
   4 (Anesthesia time units; $60 \div 15 = 4$)
   5 (Relative value)

Note:

Physical status modifier -P5 is assigned a relative value of 3, and code 99140 is assigned a relative value of 2.

$17.04 (Conversion factor, Alabama)
$323.76 (Anesthesia service payment)

Note:

The formula is $(10 + 4 + 5) \times \$17.04 = \$323.76$.

ASSIGNMENT 10.2 – ANESTHESIA MODIFIERS

1. -G8
2. -QZ
3. -AA
4. -AD
5. -P5

Note:

If the ruptured spleen was not surgically repaired or removed, the patient would have died (e.g., from hemorrhaging).

6. -P4

Note:

ESRD is a severe systemic disease that is a constant threat to life (e.g., without dialysis or a kidney transplant, the patient would die). In this case the patient undergoes a procedure unrelated to the ESRD; but since the patient has ESRD, physical status modifier -P4 is added to the anesthesia code.

7. -P2

Note:

Chronic asthma is a mild systemic disease.

8. -74
9. -23
10. -59

ASSIGNMENT 10.3 – CODING PRACTICE

Note:

ICD-9-CM (or ICD-10-CM) external cause of disease and injury (or morbidity) are not reported on anesthesia claims. Do not assign ICD-9-CM E codes (or ICD-10-CM V or Y codes) to Chapter 10 cases.

	ICD Codes	CPT Codes
1.	852.21 (S06.5x0A)	00214-P1-AA, 36620-59, 93503-59
	NOTE: Do not assign ICD codes to vertigo or headaches, which are symptoms of the subdural hematoma.	
2.	142.0, 401.9 (C07, I10)	00100-P2-QX
	NOTE: Salivary parotid malignancy medically justifies anesthesia administration, and hypertension justifies assignment of physical status modifier -P2.	
3.	925.2 (S17.0xxA)	00326-P5-AA, 99140, 36620
	NOTE: • Do not assign ICD codes to the severe breathing problems or the patient's cold and sweaty condition, which was a result of the crushed larynx injury. • Crushed larynx and trachea medically justifies anesthesia administration, and physical status modifier -P5 is assigned because the patient would not be expected to survive without the operation.	
4.	171.0 (C49.0)	00300-P4-QZ
5.	810.00 (S42.001A)	00450-P1-AA
6.	198.5, 199.1 (C79.51, C80.1)	00470-P4-AA, 99100
	NOTE: Cancer medically justifies anesthesia administration, and physical status modifier -P4 is assigned because the patient has a severe systemic disease (cancer) that is a constant threat to life.	
7.	996.01, 426.10, V45.01 (T82.198A, I44.30, Z95.0)	00530-P4-AA, 99100
	NOTE: • Twiddler syndrome is a mechanical complication of a cardiac pacemaker in which the pacemaker leads inappropriately retract, resulting in inappropriate shocks to the heart muscle. • Twiddler syndrome medically justifies anesthesia administration, and the atrioventricular block and the cardiac pacemaker status justify assignment of physical status modifier -P4.	
8.	150.9, 250.01 (C15.9, E10.9)	00500-P3-AA, 99100
	NOTE: • The esophageal malignancy medically justifies anesthesia administration, and type 1 diabetes justifies assignment of physical status modifier -P3. • It is not necessary to assign a code for history of tobacco abuse on an anesthesia case because it does not impact selection of the physical status modifier. Also do not code current tobacco abuse because that is not documented.	
9.	213.2 (D16.6)	00620-P1-QX
10.	722.0, 250.00	00600-P2-AA
	NOTE: • Do not assign an ICD code to the upper back pain because it is a symptom of the displaced cervical intervertebral disk. • Displacement of cervical intervertebral disk medically justifies anesthesia administration, and type 2 diabetes justifies assignment of physical status modifier -P2.	
11.	571.5, 303.90 (K74.0, F10.20)	00796-P4-AA, 93503
	NOTE: Cirrhosis medically justifies anesthesia administration, and alcoholism justifies assignment of physical status modifier -P2.	
12.	278.01, 401.9, 250.00, 272.0 (E66.01, I10, E11.9, E78.0)	00797-P3-AA
	NOTE: Morbid obesity medically justifies anesthesia administration; and hypertension, diabetes, and high cholesterol justify assignment of physical status modifier -P3.	

	ICD Codes	CPT Codes
13.	553.20, 413.9, 305.00 (K43.90, I20.9, F10.10)	00830-P3-QZ

NOTE:

- Do not assign an ICD code to the lump in the lower abdominal area, which was due to an abdominal hernia.
- Abdominal hernia medically justifies anesthesia administration, and angina and alcohol abuse justify assignment of physical status modifier -P3.

	ICD Codes	CPT Codes
14.	250.41, 585.6 (E10.22, N18.6)	00868-P4-AA, 36620-59, 93503-59

NOTE:

- Two ICD codes must be assigned to completely classify the diagnosis for this case.
- Diabetes with end-stage renal disease (ESRD) medically justifies anesthesia administration, and the patient has a severe systemic disease (ESRD) that is a constant threat to life.

	ICD Codes	CPT Codes
15.	752.51 (Q53.20)	00924-P1-QZ, 99100
16.	997.99, 607.84, 042, V10.49 (N99.89, N52.39, B20, Z85.49)	00938-P3-AA

NOTE:

- According to the AHA's *Coding Clinic for ICD-9-CM,* when impotence is the result of surgery performed to remove a malignancy, code 997.9 (Complications affecting other specified body systems, not elsewhere classified) is assigned, followed by code 607.84 (Impotence of organic origin) and code V10.49 (Personal history of malignant neoplasm, genital organs, other male genital organs).
- This case also indicates that the patient is HIV-infected, which is assigned ICD code 042 (B20).
- Postoperative complication (impotence) medically justifies anesthesia administration, and HIV and personal history of cancer justify assignment of physical status modifier -P3.

	ICD Codes	CPT Codes
17	808.8 (S32.9xxA)	01120-P1-AA, 99140
18.	828.0 (S42.301A, S72.92xA)	01130-P1-AA, 99140
19.	454.0 (I83.011, I83.021)	01260-P3-AA

NOTE: Varicose veins medically justifies anesthesia administration, and physical status modifier -P3 is assigned because the patient has severe systemic disease (severe varicose veins of both lower extremities with ulcers of both thighs).

	ICD Codes	CPT Codes
20.	820.8 (S72.002A)	01220-P1-QZ, 99100
21.	719.46, 401.9 (M25.562, I10)	01382-P2-AA

NOTE: Knee pain medically justifies anesthesia administration, and hypertension justifies assignment of physical status modifier -P2.

	ICD Codes	CPT Codes
22.	823.01, 250.00 (S82.831A, E11.9)	01392-P2-AA, 99100

NOTE: The fracture medically justifies anesthesia administration, and type 2 diabetes justifies assignment of physical status modifier -P2.

	ICD Codes	CPT Codes
23.	735.2 (M20.21)	01480-P2-AA

NOTE: The cocked-up fifth toe medically justifies anesthesia administration, and the history of foot problems justifies assignment of physical status modifier -P2.

	ICD Codes	CPT Codes
24.	198.5 (C79.51)	01470-P3-AA

NOTE: Cancer medically justifies anesthesia administration, and physical status modifier -P3 is assigned because the patient has severe systemic disease (metastatic cancer).

	ICD Codes	CPT Codes
25.	732.7 (M93.211)	01630-P1-AA
26.	812.00 (S42.202A)	01680-P1-AA
27.	927.11, 042 (S57.01xA, B20)	01760-P3-QX

NOTE: Crushed elbow medically justifies anesthesia administration, and HIV justifies assignment of physical status modifier -P4.

	ICD Codes	CPT Codes
28.	733.20, 579.0, 272.0 (M85.60, K90.0, E78.0)	01758-P2-AA

NOTE: Bone cyst medically justifies anesthesia administration, and celiac disease and high cholesterol justifies assignment of physical status modifier -P2.

	ICD Codes	CPT Codes
29.	813.81 (S52.91xA)	01820-P1-AA
30.	814.00 (S62.102A)	01820-P1-QX
31.	729.5 (M79.605)	01916-P1-AA
32.	724.5, 250.00 (M54.9, E11.9)	01936-P2-QX

NOTE: Back pain medically justifies anesthesia administration, and type 2 diabetes justifies assignment of physical status modifier -P2.

	ICD Codes	CPT Codes
33.	942.32, 948.00, 305.1 (T21.31xA, T31.0, F17.210)	01951-P2-AA
NOTE: Burns medically justify anesthesia administration, and tobacco abuse justifies assignment of physical status modifier -P2.		
34.	945.29, 948.00 (T24.292A, T31.0)	01952-P1-QZ
35.	669.71, 042, V27.0 (O82, B20, Z37.0)	01963-P3-AA, 99140
NOTE: Cesarean delivery medically justifies anesthesia administration, and HIV justifies assignment of physical status modifier -P4.		
36.	651.01, V27.2 (O30.003, Z37.2)	01960-P1-QX
37.	651.11, V27.5 (O30.13, V37.51)	01967-P1-AA
38.	V59.4 (Z52.4)	01990-P6-AA
NOTE: Harvesting the organ medically justifies anesthesia administration, and physical status modifier -P6 is assigned because this is a brain-dead patient whose organs are being removed for donor purposes.		
39.	332.0 (G20)	01992-P3-AA
NOTE: Parkinsonism medically justifies anesthesia administration, and physical status modifier -P3 is assigned because the patient has a severe systemic disorder (Parkinsonism).		
40.	745.5 (Q21.1)	01996-P5-AA, 99140
NOTE: Atrial septal defect medically justifies anesthesia administration, and physical status modifier -P5 is assigned because the patient was not expected to survive without the operation.		

REVIEW

Multiple Choice

1. d
2. d
3. a
4. b
5. b
6. b
7. c
8. c
9. a
10. d
11. c
12. a
13. b
14. b
15. d
16. b
17. a
18. c
19. d
20. a

Chapter 11
CPT Surgery I

ASSIGNMENT 11.1 – CODING PRACTICE

	ICD Codes	CPT Codes
1.	883.1 (S61.122A)	11760-FA
NOTE: The presence of a foreign object meets the criteria to assign a complicated wound code.		
2.	216.5 (D23.5)	11302
NOTE: To locate the ICD code, go to the Neoplasm Table in the alphabetic index and locate *skin, trunk, benign.*		
3.	172.3 (C43.39)	11644
4.	881.00, 881.02 (S51.811A, S61.511A)	12002
NOTE: Both wounds were repaired with simple closure, and they are grouped in code range 12001–12007. The wound sizes are added together to obtain a total wound size of 6.0 cm.		
5.	680.6 (L02.436)	10060

ASSIGNMENT 11.2 – CODING OPERATIVE REPORTS

	ICD Codes	CPT Codes
1.	569.49 (K62.89)	11402
NOTE: • To assign the ICD diagnosis code, locate subterm *anus* under main term *Cyst.* (There is no subterm *perianal* under main term *Cyst.*) • A cyst is a type of benign lesion. Refer to the note located above CPT code 11400, which provides examples of terms that could be used when classifying benign lesions.		
2.	686.1 (L98.0)	11421-F6
NOTE: A granuloma is a type of benign lesion. Therefore, the CPT code range for its excision is 11400–11471.		
3.	173.3 (C44.39)	14040
NOTE: CPT codes for advancement flap procedures are located in the Adjacent Tissue Transfer subheading, and the code assigned reflects the recipient site of the flap (e.g., forehead). These codes include excision of the lesion, which means that a secondary procedure code for excision of the lesion is not assigned.		
4.	707.04, 707.24, 340 (L89.224, G35)	15958, 15738-51
NOTE: A decubitus ulcer is also called a pressure ulcer, and the procedure performed requires the assignment of two CPT codes. Code 15958 is assigned for excision of the ulcer, including ostectomy, and code 15738 is assigned for the muscle flap closure of the surgical defect.		
5.	611.79 (N64.59)	19355-50
NOTE: Although the description of code 19355 contains the term *nipples* (plural of *nipple*), modifier -50 is added to the code because the CMS/Medicare physician fee schedule assigns a value of 1 in the Bilateral Surgery column for this code. The CMS definition of value 1 for Bilateral Surgery (Modifier 50) states: 1 = 150% payment adjustment for bilateral procedures applies. If the code is billed with the bilateral modifier or is reported twice on the same day by any other means (e.g., with RT and LT modifiers, or with a 2 in the units field), base the payment for these codes when reported as bilateral procedures on the lower of: (a) the total actual charge for both sides or (b) 150% of the fee schedule amount for a single code. If the code is reported as a bilateral procedure and is reported with other procedure codes on the same day, apply the bilateral adjustment before applying any multiple procedure rules.		

REVIEW

Multiple Choice

1. b

Note:

This patient's surgery requires assignment of one code for the excision of the 1.5 cm in diameter basal cell carcinoma lesion of the cheek and another code for the shaving of the 2.5 cm in diameter basal cell carcinoma lesion of the nose.

2. c
3. d
4. b
5. a
6. c
7. a
8. b
9. a
10. c

Note:

- The hand and foot wounds were repaired with an intermediate closure; the lengths of these wounds are combined based on the classification of the anatomic sites in CPT. The hand and foot wounds totaled 5.0 cm, and code 12042 is assigned.
- Based on the classification of the anatomic sites in CPT, the lengths of the scalp and neck wounds can also be combined because both required simple repairs. The scalp and neck wounds totaled 4.0 cm, and code 12002 is assigned.

11. a
12. c
13. b
14. c
15. d
16. b

Note:

This type of lesion is classified as a benign lesion and is coded in the 11400 to 11471 range of CPT codes under the Integumentary System subsection.

17. c
18. a
19. b
20. b

Chapter 12
CPT Surgery II

ASSIGNMENT 12.1 – CODING PRACTICE

	ICD Codes	CPT Codes
1.	835.01 (S73.014)	27253
NOTE: This case documents a closed hip dislocation; however, treatment was open reduction of the dislocation.		
2.	491.9 (J42)	31717
3.	754.30 (Q65.01)	27275
4.	813.43 (S52.615A)	25650
NOTE: The application of the cast is included in the code for the closed fracture treatment. Do not assign a separate code for the cast application.		
5.	511.9 (J90)	32421
6.	874.02 (S11.021A)	31800
7.	464.00 (J04.0)	31575
8.	802.0 (S02.2xxA)	21315
9.	729.71 (M79.a11)	26037
10.	578.0 (M79.a11)	31625, 31620
NOTE: • For outpatient care, do not assign codes to diagnoses stated as "rule out." Assign codes to confirmed diagnoses or signs/symptoms when there is no confirmed diagnosis. • Do not add modifier -51 to code 31620, which is an add-on code (and exempt from modifier -51).		

ASSIGNMENT 12.2 – CODING PRACTICE

	ICD Codes	CPT Codes
1.	727.03 (M65.332)	26055-F2
NOTE: To locate CPT code 26055, locate main term *Trigger finger repair* in the index.		
2.	518.89 (J98.4)	31628
NOTE: • Assign code 518.89 (or M65.332) for mucosal lesion of the bronchus because bronchi are branching passageways of the lungs. (Do not assign a code for hemoptysis, which is a symptom of the diagnosed mucosal lesion of the bronchus. • The diagnostic bronchoscopy is included in the surgical bronchoscopy code.		
3.	V54.01 (Z47.2)	20680-LT
NOTE: To assign code V54.01 (or Z47.2), use the ICD index and locate main term *Removal (of),* subterm *device*, 2nd qualifier *fixation*, and 3rd qualifier *internal*.		
4.	812.43 (S42.442A)	24575-LT
NOTE: • The abbreviation for millimeters of mercury is mmHg. • ORIF is the abbreviation for open reduction with internal fixation.		

	ICD Codes	CPT Codes
5.	162.3 (C34.11)	32480, 31622-51

NOTE:

- Do not assign a CPT code for insertion of a chest tube (code 32551) because the code description includes the phrase *separate procedure*. This means that the placement of chest tubes for drainage is considered an integral part of a thoracostomy with biopsy procedure.
- After the thoracostomy was performed, the patient underwent diagnostic bronchoscopy which is separately coded as 31622. Modifier -51 is added to this code to reflect that multiple procedures were performed during the same operative session.

6.	735.0, 726.91 (M20.11, M77.51)	28296-T5, 28288-51-T6

NOTE:

- Both ICD codes medically justify the procedure performed.
- In ICD-10-CM, main term *Spur, bone* directs the coder to *see also* Enthesopathy. Main term *Enthesopathy*, subterm *foot*, and 2nd qualifier *specified type NEC* provides direction to M77.5- (for selection of the fifth digit).
- According to the *CPT Assistant*, code 28296 is reported for an Austin, Chevron, or Mitchell bunionectomy.

7.	471.8 (J33.8)	31032-RT
8.	212.1 (D14.1)	31541
9.	784.7 (R04.0)	30905-LT, 30903-59-RT

NOTE:

- The patient underwent posterior packing and cautery, which is assigned CPT code 30905.
- The patient also underwent anterior packing after failed cautery on the right, which is assigned code 30903 to reflect a more complex treatment. Modifiers -59 (distinct procedure) and -RT are added to the code.

10.	518.82, 335.20 (J80, G12.21)	31600

NOTE:

- ALS is the abbreviation for amyotrophic lateral sclerosis, which is also known as Lou Gehrig's disease.
- Respiratory insufficiency medically justifies the procedure performed. A code for ALS is also reported because the condition contributed to the first-listed diagnosis.

REVIEW

Multiple Choice

1. c
2. c
3. b

Note:

The cast application is included in the definitive treatment code.

4. a
5. c
6. c
7. c
8. d
9. d
10. a
11. c
12. b

Note:

When a diagnostic laryngoscopy is performed during the same operative session as a surgical laryngoscopy, code only the surgical laryngoscopy. The diagnostic laryngoscopy is included in the surgical laryngoscopy code.

13. a
14. c
15. a
16. b

Note:

The fascia level is located below the subcutaneous level of skin.

17. d
18. a
19. c

Note:

The code description for 32500 indicates that the code is assigned if one wedge resection is done or if multiple wedge resections are done.

20. a

Chapter 13
CPT Surgery III

ASSIGNMENT 13.1 – CODING PRACTICE

	ICD Codes	CPT Codes
1.	454.9 (I83.92)	37722-LT
2.	785.6 (R59.0)	38510
3.	426.0 (I44.2)	33210, 71090
4.	785.6 (R59.0)	38570
5.	V46.11 (Z99.11)	36620
NOTE: Because no disease or condition was documented to justify respirator care, assign an ICD V (or ICD Z code) code by locating main term *Status* in the alphabetic index.		
6.	785.6 (R59.0)	38720
7.	397.0 (I07.1)	33464
NOTE: To assign the ICD diagnosis code, locate main term *Regurgitation* and subterm *tricuspid.* Note that the directional term see refers you to *Endocarditis, tricuspid.*		
8.	572.3 (K76.6)	38100
9.	996.04 (T82.110A)	33241, 33243-51, 33249-51
NOTE: To assign the ICD diagnosis code, locate main term *Complication,* subterm *device,* and qualifiers *cardiac* and *automatic implantable defibrillator.*		
10.	289.59, 084.1 (B51.0)	38115

ASSIGNMENT 13.2 – CODING OPERATIVE REPORTS

	ICD Codes	CPT Codes
1.	426.0, 427.89, 412 (I44.2, R00.1, I25.2)	33210, 71090
NOTE: This report documents the insertion of a temporary pacemaker electrode. It does not document or state that a permanent pacemaker with a pulse generator component was inserted.		
2.	174.9 (C50.912)	36558, 77001
NOTE: Tunneled catheters are placed through the skin in the middle of the chest. They are tunneled through the subcutaneous tissue and inserted into the superior vena cava vessel at the entrance of the right atrium of the heart. Tunneled catheters can be left in place for months or years with a low rate of infection. (Nontunneled catheters are inserted directly through the skin into the jugular or subclavian vein and are moved through the vein to the superior vena cava. Nontunneled catheters can be inserted at the bedside in a nonsurgical setting, and they are commonly used for short-term or emergency situations. Nontunneled catheters are also referred to as jugular or subclavian catheters.)		
3.	V58.81 (Z45.2)	36589
NOTE: The patient was admitted for the removal of her Hickman catheter because symptoms associated with hyperemesis gravidarum had resolved. The ICD diagnosis code can be located by referring to main term *Removal* and subterms *catheter, vascular.* A Hickman catheter is a tunneled central venous (vascular) catheter, which means that it is inserted (or tunneled) under the skin and placed in a vein. (The purpose of tunneling the catheter under the skin is to help prevent infection.)		

	ICD Codes	CPT Codes
4.	414.01 (I25.10)	33535, 33518
NOTE: • There is no documentation that the patient had previously undergone bypass surgery; therefore, ICD diagnosis code 414.01 (or I25.10) is assigned. • Code 33535 reflects the grafting of three arterial vessels. • The saphenous vein was used for two grafts; therefore, CPT code 33518 is assigned. • Cardioplegia and bypass are integral parts of a CABG, and they are not coded separately. (CABG is the abbreviation for coronary artery bypass graft.)		
5.	420.90 (I30.1)	33010, 76930
6.	785.6 (R59.0)	38525-LT
7.	289.59 (D73.4)	38120
NOTE: Because a laparoscopic spleen removal procedure was documented, code 38120 is assigned (and not code 38100).		
8.	683 (L04.0)	38300
9.	202.83 (C85.23)	38570
NOTE: The biopsied lymph nodes were located in the retroperitoneal area, which is the area behind the abdominal wall. Thus, fifth-digit 3 is assigned to the ICD diagnosis code.		
10.	V59.3 (Z52.3)	38230
NOTE: To assign the ICD diagnosis code, locate main term *Donor* in the alphabetic index.		

REVIEW

Multiple Choice

1. c

Note:

It is incorrect to assign modifier -63 to the CPT code. There is a note that directs the coder not to report modifier -63 with the code.

2. d
3. b
4. c
5. d
6. d
7. b
8. a
9. a
10. c
11. c
12. a
13. b
14. b

Note:

RBC is the abbreviation for red blood cell, and WBC is the abbreviation for white blood cell.

15. d
16. b
17. c
18. a
19. a
20. c

Chapter 14
CPT Surgery IV

ASSIGNMENT 14.1 – CODING PRACTICE

	ICD Codes	CPT Codes
1.	786.6 (R22.2)	39000
2.	211.3 (D12.3)	45385
3.	573.9 (R16.0)	47000, 76942
NOTE: To assign the ICD-9-CM diagnosis code, locate main term *Disease* and subterm *liver* in the alphabetic index. Do not go to main term *Mass* and subterm *liver* because no code is found there. However, main term *Mass* and subterm *specified disease* directs the coder to the main term *Disease*. (In the ICD-10-CM index, main term *Mass* and subterm *liver* lists code R16.0, which is classified as hepatomegaly in the tabular list.)		
4.	599.70 (R31.9)	52000
5.	553.21 (K43.91)	49560
NOTE: This case documents an incisional hernia.		
6.	212.6 (D15.0)	39400
7.	596.8 (N32.89)	52204
NOTE: There is no ICD index entry for urinary bladder or trigone below main term *Mass*. However, main term *Mass* contains subterm *specified organ NEC – see Disease, by site*, which leads to ICD-9-CM code 596.8 (or ICD-10-CM N32.89).		
8.	560.81, 197.7, V10.05 (K56.5, C78.7, Z85.030)	44005
9.	212.6 (D15.0)	39220
10.	565.0 (K60.0)	46200
11.	553.3 (K44.9)	43334
12.	998.11 (N99.820)	52214
13.	098.0 (A54.01)	53200
NOTE: To locate the ICD diagnosis code, locate main term *Urethritis* and subterm *gonococcal* in the alphabetic index.		
14.	780.60 (R50.9)	51100
15.	198.89, 199.1 (C79.89, C80.1)	39560
NOTE: This case documents cancer of the diaphragm as metastatic, which means the code is assigned from the Secondary column in the Neoplasm Table after *diaphragm* as the site is located. To assign an ICD code to the unknown primary site, go to the Neoplasm Table and locate code 199.1 (or C80.1) under the Primary column. (ICD code 199.1 is assigned as a secondary code to reflect that the primary neoplasm has a site that is not known in this case.)		

ASSIGNMENT 14.2 – CODING OPERATIVE REPORTS

	ICD Codes	CPT Codes
1.	552.20, 553.1 (K43.00, K42.9)	49561, 49585-51
NOTE: • For ICD coding purposes, the term *incarcerated* as documented in this report means that the ventral hernia resulted in an "obstruction." • The patient's age must be known to select the appropriate CPT code for an umbilical hernia repair.		
2.	540.9 (K35.80)	44950
3.	557.0, 537.89 (K55.0, K31.89)	49002
NOTE: This patient underwent a laparotomy one week prior to the laparotomy documented in this report.		

<table>
<tr><th></th><th>ICD Codes</th><th>CPT Codes</th></tr>
<tr><td>4.</td><td>211.3 (D12.3)</td><td>44140</td></tr>
<tr><td colspan="3">NOTE: Another term for a hemicolectomy is a partial colectomy.</td></tr>
<tr><td>5.</td><td>550.10 (K40.30)</td><td>49496-RT</td></tr>
<tr><td colspan="3">NOTE: The age of the patient must be known to assign the appropriate CPT code. Another factor important to assigning the correct CPT code is documentation of the incarcerated (or obstructed) small bowel.</td></tr>
<tr><td>6.</td><td>236.7, 239.4 (D41.4, D49.4)</td><td>52235, 52332-51, 74420</td></tr>
<tr><td colspan="3">NOTE:
• The physician identified the bladder tumor as a papilloma, which is assigned ICD-9-CM code 236.7 (or ICD-10-CM code D41.4) (papilloma). If a pathology report was not available, documentation from the operative report would be used to assign the ICD diagnosis code.
• A second bladder tumor was documented in the operative report, which is assigned ICD-9-CM code 239.4 (or ICD-10-CM code D49.4) because it is of unspecified nature.
• Insertion of an indwelling stent is assigned an additional procedure code. If the stent was not indwelling or had not been left in place at the conclusion of the procedure, a separate code would not be assigned.
• According to CPT Assistant, code 74420 is reported once for the bilateral retrograde pyelograms and modifier -50 is not added to the code. According to Ingenix's Encoder Pro Expert software, directional modifiers (e.g., -LT and -RT) are not added to the code.</td></tr>
<tr><td>7.</td><td>594.1, 591 (N21.0, N13.30)</td><td>52353, 52332-51</td></tr>
<tr><td colspan="3">NOTE:
• The size of the bladder stone determines the correct CPT code.
• The insertion of an indwelling stent is coded as an additional procedure code. If the stent was not indwelling or was not left in place at the conclusion of the procedure, it would not be separately coded.</td></tr>
<tr><td>8.</td><td>592.1 (N20.1)</td><td>52320-52</td></tr>
<tr><td colspan="3">NOTE: Modifier -52 is added to the CPT code to identify a reduced service for a surgical procedure that was attempted but not completed.</td></tr>
<tr><td>9.</td><td>188.4 (C67.4)</td><td>52224</td></tr>
<tr><td colspan="3">NOTE:
• ICD code 188.4 (or C67.4) is assigned for carcinoma of the bladder because documentation in the operative report indicates a posterior wall location.
• The site of the bladder tumor was not documented in the operative report, which means that the lowest code in range 52224–52240 is assigned. (The physician should be queried to provide information on the size of the tumor fulgurated on this patient.)</td></tr>
<tr><td>10.</td><td>592.1 (N20.1)</td><td>52330, 74485</td></tr>
<tr><td colspan="3">NOTE:
• The patient underwent manipulation of the ureteral stone in his bladder. Because the stone was not removed, CPT code 52330 is assigned.
• Ureteral fluoroscopy was performed to confirm the catheter's position during the operative procedure; ureteral fluoroscopy is included in CPT code 52330. Do not report a separate CPT code for ureteral fluoroscopy.
• Contrast material was injected into the catheter, and the entire left ureter and renal collecting system were outlined. Then dilatation of the ureter and collecting system was performed, which revealed presences of ureteral calculus. The fluoroscopically guided dilatation procedure is assigned CPT code 74485. (According to Ingenix's Encoder Pro Expert, directional modifiers -LT and -RT are not added to code 74485.)</td></tr>
<tr><td>11.</td><td>553.3 (K44.9)</td><td>43332</td></tr>
<tr><td>12.</td><td>782.0, 719.40, V18.3 (R20.0, M25.50, Z83.2)</td><td>39400</td></tr>
<tr><td colspan="3">NOTE: The diagnosis "sarcoidosis" is unconfirmed at the time of the procedure, which means that ICD codes for the patient's reported symptoms of numbness and joint pain are assigned along with family history of sarcoidosis (immune disorder).</td></tr>
<tr><td>13.</td><td>862.0 (S27.803A)</td><td>39501</td></tr>
<tr><td>14.</td><td>748.8 (Q34.1)</td><td>39200</td></tr>
<tr><td>15.</td><td>786.2 (R05)</td><td>39010</td></tr>
<tr><td colspan="3">NOTE:
• Because the diagnosis of lung carcinoma was not established at the time of surgery, an ICD code for the patient's symptom of cough is assigned.
• Chamberlain is an eponym for a mediastinotomy procedure, which involves incision in the third intercostal space or transthoracic space.</td></tr>
<tr><td>16.</td><td>527.2 (K11.21)</td><td>42415</td></tr>
</table>

REVIEW

Multiple Choice

1. b
2. d
3. b
4. b

Note:

ERCP is the abbreviation for endoscopic retrograde cholangiopancreatography.

5. d

Note:

EGD is the abbreviation for esophagogastroduodenoscopy.

6. c
7. a
8. a

Note:

- A TURP includes a vasectomy, meatotomy, cystourethroscopy, urethral calibration, dilation, and/or internal urethrotomy. Codes for these procedures, when performed during the same operative session as a TURP, are not reported separately.
- TURP is the abbreviation for transurethral resection of the prostate.

9. d
10. b
11. b
12. d
13. a
14. b
15. c
16. a

Note:

Cystoscopy is also known as cystourethroscopy.

17. b
18. a
19. d
20. d

Chapter 15
CPT Surgery V

ASSIGNMENT 15.1 – CODING PRACTICE

<table>
<tr><th></th><th>ICD Codes</th><th>CPT Codes</th></tr>
<tr><td>1.</td><td>186.9 (C62.12)</td><td>54520-LT</td></tr>
<tr><td>2.</td><td>246.2 (E04.1)</td><td>60300-RT</td></tr>
<tr><td>3.</td><td>956.5 (S94.8x1A)</td><td>64834-RT, 69990</td></tr>
<tr><td colspan="3">NOTE: To assign the ICD diagnosis code, locate main term Injury, subterm nerve, 2nd qualifier foot, and 3rd qualifier specified site NEC in the alphabetic index. (If main term Laceration and subterm nerve are referenced instead, the coder is directed to main term Injury.)</td></tr>
<tr><td>4.</td><td>650, V27.0 (O80, Z37.0)</td><td>59400</td></tr>
<tr><td colspan="3">NOTE:
• This is a delivery case, and ICD coding guidelines require the assignment of an outcome of delivery code to represent the status of the infant delivered. To assign this code, locate main term Outcome in the alphabetic index.
• This case documents that the physician provided antepartum, postpartum, and delivery care, which means that CPT code 59400 is assigned.</td></tr>
<tr><td>5.</td><td>245.2 (E06.3)</td><td>60271</td></tr>
<tr><td colspan="3">NOTE: Do not assign CPT code 60240 (Thyroidectomy, total or complete) because a cervical approach was used to perform the surgery, which is classified as code 60271.</td></tr>
<tr><td>6.</td><td>368.13 (H53.142)</td><td>65430-LT</td></tr>
<tr><td>7.</td><td>233.5 (D07.4)</td><td>54100</td></tr>
<tr><td colspan="3">NOTE: To assign the ICD diagnosis code, locate main term Bowen's. The coder is directed to the Neoplasm Table and subterms skin, male genital organs, penis, in situ.</td></tr>
<tr><td>8.</td><td>623.8 (N89.8)</td><td>57135</td></tr>
<tr><td>9.</td><td>355.8 (G57.9)</td><td>64555</td></tr>
<tr><td>10.</td><td>346.70 (G43.709)</td><td>64405</td></tr>
<tr><td>11.</td><td>621.8 (N81.4)</td><td>58520</td></tr>
<tr><td colspan="3">NOTE: Do not mistakenly assign CPT code 59350, which classifies hysterorrhaphy of ruptured uterus for Maternal Care and Delivery. Code 58520 correctly classifies nonobstetrical hysterorrhaphy.</td></tr>
<tr><td>12.</td><td>921.2 (S05.12xA)</td><td>67415, 77002-51</td></tr>
<tr><td colspan="3">NOTE:
• This case documents the use of a fluoroscope, which means that CPT code 77002 is assigned as an additional code.</td></tr>
<tr><td>13.</td><td>V55.8 (Z43.8)</td><td>69424-50</td></tr>
<tr><td colspan="3">NOTE:
• To locate the ICD code refer to main term Attention to and subterm artificial, opening (of) in the index because the reason for the procedure is to remove previously placed ventilation tubes.
• This case documents removal of tubes from the right and left ear; therefore, modifier -50 is added to the CPT code.</td></tr>
<tr><td>14.</td><td>608.4 (N49.2)</td><td>55100</td></tr>
<tr><td>15.</td><td>605, 607.1 (N47.1, N48.1)</td><td>54161</td></tr>
<tr><td>16.</td><td>252.01 (E21.0)</td><td>60500</td></tr>
</table>

	ICD Codes	CPT Codes
17.	606.1 (N46.11)	55300
18.	784.2 (R22.1)	60210
NOTE: To assign the ICD diagnosis code, locate main term *Mass* and subterm *neck* in the index.		
19.	227.5 (D35.5)	60600
20.	380.4 (H61.23)	69210
NOTE: The description of CPT code 69210 states one or both ears; therefore, modifier -50 is not added the CPT code.		
21.	370.00 (H16.002A)	65450-LT
NOTE: A "corneal lesion" is a corneal ulcer and is commonly caused by trauma. Main term is *ulcer* and subterm is *cornea* in the ICD index.		
22.	641.01, V27.0 (O44.03, Z37.0)	59514
NOTE: • Apgar is named after anesthesiologist Virginia Apgar, and the acronym stands for activity, pulse, grimace, appearance, and respiration. It is an assessment of newborns typically at 1 minute and 5 minutes after birth. Each area (activity, pulse, etc) is assigned a score of 0, 1, or 2. The five areas are combined to achieve a total score. A total score of 7 to 10 is normal. • This case documents a delivery, which means that an outcome of delivery ICD code is assigned.		
23.	354.0 (G56.02)	64721-LT
24.	173.2 (C44.22)	69100
NOTE: To assign the code refer to the Neoplasm Table in the ICD index and locate subterm *ear (external).*		
25.	626.8 (N93.8)	57180
26.	351.8 (G51.8)	64732
NOTE: To assign the code locate main term *Neuritis* and subterm *facial* in the ICD index. Notice that there is no subterm for *orbital, supraorbital,* or *frontal.* The supraorbital nerve is a branch of the frontal nerve, which passes through the supraorbital notch of the forehead. It controls sensory functions of the upper eyelid, eyebrow, forehead, scalp up to the occipital bone, and conjunctiva. It is classified as a facial nerve.		
27.	365.22 (H40.211)	66762
28.	634.91 (O03.4)	59812
NOTE: In ICD, a miscarriage is a spontaneous abortion.		
29.	216.1 (D22.12)	67850-E1
30.	614.4 (N73.1)	58823
31.	385.30 (H71.91)	69540
32.	634.90 (O03.9)	59425
33.	380.10 (H60.02)	69020
34.	131.01 (A59.01)	57105
35.	744.29 (Q17.5)	69300-LT

ASSIGNMENT 15.2 – CODING OPERATIVE REPORTS

	ICD Codes	CPT Codes
1.	185 (C61)	52601
NOTE: • Cystoscopy is a diagnostic procedure that is not be coded or reported separately for this surgical case.		
2.	600.00 (N40.0)	55700, 76872
3.	V25.2 (Z30.2)	55250
NOTE: This patient was admitted for the sterilization procedure. In the ICD-9-CM index, go to main term *Admission (for)*, subterm *sterilization*. In the ICD-10-CM index, go to main term *Encounter (for)* and subterm *sterilization*.		

<table>
<tr><th></th><th>ICD Codes</th><th>CPT Codes</th></tr>
<tr><td>4.</td><td>603.9 (N43.3)</td><td>55040</td></tr>
<tr><td colspan="3">NOTE: According to Ingenix's Encoder Pro Expert software, directional modifiers (e.g., -LT and -RT) are not added to the CPT code.</td></tr>
<tr><td>5.</td><td>198.82 (C79.82)</td><td>54520-50</td></tr>
<tr><td colspan="3">NOTE: The patient has metastatic carcinoma from the prostate gland to the testicles. There is no documentation that the patient had previous prostatectomy or is undergoing chemotherapy or radiation treatment for the primary site. If this information was provided, ICD code 185 would be assigned to classify the primary prostate cancer (still under treatment or not removed). If documentation was present that the patient had previously undergone a prostatectomy and was no longer receiving treatment for prostate cancer, ICD code V10.46 could be assigned to reflect the patient's history of malignant neoplasm.</td></tr>
<tr><td>6.</td><td>618.6 (N81.5)</td><td>57268</td></tr>
<tr><td>7.</td><td>218.9 (D25.9)</td><td>58150, 44950-51-52</td></tr>
<tr><td colspan="3">NOTE: This operative report documents that the patient's appendix was also removed. There is no documentation that the appendix was diseased; therefore, it is coded as an incidental appendectomy. Modifiers -51 (additional procedure) and -52 (reduced services) are added to the appendectomy code.</td></tr>
<tr><td>8.</td><td>626.6, 614.2, V13.29 (N92.1, N70.01, Z87.59)</td><td>58120, 58661-50-51</td></tr>
<tr><td colspan="3">NOTE: CPT code 58120 is reported for dilation and curettage of the endometrium of this patient. CPT code 58661 is reported for removal of the patient's fallopian tubes, which was done bilaterally. Modifiers -50 (bilateral procedure) and -51 (additional procedure) are added to the laparoscopic salpingectomy, bilateral, code.</td></tr>
<tr><td>9.</td><td>654.21, V27.0 (O34.21, Z37.0)</td><td>59514</td></tr>
<tr><td colspan="3">NOTE:
• An outcome of delivery code is assigned for the single liveborn infant.
• If this physician had provided routine antepartum and postpartum care, CPT code 59510 would have been assigned instead of 59514.
• Treatment of omentum adhesions is not separately coded unless lysis of adhesions takes significant time and effort and is reflected in the operative note as being extensive.</td></tr>
<tr><td>10.</td><td>642.41, V27.0 (O14.03, Z37.0)</td><td>59514</td></tr>
<tr><td colspan="3">NOTE: If this physician had provided routine antepartum and postpartum care, CPT code 59510 would have been assigned instead of 59514.</td></tr>
<tr><td>11.</td><td>650, V27.0 (O80, Z37.0)</td><td>59409</td></tr>
<tr><td colspan="3">NOTE:
• The bradycardia condition was not treated and is not assigned an ICD diagnosis code.
• If this physician had provided routine antepartum and postpartum care, CPT code 59400 would have been assigned instead of 59409.
• The episiotomy, including repair, and artificial rupture of membranes are included in code 59409. Do not assign separate CPT codes for these procedures.</td></tr>
<tr><td>12.</td><td>226 (D34)</td><td>60220-RT</td></tr>
<tr><td>13.</td><td>351.8 (G51.8)</td><td>64732</td></tr>
<tr><td>14.</td><td>355.6 (G57.62)</td><td>64776-LT</td></tr>
<tr><td>15.</td><td>998.89, 349.81 (G97.82, G96.0)</td><td>62100, 69990</td></tr>
<tr><td colspan="3">NOTE:
• This report documents a complication of surgical care. To assign the ICD-9-CM diagnosis code, locate index main term Complication.
• This report documents a postoperative complication because the patient's previous surgery at a different facility was unsuccessful in resolving his rhinorrhea of cerebrospinal fluid. Thus, the patient is undergoing repeat surgery.
• To locate the ICD-9-CM code, in the index, go to main term Complication, subterm surgical procedure, and second qualifier specified complication NEC.
• To locate the ICD-10-CM code, in the index, go to main term Complication, subterm nervous system, and second qualifier postprocedural. (In ICD-10-CM, the code is classified in the Nervous System chapter.)
• Assign CPT code 69990 to indicate use of the operating microscope during surgery. The operating microscope code is an add-on code; therefore, modifier -51 (additional procedure) is not added to the code.</td></tr>
</table>

REVIEW

Multiple Choice

1. b
2. c
3. b

Note:

The medical term for the condition ingrown eyelashes is trichiasis.

4. c
5. a
6. b
7. b
8. d
9. a
10. d
11. c
12. d
13. c

Note:

The operating microscope code is an add-on code; therefore, modifier -51 (additional procedure) is not added to the code.

14. a
15. b
16. a
17. c

Note:

The lesion was removed using cryosurgery; therefore, code 54056 is assigned. If the lesion had been excised, code 11421 could have been assigned.

18. c
19. b
20. c

Note:

This procedure was performed on an infant; however, the note states that modifier -63 is not assigned to codes 63704 and 63706.

Chapter 16
CPT Radiology

ASSIGNMENT 16.1 – CODING PRACTICE

	ICD Codes	CPT Codes
1.	789.01 (R10.11)	76700
2.	724.2 (M54.5)	72040, 72110
NOTE: No fracture was found on x-ray; therefore, assign an ICD code to the symptom only.		
3.	786.50 (R07.81)	71100-RT
4.	719.41, V54.89 (M25.512, Z47.81)	73100-LT, 73030-LT
5.	786.05 (R06.02)	71020
6.	526.9 (M27.8)	70100
7.	794.8 (R94.5)	78216
8.	722.10 (M51.26)	72131
9.	719.42 (M25.522)	73070-LT
10.	812.01 (S42.215A)	73030-LT
11.	813.44 (S52.325A)	73110-LT
12.	786.50 (R07.9)	71010
13.	719.45 (M25.551)	72170
14.	787.20 (R13.10)	74230
15.	789.07 (R10.84)	74022
NOTE: Do not code the single view chest x-ray separately because it is included in CPT code 74022.		
16.	784.2 (R22.0)	70487
NOTE: • A mass was found on radiological exam. To assign the ICD-9-CM diagnosis code, locate main term *Mass* and subterm *nose and sinus* in the index. In the ICD-10-CM index, locate main term *Mass* and subterm *head*. • This case documents the use of a contrast agent, which means that CPT code 70487 is assigned.		
17.	786.05, 786.50 (R06.02, R07.9)	71022
18.	620.2, 620.5 (N83.20, N83.52)	76856
NOTE: There is no documentation that this pelvic ultrasound was an obstetrical ultrasound. Therefore, refer to the nonobstetrical ultrasound code range (CPT codes 76830–76857). Documentation also supports the assignment of a complete code (instead of a limited or follow-up code).		
19.	185 (C61)	77327
20.	193 (C73)	79403

ASSIGNMENT 16.2 – CODING RADIOLOGY REPORTS

	ICD Codes	CPT Codes
1.	722.4, 807.2 (M50.30, S22.20xA)	72040, 71020, 71120
2.	434.91, 784.3 (I63.50, R47.01)	70470
3.	786.50 (R07.9)	71260
4.	794.4 (R94.4)	74400
NOTE: To assign the CPT procedure code, locate main term *Urography* and subterm *intravenous* in the CPT index.		
5.	747.81 (Q28.2)	77432, 70450
6.	789.06 (R10.13)	74246
7.	786.50, 724.5, 473.0, 473.1, 789.2 (R07.9, M54.9, J32.0, J32.1, R16.1)	71015, 70210, 74400
8.	786.50 (R07.9)	78453
9.	789.1 (R16.0)	76700
10.	438.11 (I69.920)	70460
11.	493.90 (J45.909)	71030
12.	816.01 (S62.625A)	73120-LT
NOTE: According to Ingenix's Encoder Pro Expert, modifier -LT (or -RT) is added to code 73120. HCPCS level II modifier(s) specifying digits of the hand are not added to the code.		
13.	782.0, 723.1 (R20.0, M54.2)	72240
14.	807.02, 733.00, 786.50, 719.45 (S22.42xA, M81.8, R07.9, M25.552)	72170, 73500-LT, 71010, 71100-LT
15.	240.9 (E04.9)	70360
16.	794.4 (R94.4)	74420
17.	553.3, 532.90, 562.00 (K44.9, K26.9, K57.10)	74245
18.	346.90 (G43.909)	70450
19.	241.1 (E04.2)	78006
20.	733.00 (M81.8)	73562-LT

REVIEW

Multiple Choice

1. c
2. c
3. b
4. d
5. a
6. b
7. b
8. d
9. b
10. c
11. d
12. b
13. d
14. c

Note:

According to CPT, ribbons are considered temporary interstitial placement during clinical brachytherapy.

15. b
16. b
17. a
18. a

Note:

The abbreviation r/o means "rule out."

19. b

Note:

Because the physician provided an interpretation and report only, modifier -26 is added to the code.

20. c

Chapter 17
CPT Pathology and Laboratory

ASSIGNMENT 17.1 – CODING PRACTICE

	ICD Codes	CPT Codes
1.	783.21 (R63.4)	80076, 85027
NOTE: • The albumin, bilirubin total and direct, phosphatase, protein, ALT, and AST tests constitute a panel code (CPT code 80076); however, this panel does not include a CBC. Therefore, code 80076 is also assigned.		
2.	V70.8 (Z00.5)	86022
NOTE: To assign the diagnosis code, locate main term *Examination* and subterm *donor (potential)* in the ICD index.		
3.	780.79 (R53.83)	88371
4.	659.53 (009.511)	88271
NOTE: • Gravida indicates the number of times this patient has been pregnant including the current pregnancy, and para indicates how many times the patient has delivered one or more fetuses. In this case, because the patient is gravida 1, para 0, she is still pregnant. • Because the patient is age 46, she is considered an elderly primigravida (first pregnancy).		
5.	474.10 (J35.3)	88304
NOTE: • To assign the ICD diagnosis code, the coder is directed by the index to a combination code that reflects enlarged tonsils and adenoids. • Tonsils and adenoids are located in level III of the surgical pathology codes in the Pathology and Laboratory section of CPT.		
6.	782.1, 285.9 (R21, D64.9)	86039
7.	787.91 (R19.7)	87045
8.	786.05, 780.79 (R06.02, R53.83)	88237
9.	599.70 (R31.9)	88305
NOTE: Kidneys are located under level IV of the surgical pathology codes in the Pathology and Laboratory section of CPT.		
10.	V70.5 (Z02.1)	80100
11.	V72.83 (Z01.818)	80061, 82947
NOTE: CPT classifies total cholesterol, HDL, and triglycerides as a lipid panel.		
12.	788.41 (R35.0)	87086
13.	225.0 (D33.0)	88037
14.	197.7 (C78.7)	88307
NOTE: • To assign the ICD code, go to the Neoplasm Table in the index and locate the Malignant secondary columns. • The liver is located under level V of the surgical pathology codes in the Pathology and Laboratory section of CPT.		
15.	V73.3 (Z11.59)	86762
NOTE: To assign the ICD code, locate main term *Screening* and subterm *rubella* in the index.		

	ICD Codes	CPT Codes
16.	V81.5 (Z13.89)	82565
NOTE: • To assign the ICD code, locate main term *Screening* and subterm *renal disease* in the index. • The renal insufficiency diagnosis was not confirmed as a disease, and it is incorrect to assign an ICD diagnosis code.		
17.	V72.31 (Z01.419)	88142
18.	783.43 (R62.52)	86277
19.	606.9 (N46.9)	89321
20.	704.00 (L64.9)	87101

ASSIGNMENT 17.2 – CODING PATHOLOGY AND LABORATORY REPORTS

	ICD Codes	CPT Codes
1.	786.50 (R07.9)	82550, 83625
NOTE: Cardiac isoenzymes test CPK and LDH levels in blood serum and help determine the location of tissue damage, such as heart tissue. CPK is the abbreviation for creatine phosphokinase, and LDH is the abbreviation for lactate (or lactic) dehydrogenase.		
2.	780.79 (R53.83)	85027
NOTE: Because this CBC laboratory test did not include a differential WBC count, CPT code 85027 is assigned (instead of 85025).		
3.	V08 (Z21)	87075
4.	788.1 (R30.0)	81005
5.	518.82 (J80)	82805
6.	782.1 (R21)	86592
7.	532.50 (K26.5)	87070
8.	788.1, 599.70 (R30.0, R31.9)	87086
9.	496 (J44.9)	82803
10.	595.9 (N30.90)	88305
NOTE: To assign the CPT procedure code, locate main term *Urinary bladder* and subterm *biopsy* in the alphabetic index.		
11.	685.0 (L05.01, L05.02)	88304
12.	V25.2 (Z30.2)	88302
NOTE: CPT code 88302 reflects the fallopian tube submitted as a part of sterilization procedure.		
13.	366.9 (H26.9)	88300
14.	780.8 (N95.1, R61)	80053, 82465, 84550
NOTE: The CPT panel code does not include the uric acid and cholesterol laboratory tests, which are assigned separate codes.		
15.	719.50 (M25.60)	85025
NOTE: Assign CPT code 85025 to a complete blood count (CBC) with differential (not code 85027).		
16.	V72.83 (Z01.818)	81007
17.	226 (D34)	88307
18.	634.91 (O03.4)	88305
19.	709.2, V54.01 (L90.5, Z47.2)	88304, 88300
NOTE: CPT code 88304 is assigned for gross and microscopic examination of scar from left lower leg and debridement tissue. CPT code 88300 is assigned for gross examination of the metal rod that was removed.		
20.	594.1 (N21.0)	88300

REVIEW

Multiple Choice

1. a

> **Note:**
>
> *Hep is the abbreviation for hepatitis.*

2. c
3. b
4. a
5. c
6. b
7. c
8. c
9. d

> **Note:**
>
> *CPT code 80048 is assigned for a basic metabolic blood panel only when all laboratory tests associated with the panel are performed. In this case, because just three of the tests were performed, a separate CPT code is assigned for each.*

10. b
11. c
12. c
13. d
14. c

> **Note:**
>
> *Brachytherapy is the application of radioactive isotopes (e.g., Cobalt isotope) for internal radiation, and radioactive material is encapsulated for intracavitary implantation (e.g., ribbons). Code 77777 is reported for the for intermediate interstitial application of 5 to 10 ribbons.*

15. d

> **Note:**
>
> *Chickenpox is also known as varicella zoster.*

16. b
17. b

> **Note:**
>
> *Sed is the abbreviation for sedimentation.*

18. a
19. a
20. d

Chapter 18
CPT Medicine

ASSIGNMENT 18.1 – CODING PRACTICE

	ICD Codes	CPT Codes
1.	492.8 (J43.9)	94621
2.	368.8, 250.00 (H53.8, E11.9)	92235
3.	V56.0, 585.9 (N18.9, Z99.2)	90937
4.	V58.11, 174.9 (Z51.11, C50.911)	96413, 96415

NOTE: CPT code 96415 is an add-on code that reflects the additional hours of chemotherapy treatment via infusion. Modifier -51 is not added to add-on codes.

	ICD Codes	CPT Codes
5.	311 (F32.9)	90847
6.	388.30 (H93.13)	92625
7.	427.9 (I49.9)	92960
8.	367.4 (H52.4)	92342
9.	892.0, E920.5, E849.7 (S91.341A, W46.0, Y92.239)	90471, 90703

NOTE:

- For coding purposes, a retained foreign object or foreign body is classified as a complicated open wound. However, in this case, the patient removed the object (needle) and brought it with him to the clinic; so, this is not a *complicated* open wound.
- CPT code 90471 is assigned for the administration of the injection via intramuscular (IM) route, and code 90703 is assigned for the vaccine (that is located in the syringe).
- Because this patient is over age 7, code 90702 is not assigned.
- Because there is no documentation that this vaccine was preservative-free, code 90714 is not assigned.

	ICD Codes	CPT Codes
10.	V71.89 (Z03.89)	99173

NOTE: This child was lavaged due to suspected ingestion of a poison. However, documentation does not confirm that this case is a poisoning. Therefore, assign an ICD-9-CM diagnosis code for observation of specified suspected condition.

ASSIGNMENT 18.2 – CODING MEDICINE REPORTS

	ICD Codes	CPT Codes
1.	V81.2 (Z13.6)	93880
2.	780.39 (R56.9)	95816
3.	784.3 (R47.01)	92506
4.	427.0, 786.59, 401.9 (I47.1, R07.89, I10)	93015

NOTE:

- METs is the abbreviation for metabolic equivalents.
- This patient has a documented history of chest discomfort and medical history of hypertension. During the exam, the patient experienced weakness and dizziness; therefore, codes for those symptoms are also assigned. Do not assign a code to *rule out coronary artery disease* because it is a qualified diagnosis, which is not reported for an outpatient encounter.

	ICD Codes	CPT Codes
5.	786.05 (R06.02)	94660

NOTE: CPAP is the abbreviation for continuous positive airway pressure.

	ICD Codes	CPT Codes
6.	724.5, 724.8, 782.0 (M54.9, M62.830, R20.8)	97001
NOTE: • RLE is the abbreviation for right lower extremity, and RLQ is the abbreviation for right lower quadrant. • For ICD-9-CM coding, because the patient complains of back pain and muscle spasms, codes are assigned for each. During the evaluation, the patient reported numbness, which is also coded.		
7.	704.00 (L65.9)	96902
8.	250.01 (E10.9)	96522
9.	747.22 (Q25.3)	93315
NOTE: • TEE is the abbreviation for transesophageal echocardiography, and NICU is the abbreviation for neonatal intensive care unit. • This test was performed on a 5-day-old infant, which means that the diagnosis code for congenital aortic stenosis is assigned.		
10.	787.01 (R11.2)	91132

REVIEW

Multiple Choice

1. c

Note:

IM is the abbreviation for intramuscular.

2. b
3. b
4. b
5. b

Note:

Although five manipulations were performed, just three regions were manipulated.

6. c
7. d
8. d
9. b

Note:

SAECG is the abbreviation for signal-averaged electrocardiography. Modifier –26 is added to CPT code 93278 to report the physician interpretation and reporting.

10. a
11. c
12. a
13. d
14. a
15. b

Note:

HepA is the abbreviation for hepatitis A, and HepB is the abbreviation for hepatitis B.

16. d
17. a
18. d
19. b
20. b

Chapter 19
Insurance and Reimbursement

ASSIGNMENT 19.1 – CHARGEMASTER REVIEW PROCESS

1. No, the street address is missing.
2. No, the chargemaster is dated April 5, YYYY.
3. Yes, the service descriptions listed in Column 2 describe services provided by the radiology department.
4. No.
   - Code 71012 should be changed to 71020.
   - Code 71034 is for four views.
   - Code 74214 should be changed to 74241.
   - Code 74274 is not a valid code.
   - Code 74250 does not have “separate procedure” in its CPT description.
5. Yes.

ASSIGNMENT 19.2 – INTERPRETING A REMITTANCE ADVICE

1. The check number is 9568547, and the amount is $905.
2. 0405YY
3. $20
4. When the student looks up the CPT code for Joseph Lynch’s visit, he or she will see that it is a code for preventive services. The student could determine that the payer requires no coinsurance payment for preventive services.
5. FISC1234567-01
6. Each patient had a place of service (POS) code of 11.
7. 99212
8. $905
9. $60
10. $750

ASSIGNMENT 19.3 – INTERPRETING A MEDICARE FEE-FOR-SERVICE PAYMENT ERROR REPORT

1. Yes, FY 2004 is down by 1.3 percent in the Insufficient Documentation category. The area of nonresponse increased from FY 2003 at 18.5 percent to FY 2004 at 29.7 percent, which is an increase of 11.2 percent.
2. c
3. Yes, this category has seen improvement. In FY 2002, the percentage was 14.3; and in FY 2004, the percentage was 7.7, which is a decrease of 6.6 percent.

4. When comparing FY 2004 to FY 2003, the medically unnecessary type of error improved, decreasing by 4.5 percent (from 21.7 percent to 17.2 percent).
5. There is a decrease of 4.4 percent (12.1% to 7.7%).

ASSIGNMENT 19.4 – AMBULATORY PAYMENT CLASSIFICATIONS

Note:

APC grouper software with ICD-10-CM codes was not available upon publication of this workbook, which means ICD-10-CM codes are not included in the answer key for these cases.

1. a.

First-Listed diagnosis code:	553.1 (K42.9)
Additional diagnosis code:	
Additional diagnosis code:	
Procedure code:	49585

   b.
   i. 00154
   ii. $1690.75

2. a.

First-Listed diagnosis code:	599.70 (R31.9)
Additional diagnosis code:	
Additional diagnosis code:	
Procedure code:	52000

   b.
   i. 00160
   ii. $407.54

3. a.

First-Listed diagnosis code:	780.79 (R53.83)
Additional diagnosis code:	794.5 (R94.6)
Additional diagnosis code:	
Procedure code:	10021

   b.
   i. 00002
   ii. $83.60

4. a.

First-Listed diagnosis code:	366.14 (H25.012)
Additional diagnosis code:	
Additional diagnosis code:	
Procedure code:	66984-LT

   b.
   i. 00246
   ii. $1405.02
   ii. $880.88

5. a.

First-Listed diagnosis code:	574.00 (K80.00)
Additional diagnosis code:	574.10 (K80.10)
Additional diagnosis code:	
Procedure code:	47563

b.

i. 00131 and 00263. The APC of 00263 is for the intraoperative choliagogram.
ii. $2686.08
ii. $1733.39

ASSIGNMENT 19.5 – INTERPRETING DIAGNOSIS-RELATED GROUPS DECISION TREES

Medical Partitioning DRG Decision Tree (Figure 19-4 in the Workbook)

1. DRG 14
2. DRG 19
3. DRG 18
4. DRG 11
5. DRG 17

Surgical Partitioning DRG Decision Tree (Figure 19-5 in the Workbook)

6. DRG 6
7. DRG 531
8. DRG 3
9. DRG 533
10. DRG 529

ASSIGNMENT 19.6 – ASSIGNING DIAGNOSIS-RELATED GROUPS

Note:

Estimated Medicare reimbursement amounts included in each answer are based on the Medicare DRG calculator results at the IRP.com Web site. You may notice different reimbursement amounts if other DRG groupers (e.g., 3M or QuadraMed) are used and/or as the IRP.com Web site is updated to reflect revised case mix weights and other data.

Note:

DRG grouper software with ICD-10-CM/PCS codes was not available upon publication of this workbook, which means ICD-10-CM/PCS codes are not included in the answer key for these cases.

1a.

Principal diagnosis code:	428.0
Comorbidity code:	482.0
Comorbidity code:	404.91
Comorbidity code:	250.00
Comorbidity code:	272.4

Comorbidities of type 2 diabetes mellitus and hyperlipidemia were treated during this inpatient admission.

1b.

- 05
- 127 HEART FAILURE & SHOCK
- Estimated Medicare Reimbursement = $4,975.90

1c.

- 04
- 079 RESPIRATORY INFECTIONS & INFLAMMATIONS AGE >17 W CC
- Estimated Medicare Reimbursement = $7,810.41
- Either condition could be sequenced as the principal diagnosis based on the information presented in the case and ICD-9-CM coding guidelines.
- Yes. Changing the principal diagnosis from "congestive heart failure" to "pneumonia due to *Klebsiella pneumoniae*" increases the estimated DRG reimbursement amount.

2a.

Principal diagnosis code:	480.9
Comorbidity code:	438.82
Comorbidity code:	250.00
Comorbidity code:	401.9
Principal procedure code:	43.11

The patient's comorbidities of type 2 diabetes mellitus and hypertension were treated as an inpatient.

2b.

- 04
- 090 SIMPLE PNEUMONIA & PLEURISY AGE >17 W/O CC
- Estimated Medicare Reimbursement = $3,100.86

2c.

- 01
- 012 DEGENERATIVE NERVOUS SYSTEM DISORDERS
- Estimated Medicare Reimbursement = $4,589.99
- The late effect of cerebrovascular accident (CVA) with dysphagia should not be sequenced as the principal diagnosis because it was not treated during the inpatient admissions (e.g., speech therapy); viral pneumonia is the principal diagnosis.
- No. Changing the principal diagnosis to late effect of cerebrovascular accident (CVA) with dysphagia maximizes the DRG reimbursement rate, which is fraud. It is also an example of DRG creep.

3a.

Principal diagnosis code:	784.7
Comorbidity code:	285.1
Comorbidity code:	250.00
Comorbidity code:	401.9
Comorbidity code:	272.4
Principal procedure code:	21.03
Additional procedure code:	99.04

This patient's comorbidities of type 2 diabetes mellitus and hypertension were treated during this admission. All transfusions are coded on inpatient hospital stays due to training required to perform this procedure.

Under UHDDS guidelines, all significant procedures that are surgical in nature carry an anesthetic risk; or if the procedures require specialized training to perform, they should be reported.

3b.

- 03
- 066EPISTAXIS
- Estimated Medicare Reimbursement = $2,944.61

3c.

- 16
- 395 RED BLOOD CELL DISORDERS AGE >17
- Estimated Medicare Reimbursement = $4,219.72
- The sequencing of diagnoses in 3c results in a higher estimated Medicare reimbursement.
- No. Changing the principal diagnosis to "acute posthemorrhagic anemia" maximizes the DRG reimbursement rate, which is fraud. It is also an example of DRG creep.

4a.

Principal diagnosis code:	996.73
Complication code:	403.91
Comorbidity code:	997.1
Comorbidity code:	E878.8
Principal procedure code:	39.50
Additional procedure code:	88.60

The sinus tachycardia developed postoperatively and is coded.

4b.

- 05
- 554 OTHER VASCULAR PROCEDURES W CC WITHOUT MAJOR CV DIAGNOSIS
- Estimated Medicare Reimbursement = $9,966.72

4c.

- 11
- 315 OTHER KIDNEY & URINARY TRACT PROCEDURES
- Estimated Medicare Reimbursement = $10,015.78
- The sequencing of diagnoses in 3c results in a higher estimated Medicare reimbursement.
- No. Changing the principal diagnosis to "hypertensive renal disease" maximizes the DRG reimbursement rate, which is fraud. It is also an example of DRG creep.

5a.

Principal diagnosis code:	424.1
Comorbidity code:	V45.81
Comorbidity code:	274.9
Comorbidity code:	V10.05
Principal procedure code:	35.22
Additional procedure code:	37.23

Assigning V codes for this case is valid. The patient's history of bypass surgery was a clinical reason for the cardiac catheterization procedure that was performed during this admission. The history of colon neoplasm code is reported for statistical purposes.

5b.

- 05
- 104 CARDIAC VALVE & OTHER MAJOR CARDIOTHORACIC PROC W CARDIAC CATH
- Estimated Medicare Reimbursement = $39,780.59

5c.

- 05
- 105 CARDIAC VALVE & OTHER MAJOR CARDIOTHORACIC PROC W/O CARDIAC CATH
- Estimated Medicare Reimbursement = $29,107.95
- The sequencing of diagnoses in 3c results in a higher estimated Medicare reimbursement.
- If the cardiac catheterization code is not reported, a loss of $10,672.64 results.

ASSIGNMENT 19.7 – RESOURCE UTILIZATION GROUPS

1. b

Note:

Divide each RUG-53 category nonlabor rate into the total rate to calculate the approximately 24 percent. For example, RUX = 136/564.83 × 100 = 24%.

2. c

Note:

Divide each RUG-53 category labor rate into the total rate to calculate the approximately 76 percent. For example, RUX = 428.83/564.83 × 100 = 76%.

3. c

Note:

The total rate for RUC is $479.53, and the total rate for RUX is $564.83. The percentage increase from RUC to RUX is calculated by subtracting $479.53 from $564.83, dividing that calculated figure into $564.83, and multiplying by 100 to calculate the percentage. Thus,

- 479.53 − 564.83 = 85.30
- 85.30/564.83 = 0.1510
- 0.1510 × 100 = 15%

4. Upon entry of all data, the student's spreadsheet should look similar to the following:

RUG-53 Category	Total Rate	Labor Portion	Nonlabor Portion
Rehabilitation Ultra High plus Extensive Services High (RUX)	564.83	428.83	136
Rehabilitation Ultra High plus Extensive Services Low (RUL)	496.04	376.6	119.44
Rehabilitation Very High plus Extensive Services High (RVX)	428.24	325.13	103.11
Rehabilitation Very High plus Extensive Services Low (RVL)	399.34	303.19	96.15
Rehabilitation High plus Extensive Services High (RHX)	363.02	275.61	87.41
Rehabilitation High plus Extensive Services Low (RHL)	356.14	270.39	85.75
Rehabilitation Medium (RMC)	308.25	234.03	74.22
Rehabilitation Medium (RMB)	299.99	227.76	72.23
Rehabilitation Medium (RMA)	293.11	222.53	70.58
Rehabilitation Low (RLB)	271.64	206.23	65.41
Rehabilitation Low (RLA)	231.74	175.94	55.8

5. Upon completion of the chart wizard, the student's pie chart should look similar to the following:

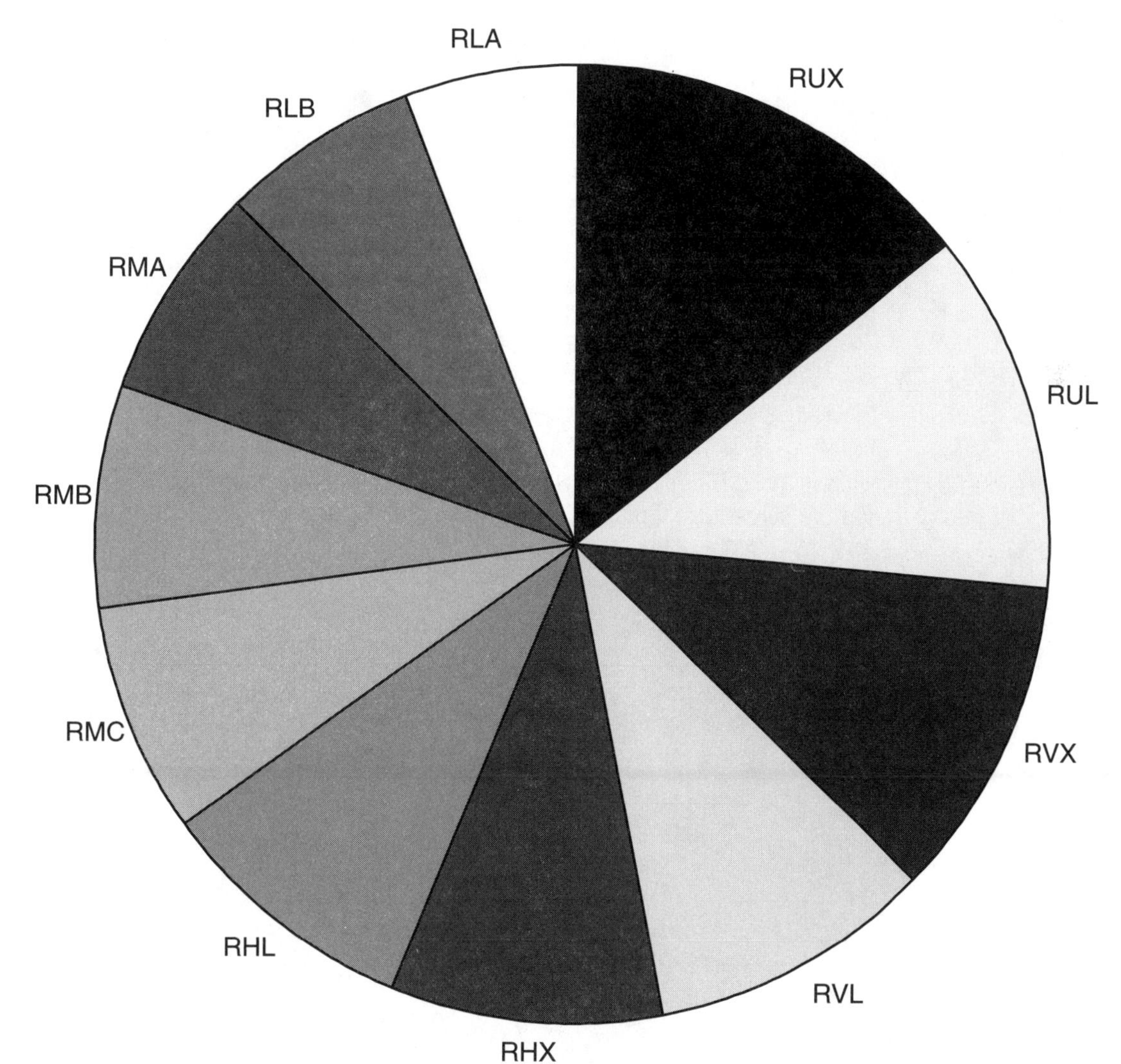

REVIEW

Multiple Choice

1. a
2. d
3. b
4. a
5. a
6. d
7. a
8. b
9. a
10. d
11. d
12. c
13. c
14. b
15. d
16. b
17. a
18. c
19. c
20. c

SECTION V

Answer Keys to Workbook Coding Cases

CODING ANSWER KEYS

- Ambulatory Surgery Unit Coding Cases Answer Key (for Workbook Appendix A)
- Emergency Department Coding Cases Answer Key (for Workbook Appendix B)
- Physician Office Coding Cases Answer Key (for Workbook Appendix C)
- Inpatient Coding Cases Answer Key (for Workbook Appendix D)

Note:

- Coding answers are from 2011 ICD-9-CM, CPT, and HCPCS level II.
- Coding answers from 2010 ICD-10-CM and ICD-10-PCS, and 2011 CPT and HCPCS level II are located at the textbook's online companion (OLC).
  - Go to http://www.delmarlearning.com/companions, enter Green in the Companion Search box, and click Enter.
  - Scroll down to locate the *3-2-1 Code It! 3e* link, and click on it.
  - Click on *Instructor Resources*, and enter the username and password (located in the Preface of the Instructor's Manual).
  - Locate the *3-2-1_3e_OLC_Instructor_Resources_ICD-10_Answer_Keys_to_Workbook_Appendices_A-D.pdf* file, and click on it.

Workbook Appendix A: Ambulatory Surgery Unit Coding Cases

ASUCASES ANSWER KEY

ASUCase001	Admission Diagnosis	First-Listed Diagnosis	Secondary Diagnosis	Secondary Diagnosis	Secondary Diagnosis
	354.0	354.0	727.05		
	First-Listed Procedure	Secondary Procedure	Secondary Procedure	Secondary Procedure	Secondary Procedure
	64721-RT	26145-51-F8	26145-F9	25115-51	

The reference to "4½ loupe magnification" is not microscopic surgery, which means that CPT code 64727 is not assigned in addition to code 64721-RT.

Add modifier -51 to the first reporting of secondary procedure code 26145, but not to subsequent reporting (due to the word "each" in the code description). A third-party payer knows to pay 26145 at a certain rate; and if the code (26145) is reported multiple times, the payer discounts subsequent reportings. Don't forget to add HCPCS alphanumeric modifiers (e.g., RT and F8) where appropriate. Report 26145-51-F8 for the right ring finger surgery and 26145-F9 for the right little finger surgery. (Reference to the ring and little fingers can be found in the operative report.)

Code 25115 is assigned to report tenosynovectomy of wrist, which is documented in the narrative of the operative report. Add modifier -51 to this code.

NOTE: Code 88304 would be assigned by the pathologist who examines tissue removed during surgery. Code 01810 would be assigned by the anesthesiologist.

ASUCase002	Admission Diagnosis	First-Listed Diagnosis	Secondary Diagnosis	Secondary Diagnosis	Secondary Diagnosis	Secondary Procedure
	622.11	622.11	623.8			
	First-Listed Procedure	Secondary Procedure	Secondary Procedure	Secondary Procedure	Secondary Procedure	Secondary Procedure
	57513	57010-51	80048	85027	85610	

CPT coding rules require reporting of chemistry panel code 80048 (Basic Metabolic, which covers calcium, CO2, chloride, creatinine, glucose, potassium, sodium, and BUN). CPT code 85027 is reported for a complete blood count (CBC), which includes WBC, RBC, Hgb, Hct, and platelets. Code 85610 is reported for the prothrombin time (PT).

ASUCase003	Admission Diagnosis	First-Listed Diagnosis	Secondary Diagnosis	Secondary Diagnosis	Secondary Diagnosis	Secondary Procedure
	724.4	724.4	729.1			
	First-Listed Procedure	Secondary Procedure	Secondary Procedure	Secondary Procedure	Secondary Procedure	Secondary Procedure
	64483					

To locate code 724.4, go to main term *Radiculopathy* in the ICD-9-CM Index to Diseases and follow the instruction to "see also Radiculitis." Then go to main term *Radiculitis* and subterm *lumbosacral* to locate code 724.4.

ASUCase004	Admission Diagnosis	First-Listed Diagnosis	Secondary Diagnosis			
	625.9	628.9	625.9			
	First-Listed Procedure	Secondary Procedure	Secondary Procedure	Secondary Procedure	Secondary Procedure	Secondary Procedure
	49320	80048	85027	85610		

Do not assign code 58350-51 for hydrotubation of uterus. Code 58350 is reported for chromotubation of oviduct (fallopian tube). Hydrotubation of the uterus is included as part of the diagnostic laparoscopy and not separately coded.

ASUCase005	Admission Diagnosis	First-Listed Diagnosis	Secondary Diagnosis	Secondary Diagnosis	Secondary Diagnosis	Secondary Procedure
	V25.2	V25.2	V58.69			
	First-Listed Procedure	Secondary Procedure	Secondary Procedure	Secondary Procedure	Secondary Procedure	Secondary Procedure
	58671	80048	85027	85610		

Code V58.69 is assigned for the documented long-term use of lithium.

ASUCase006	Admission Diagnosis	First-Listed Diagnosis	Secondary Diagnosis	Secondary Diagnosis	Secondary Diagnosis	Secondary Procedure
	654.53	654.53				
	First-Listed Procedure	Secondary Procedure	Secondary Procedure	Secondary Procedure	Secondary Procedure	Secondary Procedure
	59320	80048	85027	85610		

ICD code 654.53 is reported because this is an antepartum condition for a patient who is at 13 weeks' gestation. The patient previously had a 23-week loss of twins secondary to cervical incompetence; but that is in her past history; however, that is documented in her past history and is, thus, not coded.

ASUCase007	Admission Diagnosis	First-Listed Diagnosis				
	078.11	078.11				
	First-Listed Procedure	Secondary Procedure	Secondary Procedure	Secondary Procedure	Secondary Procedure	Secondary Procedure
	56620	80048	85027	85610		

CPT code 56620 (Vulvectomy, simple; partial) is reported for "vulvar excisional biopsy." Do not report a code from the CPT Integumentary section for that surgery.

ASUCase008	Admission Diagnosis	First-Listed Diagnosis	Secondary Diagnosis	Secondary Diagnosis	Secondary Diagnosis	Secondary Procedure
	620.2	620.2				
	First-Listed Procedure	Secondary Procedure	Secondary Procedure	Secondary Procedure	Secondary Procedure	Secondary Procedure
	58662	80048	85027	85610		

ASUCase009	Admission Diagnosis	First-Listed Diagnosis	Secondary Diagnosis	Secondary Diagnosis	Secondary Diagnosis	Secondary Procedure
	V54.01	V54.01				
	First-Listed Procedure	Secondary Procedure	Secondary Procedure	Secondary Procedure	Secondary Procedure	Secondary Procedure
	20680-RT	80048	85027	85610		

CPT code 88307 would be reported by the pathologist for gross and microscopic examination of specimen(s) removed during surgery.

ASUCase010	Admission Diagnosis	First-Listed Diagnosis	Secondary Diagnosis	Secondary Diagnosis	Secondary Diagnosis	Secondary Procedure
	727.03	727.03				
	First-Listed Procedure	Secondary Procedure	Secondary Procedure	Secondary Procedure	Secondary Procedure	Secondary Procedure
	26055-F2	80048	85027	85610		

Don't forget to add HCPCS modifier -F2 to indicate "middle finger."

Do not mistakenly assign code 26440-F2, which is reported for tenolysis of a trigger finger. This patient underwent incision of the tendon sheath to release the trigger finger. Per documentation in the operative report, the more invasive tenolysis procedure was not required.

Workbook Appendix B: Emergency Department Coding Cases

EDCASES ANSWER KEY

EDCase001	First-Listed Diagnosis	Secondary Diagnosis	Secondary Diagnosis	Secondary Diagnosis	Secondary Diagnosis	Secondary Diagnosis
	891.0	E920.8	E849.0			
	First-Listed Procedure	Secondary Procedure	Secondary Procedure	Secondary Procedure	Secondary Procedure	Secondary Procedure
	99281	90703	90471			

EDCase002	First-Listed Diagnosis	Secondary Diagnosis	Secondary Diagnosis	Secondary Diagnosis	Secondary Diagnosis	Secondary Diagnosis
	883.0	E920.8	E849.0			
	First-Listed Procedure	Secondary Procedure	Secondary Procedure	Secondary Procedure	Secondary Procedure	Secondary Procedure
	99281-25	12002-F6	90703	90471		

EDCase003	First-Listed Diagnosis	Secondary Diagnosis	Secondary Diagnosis	Secondary Diagnosis	Secondary Diagnosis	Secondary Diagnosis
	881.22	881.02	882.0	883.0	E920.8	E849.0
	First-Listed Procedure	Secondary Procedure	Secondary Procedure	Secondary Procedure	Secondary Procedure	Secondary Procedure
	99281-25	25260-RT	12001-59	90703	90471	

Coding guidelines indicate that tendon repair should be reported with a code associated with the appropriate system. Thus, code 25260-RT is reported for the tendon repair.

Code 12001 is also reported for the simple repair of the additional wound that required suturing. Modifier -RT is not added to code 12001. (Do *not* report CPT code 12032, which is reported for wounds affecting the deeper layers of the subcutaneous tissue and nonmuscle fascia.)

EDCase004	First-Listed Diagnosis	Secondary Diagnosis	Secondary Diagnosis	Secondary Diagnosis	Secondary Diagnosis	Secondary Diagnosis
	870.8	368.8	E914	E917.9	E849.0	
	First-Listed Procedure	Secondary Procedure	Secondary Procedure	Secondary Procedure	Secondary Procedure	Secondary Procedure
	99282	90703	90471			

EDCase005	First-Listed Diagnosis	Secondary Diagnosis	Secondary Diagnosis	Secondary Diagnosis	Secondary Diagnosis	Secondary Diagnosis
	810.02	922.1	807.03	E820.0	E849.4	
	First-Listed Procedure	Secondary Procedure	Secondary Procedure	Secondary Procedure	Secondary Procedure	Secondary Procedure
	99282	71100-RT	73000-RT	73030-RT	A4565	

Although the chest x-ray report documents "thickening of the pleura in this region suggesting associated hemorrhage," do not assign codes to these conditions because the emergency department (ED) physician did not document them on the face sheet. In the real world, a coder would generate a physician query to ask the ED physician if diagnoses should be added to the face sheet based on documentation in the x-ray report.

EDCase006	First-Listed Diagnosis	Secondary Diagnosis	Secondary Diagnosis	Secondary Diagnosis	Secondary Diagnosis	Secondary Diagnosis
	891.0	E880.9	E849.0			
	First-Listed Procedure	Secondary Procedure	Secondary Procedure	Secondary Procedure	Secondary Procedure	Secondary Procedure
	99281-25	12002	90471	90703	73562-RT	

According to Ingenix's www.EncoderPro.com software, directional modifier -RT is not added to CPT code 12002.

EDCase007	First-Listed Diagnosis	Secondary Diagnosis	Secondary Diagnosis	Secondary Diagnosis	Secondary Diagnosis	Secondary Diagnosis
	873.44	E885.9	E849.0			
	First-Listed Procedure	Secondary Procedure	Secondary Procedure	Secondary Procedure	Secondary Procedure	Secondary Procedure
	99281-25	12011				

EDCase008	First-Listed Diagnosis	Secondary Diagnosis	Secondary Diagnosis	Secondary Diagnosis	Secondary Diagnosis	Secondary Diagnosis
	873.0	924.8	919.8	E819.1	E849.5	
	First-Listed Procedure	Secondary Procedure	Secondary Procedure	Secondary Procedure	Secondary Procedure	Secondary Procedure
	99282-25	12002	70260	90703	90471	

There is no CPT or HCPCS level II code for the oral administration of Tylenol. That service is included in the CPT E/M code (99283).

EDCase009	First-Listed Diagnosis	Secondary Diagnosis	Secondary Diagnosis	Secondary Diagnosis	Secondary Diagnosis	Secondary Diagnosis
	883.0	881.00	E920.8	E917.3	E849.0	
	First-Listed Procedure	Secondary Procedure	Secondary Procedure	Secondary Procedure	Secondary Procedure	Secondary Procedure
	99282	12002				

When coding lacerations (12002), add like areas together that are treated using the same method and assign one CPT code. Do not assign separate codes for multiple lacerations of the same site.

The nurse's notes state that the patient's last tetanus shot was 6–7 years ago; there is no documentation that tetanus toxoid was administered during this encounter.

EDCase010	First-Listed Diagnosis	Secondary Diagnosis	Secondary Diagnosis	Secondary Diagnosis	Secondary Diagnosis	Secondary Diagnosis
	V58.43	E906.8				
	First-Listed Procedure	Secondary Procedure	Secondary Procedure	Secondary Procedure	Secondary Procedure	Secondary Procedure
	99281					

This case is a recheck of a previously treated injury, which means that a V code is assigned first-listed diagnosis.

Workbook Appendix C: Physician Office Coding Cases

POCASES ANSWER KEY

POCase001	First-Listed Diagnosis	Secondary Diagnosis	Secondary Diagnosis	Secondary Diagnosis	Secondary Diagnosis	Secondary Diagnosis
	296.40					
	First-Listed Procedure	Secondary Procedure	Secondary Procedure	Secondary Procedure	Secondary Procedure	Secondary Procedure
	99212	90862				

Report 296.40 because documentation indicates that this patient suffers from the manic type of bipolar disorder. The description in ICD for 296.4x indicates "most recent episode," and documentation in the patient's record is of manic type.

This provider is a psychiatrist, which is a medical doctor who reports appropriate level E/M codes for office visits. (If psychotherapy had been provided during the encounter in addition to or instead of an E/M service, the physician would also report an appropriate medicine code, such as code 90805.)

The statement in the notes "Patient seen today for regular appointment" indicates that this is an established patient. The levels of history and exam are problem focused, and medical decision making is straightforward.

POCase002	First-Listed Diagnosis	Secondary Diagnosis	Secondary Diagnosis	Secondary Diagnosis	Secondary Diagnosis	Secondary Diagnosis
	715.90	719.7				
	First-Listed Procedure	Secondary Procedure	Secondary Procedure	Secondary Procedure	Secondary Procedure	Secondary Procedure
	99212					

The degenerative joint disease described is not specified as "generalized or localized." Also, the abnormality in walking is related to the joint disease, not a gait disorder.

The statement in the notes "Patient seen for regular appointment today" indicates that this is an established patient. The levels of history and exam are problem focused, and medical decision making is straightforward. Because *degenerative joint disease* was not specified as localized or generalized, the unspecified (715.9) code is appropriate.

POCase003	First-Listed Diagnosis	Secondary Diagnosis	Secondary Diagnosis	Secondary Diagnosis	Secondary Diagnosis	Secondary Diagnosis
	250.00	272.4				
	First-Listed Procedure	Secondary Procedure	Secondary Procedure	Secondary Procedure	Secondary Procedure	Secondary Procedure
	99212					

The statement in the notes "This is a 78-year-old white male veteran who is seen for his regular appointment" indicates that this is an established patient. The levels of history and exam are problem focused, and medical decision making is straightforward. Since the patient was seen for a regular appointment, and received refills for both medications, both the diabetes mellitus and hyperlipidemia are assigned codes.

POCase004	First-Listed Diagnosis	Secondary Diagnosis	Secondary Diagnosis	Secondary Diagnosis	Secondary Diagnosis	Secondary Diagnosis
	312.00	555.9				
	First-Listed Procedure	Secondary Procedure	Secondary Procedure	Secondary Procedure	Secondary Procedure	Secondary Procedure
	99212					

Do not assign ICD code E932.0 (Adrenal cortical steroids causing adverse effect in therapeutic use) because "Possible reaction to Prednisone" is a qualified diagnosis that is not reported for outpatient care. However, it is important to code the result of the "possible" reaction by coding the Anger reaction and Crohn's Disease (as the reason for taking the Prednisone).

POCase005	First-Listed Diagnosis	Secondary Diagnosis	Secondary Diagnosis	Secondary Diagnosis	Secondary Diagnosis	Secondary Diagnosis
	627.0					
	First-Listed Procedure	Secondary Procedure	Secondary Procedure	Secondary Procedure	Secondary Procedure	Secondary Procedure
	99212					

Do not assign ICD code 256.31 (Premature, or early, menopause) because the term *probable* (in the "notes") indicates that this is a qualified diagnosis, which is not assigned a code for outpatient care. However, there are two definitive diagnoses present (627.0 and 780.79).

POCase006	First-Listed Diagnosis	Secondary Diagnosis	Secondary Diagnosis	Secondary Diagnosis	Secondary Diagnosis	Secondary Diagnosis
	414.00		437.9	530.81	272.4	
	First-Listed Procedure	Secondary Procedure	Secondary Procedure	Secondary Procedure	Secondary Procedure	Secondary Procedure
	99213					

The statement "Mr. Hall is an 80-year-old white male who was last seen in June of this year for the above problems" indicates that he is an established patient. The levels of history and exam are expanded problem focused, and medical decision making is straightforward.

POCase007	First-Listed Diagnosis	Secondary Diagnosis	Secondary Diagnosis	Secondary Diagnosis	Secondary Diagnosis	Secondary Diagnosis
	781.2	721.0	356.9			
	First-Listed Procedure	Secondary Procedure	Secondary Procedure	Secondary Procedure	Secondary Procedure	Secondary Procedure
	99212					

The phrase "Patient returns for recheck" indicates an established patient. The level of history and exam are problem focused, and medical decision making is moderate complexity.

POCase008	First-Listed Diagnosis	Secondary Diagnosis	Secondary Diagnosis	Secondary Diagnosis	Secondary Diagnosis	Secondary Diagnosis
	355.8					
	First-Listed Procedure	Secondary Procedure	Secondary Procedure	Secondary Procedure	Secondary Procedure	Secondary Procedure
	99212					

To locate ICD code 355.8, go to main term *Neuropathy, neuropathic* and follow the instruction that says "*see also* Disorder, nerve." Then go to main term *Disorder* and subterm *lower limb* to locate code 355.8.

Do not assign ICD code E939.0 as a secondary diagnosis. The statement "symptomatic response to prescribed amitriptyline" in the assessment portion of the SOAP note is not documenting an adverse reaction to medication case. The patient was prescribed the medication (amitriptyline), and the physician documents that the patient's condition (paresthesias) has improved as a result of taking the medication.

Do not assign ICD code 782.0 (Disturbance of skin sensation) because paresthesias are symptoms of the patient's established diagnosis, distal sensorimotor neuropathy.

The phrase as "per previous visit" indicates an established patient. The level of history and exam are problem focused, and medical decision making is straightforward.

POCase009	First-Listed Diagnosis	Secondary Diagnosis	Secondary Diagnosis	Secondary Diagnosis	Secondary Diagnosis	Secondary Diagnosis
	333.1	401.9	434.91			
	First-Listed Procedure	Secondary Procedure	Secondary Procedure	Secondary Procedure	Secondary Procedure	Secondary Procedure
	99212					

Hypertensive vascular disease is coded as hypertension. In the ICD-9-CM Index to Diseases, go to main term *Disease*, subterm *Vascular*, and second qualifier *hypertensive* to locate the instruction to "*see* Hypertension."

To locate code 434.91, go to main term *Infarct, infarction* and subterm *cortical* in the ICD-9-CM Index to Diseases.

The phrase "upon recheck" indicates an established patient. The level of history is expanded problem focused, level of exam is problem focused, and medical decision making is moderate.

POCase010	First-Listed Diagnosis	Secondary Diagnosis	Secondary Diagnosis	Secondary Diagnosis	Secondary Diagnosis	Secondary Diagnosis
	110.1	701.1	250.61	357.2		
	First-Listed Procedure	Secondary Procedure	Secondary Procedure	Secondary Procedure	Secondary Procedure	Secondary Procedure
	11721	11056-59				

Report modifier -51 with 11056 to indicate that multiple procedures were performed during this office visit. (The payer will reimburse code 11721 at 100 percent and code 11056-51 at 50 percent.) If modifier -51 is not added to multiple procedure code(s) when the claim is submitted, the payer will reject the claim. The provider will not receive reimbursement until a corrected claim is submitted.

According to Ingenix's Encoder Pro Expert software, directional modifiers are not added to CPT code 11721 or 11056 (e.g., T7 and T8). (After entering a CPT code in Encoder Pro Expert, click the M button on the toolbar to determine which modifiers can be added to the code.) Codes 11721 and 11056 are classified in the CPT Surgery section, Integumentary System subsection; the integumentary system (skin) does not contain paired organs or anatomic sites, although surgery is performed on the skin of a paired anatomic site (e.g., foot).

Do not assign a CPT E/M code because evaluation and management services were not provided.

Workbook Appendix D: Inpatient Coding Cases

IPCASES ANSWER KEY

IPCase001	Admission Diagnosis	Principal Diagnosis	Secondary Diagnosis	Secondary Diagnosis	Secondary Diagnosis
	780.60	590.10	041.4	276.51	
	Principal Procedure	Secondary Procedure	Secondary Procedure	Secondary Procedure	Secondary Procedure
	MS-DRG: 690 (Kidney and urinary tract infections w/o MCC)				

Do not report code 305.x for tobacco abuse because it was not medically managed (e.g., treatment or patient counseling).

Ancillary tests (e.g., IVP, EKG, and chest x-ray) are not usually coded for inpatient cases because the ICD-9-CM codes do not impact DRG grouping. However, your instructor (or the facility at which you become employed) may require you to assign such codes.

IPCase002	Admission Diagnosis	Principal Diagnosis	Secondary Diagnosis	Secondary Diagnosis	Secondary Diagnosis
	366.9	366.9	496		
	Principal Procedure	Secondary Procedure	Secondary Procedure	Secondary Procedure	Secondary Procedure
	13.59	13.71			
	MS-DRG: 117 (Intraocular procedures w/o CC/MCC)				

Do not assign 13.41 for this case because there is no documentation of *phacoemulsification* technique, which is "a method of emulsifying and aspirating a cataract with a low frequency ultrasonic needle." (Stedman's Medical Dictionary) In this case, the patient underwent extracapsular cataract extraction (13.59) with implantation of a lens (13.71).

IPCase003	Admission Diagnosis	Principal Diagnosis	Secondary Diagnosis	Secondary Diagnosis	Secondary Diagnosis
	523.9	521.00	525.8	428.0	287.30
			414.00	303.90	571.5
	Principal Procedure	Secondary Procedure	Secondary Procedure	Secondary Procedure	Secondary Procedure
	23.19	24.5			
	MS-DRG: 138 (Mouth procedures w/o CC/MCC)				

Sequence 428.0 in the top five secondary diagnoses, below the principal diagnosis, because it is a comorbidity that impacts the DRG assignment. Under MS-DRGs, code 428.0 is not considered a comorbidity, which means that it does not impact the MS-DRG assignment (or payment). The "unspecified" fifth-digit 0 is added to code 303.9 because the physician did not document whether the condition is continuous, episodic, or in remission.

Do not assign ICD-9-CM diagnosis codes for ingrown toenail or abscess (or ICD-9-CM procedure codes for treatment of the conditions); that surgery was performed prior to inpatient admission. Postsurgical care is provided during this inpatient admission and is included in the global period.

IPCase004	Admission Diagnosis	Principal Diagnosis	Secondary Diagnosis	Secondary Diagnosis	Secondary Diagnosis
	332.0	276.8	332.0	276.51	
	Principal Procedure	Secondary Procedure	Secondary Procedure	Secondary Procedure	Secondary Procedure
	MS-DRG: 641 (Nutritional and miscellaneous metabolic disorders w/o MCC)				

IPCase005	Admission Diagnosis	Principal Diagnosis	Secondary Diagnosis	Secondary Diagnosis	Secondary Diagnosis
	303.00	303.00	303.90		
	Principal Procedure	Secondary Procedure	Secondary Procedure	Secondary Procedure	Secondary Procedure

Although a physician order indicates medical management of the previous fracture (V66.4), it was not documented as a final diagnosis and cannot be coded on this case.

MS-DRG: 897 (Alcohol/drug abuse or dependence w/o rehabilitation therapy w/o MCC)

IPCase006	Admission Diagnosis	Principal Diagnosis	Secondary Diagnosis	Secondary Diagnosis	Secondary Diagnosis
	486	482.81	041.84	429.2	
	Principal Procedure	Secondary Procedure	Secondary Procedure	Secondary Procedure	Secondary Procedure

MS-DRG: 179 (Respiratory infections and inflammations w/o CC/MCC)

IPCase007	Admission Diagnosis	Principal Diagnosis	Secondary Diagnosis	Secondary Diagnosis	Secondary Diagnosis
	332.0	332.0			
	Principal Procedure	Secondary Procedure	Secondary Procedure	Secondary Procedure	Secondary Procedure

MS-DRG: 057 (Degenerative nervous system disorders w/o MCC)

IPCase008	Admission Diagnosis	Principal Diagnosis	Secondary Diagnosis	Secondary Diagnosis	Secondary Diagnosis
	998.59	998.59	682.2	041.4	041.82
			E878.6	112.0	V10.05
	Principal Procedure	Secondary Procedure	Secondary Procedure	Secondary Procedure	Secondary Procedure
	86.04	97.83			

MS-DRG: 863 (Postoperative and post-traumatic infections w/o MCC)

Assign code 97.83 for removal of staples, as documented in progress note dated 11-18. (The patient was admitted due to a postoperative complication, which was an infection of the surgical wound, and the surgical treatment was performed during a previous admission. The staples were removed during this admission, which means that a code is assigned for staple removal.)

IPCase009	Admission Diagnosis	Principal Diagnosis	Secondary Diagnosis	Secondary Diagnosis	Secondary Diagnosis
	345.90	345.90	780.2		
	Principal Procedure	Secondary Procedure	Secondary Procedure	Secondary Procedure	Secondary Procedure

MS-DRG: 101 (Seizures WO MCC)

The principal diagnosis is the qualified diagnosis, "rule out seizure disorder." The secondary diagnosis is "syncopal episode." You might be tempted to assign code 460 for the treatment of the patient's worsening cold. Note that treatment was Tylenol only and that no documentation indicates that the patient's having a cold impacted treatment of the principal diagnosis. Therefore, don't assign code 460.

IPCase010	Admission Diagnosis	Principal Diagnosis	Secondary Diagnosis	Secondary Diagnosis	Secondary Diagnosis
	466.19	466.19			
	Principal Procedure	Secondary Procedure	Secondary Procedure	Secondary Procedure	Secondary Procedure

MS-DRG: 203 (Bronchitis and asthma w/o CC/MCC)

SECTION VI

Answer Key to Workbook Appendix E: Mock Certified Professional Coder (CPC) Certification Examination

1. a
2. b
3. c
4. a
5. d
6. d
7. c
8. a
9. d
10. c
11. d
12. d
13. d
14. b
15. a
16. a
17. b
18. b
19. c
20. d
21. d
22. b
23. d
24. c
25. b
26. b
27. b
28. c
29. d
30. c
31. a
32. b
33. c
34. b
35. b
36. c
37. a, b
38. a
39. d
40. c
41. c
42. b
43. a
44. a
45. d
46. b
47. b
48. c
49. c
50. d
51. c
52. d
53. d
54. c
55. a
56. a
57. c
58. a
59. c
60. c
61. b
62. c
63. a
64. b
65. b
66. c
67. a
68. d
69. d
70. c
71. c
72. a
73. b
74. c
75. a
76. c
77. c
78. b
79. b
80. b
81. b
82. a
83. d
84. c
85. c
86. a
87. d
88. a
89. a
90. c
91. c
92. d
93. a
94. a
95. b
96. d
97. b
98. d
99. b
100. b
101. c
102. a
103. a
104. c
105. c
106. b
107. a
108. a
109. b
110. d
111. c
112. b
113. c
114. b
115. a
116. c
117. c
118. a
119. a
120. c
121. b
122. b
123. a
124. c
125. b
126. d
127. a
128. b
129. d
130. c
131. b
132. a
133. b
134. a
135. d
136. c
137. b
138. a
139. b
140. b
141. b
142. d
143. b
144. a
145. b
146. b
147. a
148. b
149. b
150. c

SECTION VII

Answer Key to Workbook Appendix F: Mock Certified Coding Specialist-Physician (CCS-P) Certification Examination

PART I: CERTIFIED CODING SPECIALIST—PHYSICIAN (CCS-P)

1. b

Note:

HCPCS (CPT and HCPCS level II) and ICD-9-CM (or ICD-10-CM) are used to completely code this case. ICD-9-CM (or ICD-10-CM) is used to code the diagnosis, and CPT (level I of HCPCS) is used to code the procedure.

2. d
3. a
4. b
5. a

Note:

The information associated with this question are data elements collected by hospital emergency departments for the Data Elements for Emergency Systems (DEEDS) data set.

6. d
7. d
8. b
9. c
10. d

Note:

CMS's official ICD-9-CM (or ICD-10-CM) coding guidelines state that when a patient presents for scheduled chemotherapy, a code from category V58 (or ICD-10-CM Z51.11) is reported as the first-listed diagnosis code, followed by the cancer code. ICD-9-CM V10.11 (or ICD-10-CM Z85.118) is not reported when the patient is undergoing active treatment for a diagnosis such as lung cancer.

11. c
12. a
13. d
14. c
15. a
16. c
17. b
18. a
19. c
20. b
21. c
22. c
23. b

Note:

Review the operative report to locate the depth of the abscess, such as documentation that the surgeon penetrated the fascia. (The fascia is the layer of tissue that connects muscle to skin.) If the fascia is penetrated, determine how far (e.g., muscle, or muscle and bone) and locate the appropriate code in the Musculoskeletal subsection of CPT Surgery. If the surgeon did not penetrate the fascia, report a code from the Integumentary subsection of CPT Surgery instead.

24. a
25. c

Note:

ICD-9-CM contains E codes (and ICD-10-CM contains external cause of injuries and diseases codes), which are assigned for mechanism of injury data.

26. a
27. c
28. c
29. d
30. c
31. c
32. b
33. d

Note:

Per the 1995 guidelines, a level 5 E/M code would be reported based on the presenting nature of this patient and the severe life-threatening femoral artery injury. Also, the patient is unable to provide his or her own medical history due to the documented fact that he or she is in and out of consciousness.

34. c

Note:

The physician documented range of motion (ROM) and neurological reflexes. The physician also documented the condition of the patient's skin for the areas of the patient's complaint. This would be an expanded problem focus due to the neurological component and the Integumentary component that is documented.

35. d
36. c

Note:

An open tube bronchoscopy is used to remove foreign objects from the bronchial area.

37. c
38. c
39. a

Note:

No CPT modifier is added, the nose/nares is not a paired organ; therefore, it would be incorrect to assign a modifier -50 to the code for this procedure.

40. a
41. a
42. d
43. b
44. c
45. c
46. b
47. a
48. d

Note:

RAC, or Recovery Audit Contractor, is a program implemented in 2009 under the MMA Act of 2003. CoP is the abbreviation for conditions of participation, NCCI is the abbreviation for National Correct Coding Initiative, and POA is the abbreviation for present on admission. POA is part of the MS-DRG system, which is focused on inpatient services. NCCI provides information on CPT codes to prevent the practice of unbundling. RAC is the most recent of Medicare's initiatives and is focused particularly on overpayments and underpayments.

49. b
50. c
51. b
52. d
53. a
54. a
55. c
56. c

Note:

Category III CPT codes are temporary codes for emerging technology

57. c

Note:

Appendix A of CPT lists level I modifiers. Also in this appendix is a listed of modifiers that are approved for use in ASU outpatient centers. These include modifiers -25, -27, -50, -52, -58, -59, -73, -74, -76, -77, -78, -79, and -91.

58. b

Note:

Appendix B of CPT contains a summary of additions, deletions, and revisions for the current CPT coding manual.

59. a

60. b

Note:

Appendix I of CPT contains the genetic testing modifiers that are alphabetic or alphanumeric in format and can be added to both CPT and HCPCS level codes.

PART II: CODING PATIENT CASES

Hospital

1. ICD: 385.30 (H71.91)
   CPT: 88304
2. ICD: 492.8 (J43.9)
   CPT: 94150
3. ICD: 585.1 (N18.1)
   CPT: 90997, 36000

Note:

The "blood transfused back into the patient using a needle and catheter" procedure is included in the code reported for the hemoperfusion.

4. ICD: V72.11 (Z01.10)
   CPT: 92551

Emergency Department

5. ICD: 008.8, 276.41 (A08.3, E86.0)
   CPT: 99281

6. ICD: 873.0, 913.0 (S01.01xA, S50.311A)
   CPT: 99282-57, 12002
7. ICD: 599.0 (N39.0)
   CPT: 99283
8. ICD: 296.30 (F33.9, T14.91)
   CPT: 99283

Operating Room

9. ICD: 173.3 (C44.39)
   CPT: 11642, 14040

Note:

- In ICD-10-CM, the suicide attempt is classified to Chapter 19, Injury, Poisoning and Certain Other Consequences of External Causes (S00-T98); thus, assigning code T14.91 is permitted.
- A rhomboid flap is a local tissue advancement flap, classified as "adjacent tissue transfer or rearrangement" in the CPT coding manual.
- Per instructions for assigning CPT codes to case studies, do not assign modifier -51.

10. ICD: 622.12 (N87.9)
    CPT: 57520
11. ICD: 836.0, 715.36, 727.51 (S83.232D, M17.9, M71.21)
    CPT: 29881

Note:

- Do not report a separate code for the chondroplasty because that procedure is included in the arthroscopic medical meniscectomy.
- Do not assign a separate CPT code for surgical treatment of the Baker's cyst because, as stated in the operative report, "It was felt that by addressing the intra-articular pathology, the synovial fluid would be hopefully alleviated, the Baker's cyst would return back to a normal configuration and not require a separate operative procedure."

12. ICD: 706.2 (L72.1)
    CPT: 11424

Note:

The natal cleft is the anatomical term for groove or crack between the buttocks; it is also called the gluteal cleft or anal cleft, and it is located just above the anus. A sebaceous cyst is a closed sac that forms as the result of obstruction of an excretory gland and is located below the skin's surface. A sebaceous cyst of the natal cleft is not the same as a pilonidal cyst, which is entrapped epithelial tissue located in the sacrococcygeal region above the buttocks, usually associated with ingrown hair.

Physician Office/Clinic Setting

13. ICD: 216.3 (D23.30)
    CPT: 11441

Note:

Do not assign a CPT evaluation and management code to this case because the patient underwent a surgical procedure during the encounter.

14. ICD: 227.1, 252.02 (D35.1, E21.1)
    CPT: 99213
15. ICD: 786.5, 401.9, V45.81, V17.3 (R07.9, I10, Z95.1, Z82.49)
    CPT: 99243, 93000

Note:

Do not assign an ICD code for "possible angina," which is a qualified diagnosis and not reported for outpatient encounters. Instead of reporting a qualified diagnosis, report the symptom (in this case, chest pain).

16. ICD: 726.73 (M77.32)
    CPT: 99202

SECTION VIII

Answer Key to Workbook Appendix G: Mock Certified Coding Specialist (CCS) Certification Examination

1. a
2. d
3. c
4. b
5. b
6. c
7. c
8. a
9. d
10. a
11. b
12. d
13. b
14. b
15. b
16. d
17. b
18. b
19. a
20. a
21. a
22. b
23. b
24. a
25. d
26. c
27. b
28. a
29. d
30. b
31. a
32. c
33. b
34. a
35. b
36. a
37. a
38. d
39. d
40. b
41. c
42. c
43. c
44. a
45. a
46. d
47. d
48. c
49. c
50. d
51. d
52. d
53. c
54. d
55. b
56. c
57. c
58. b
59. c
60. d